MEDICAL INFORMATICS EUROPE '97

Studies in Health Technology and Informatics

Editors

Jens Pihlkjaer Christensen, European Commission DG XIII/C-5, Brussels; Tim De Dombal †, University of Leeds;
Ilias Iakovidis, EC DG XIII Health Telematics, Brussels; Zoi Kolitsi, University of Patras;
Jaap Noothoven van Goor †, ACOSTA, Brussels; Antonio Pedotti, Politecnico di Milan; Otto Rienhoff,
Georg-August-Universität Göttingen; Francis H. Roger-France, Centre for Medical Informatics, UCL, Brussels;
Niels Rossing, Centre for Clinical Imaging and Engineering, National University Hospital, Copenhagen;
Faina Shtern, National Institute of Health, Bethesda, MD; Viviane Thévenin, CEC DG XII/F BIOMED-I, Brussels

Volume 43

Earlier published in this series

ISSN: 0926-9630

Medical Informatics Europe '97

Part A

Edited by

C. Pappas
Laboratory of Medical Informatics
Aristotelian University of Thessaloniki, Greece

N. Maglaveras
Laboratory of Medical Informatics
Aristotelian University of Thessaloniki, Greece

and

J.-R. Scherrer
Division d'Informatique Médicale, Hôpital Cantonal Universitaire
Geneva, Switzerland

IOS
Press

Ohmsha

Amsterdam • Berlin • Oxford • Tokyo • Washington, DC

© 1997, The authors mentioned in the table of contents

ISBN: 90 5199 343 9 (IOS Press)
ISBN 4 274 90169 6 C3047 (Ohmsha)
Library of Congress Catalog Card Number 97-72896

Publisher
IOS Press
Van Diemenstraat 94
1013 CN Amsterdam
Netherlands

Distributor in the UK and Ireland
IOS Press/Lavis Marketing
73 Lime Walk
Headington
Oxford OX3 7AD
England

Distributor in Germany
IOS Press
Spandauer Strasse 2
D-10178 Berlin
Germany

Distributor in the USA and Canada
IOS Press, Inc.
5795-G Burke Centre Parkway
Burke, VA 22015
USA

Distributor in Japan
Ohmsha, Ltd.
3-1 Kanda Nishiki-cho
Chiyoda-ku
Tokyo 101
Japan

LEGAL NOTICE
The publisher is not responsible for the use which might be made of the following information.

PRINTED IN THE NETHERLANDS

Preface

The MIE'97 Conference (Medical Informatics Europe) is the fourteenth conference in the area of medical informatics that commenced in 1978 in Cambridge. This conference is held for two consecutive years in Europe before migrating in the third year to a country outside Europe where it is held under the name of MEDINFO. Through the years this conference has evolved into the major international event in the medical informatics area.

The proceedings contain 192 high quality papers in the area of medical informatics that set the tone for future developments in this field of science. These papers were selected from 255 submissions based on reviews by two or more impartial reviewers. The paper selection criteria were based on 1) significance to medical informatics, healthcare and/or medicine, 2) quality of scientific and/or technical content, 3) originality and innovativeness, 4) reference to related prior work, and 5) organisation and clarity of presentation.

Since the main theme of the conference is *Information Highways in Medicine*, the conference contents were broken up into four major themes related to this main theme. These themes are 1) health care information systems, 2) computer based patient records, 3) images and PACS, and 4) education/technology assessment. Thus the contents of these proceedings follow these four categories, although there are papers that belong to more than one category. In these cases, the papers were placed in the category that was considered by the editors as being closest to the contents of the papers. It is believed that these papers will provide a solid basis for the further development of medical informatics in the future through the information highways.

We wish to thank all who contributed to these proceedings, namely 1) the authors, 2) the reviewers and the EFMI board for their valuable advice, 3) the Laboratory of Medical Informatics for providing the editorial and E-mail facilities, and 4) IOS Press for giving advice during the preparation process and for their flexibility in the planning and printing of this book.

Costas Pappas, Chief Editor   Nicos Maglaveras   Jean-Raoul Scherrer
Greece   Greece   Switzerland

Contents

Medical Informatics Europe '97
C. Pappas et al. (Eds.)
IOS Press, 1997

System integrational and migrational concepts and methods within Healthcare

Frederik Endsleff, MD, MSc. E
Per Loubjerg, MSc, Head of Dept.
The Biomedical Engineering and IT Dept., Hvidovre Hospital,
Kettegaard Alle' 30, 2650, Hvidovre, Denmark

Abstract. In this paper an overview and comparison of the basic concepts and methods behind different systemintegrational implementations is given, including the DHE, which is based on the coming Healthcare Information Systems Architecture pre-standard HISA, developed by CEN TC251. This standard and the DHE (Distributed Healthcare Environment) not only provides highly relevant standards, but also provides an efficient and wellstructured platform for Healthcare IT Systems

1. Introduction

Traditionally, system integration strategies are based on one of two concepts:
- Sharing of Database
- Sharing of Information

In the next paragraphs these concepts and available related methods for integration will be examined, including the DHE, which will also be regarded in relation to user requirements.

2. Integration based on Database Sharing

Each application is build on top of the same database, which is common for the applications. This gives every application access to all data in the database, according to the scope of the application.

The concept has the following advantages:
- Unambiguous non-redundant data
- Synchronous, fast data access
- Direct access to all data

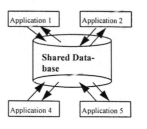

The concept has the following disadvantages:
- All applications has to know the database-structure. If an application is added or changed, thereby affecting the database-structure, other applications might need to be changed accordingly. Development implies a thorough and skilled database-design. The database-dependency thereby easily inflicts dependency between the applications.
- Existing applications will have to be migrated to the shared database.

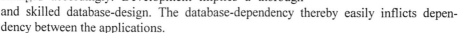

3. Integration based on the Sharing of Information

Each application has basically its own database. Data relevant for the other applications, who are not the owner of the data, are replicated from or directly requested in the owner application and its database, via the Integration/Interface Engine or Middleware/Gateway.

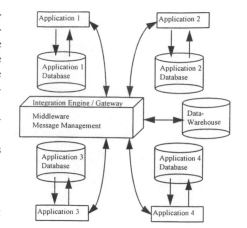

    The concept provides 'data interchange', and implies:

- Asynchronous exchange of messages between the applications
- Message management
- 'Events', which can be:
  - ☞ A change in the database content of one of the applications
  - ☞ A message
  - ☞ A request/response
- Events are able to 'trig' other events.
- Applications 'subscribe' on specific events, in order to receive specific messages trigged by certain events.
- Transformation of syntax (HL7/Edifact/Inhouse)
- Other message manipulation
- DataWarehouse for the storage of replicated data from all databases

The concept has the following advantages:

- It is simple to interface different systems with widely different architectures, via the IE/Middleware, thereby achieving integration to some extent.

The concept has the following disadvantages:

- Data redundancy
- Synchronisation of databases to maintain dataintegrity
- Only asynchronous communication between systems. Not always appropriate.
- The complexity in the handling of messages and events grows exponentially, with the degree of integration and the number of systems
- Message acknowledgements on several levels, and database storage of messages are required, raising considerable demands on the HW
- System adjustment/development has to be done manually

4. Integration on the Workstation

The concept relies on:

TCP/IP   -   Transmission Control Protocol / Internet Protocol
HTTP   -   Hyper Text Transfer Protocol
HTML   -   Hyper Text Mark-up Language
Web-browsers   -   such as Netscape, Microsoft Explorer
Web-applications

The user is provided with a homogeneous Internet-browser like environment, which makes it possible to access data from one system and jump to another, without the user having to deal with different user-interfaces, because the different systems are handled under the Intranet/Web 'shell'.

The concept has the following advantages:

- The simplicity in connecting widely different systems to the Intranet, if provided with an Intranet 'front-end', for example on a UNIX Server already running TCP/IP. The Intranet and the UNIX environment from which it has originated, are open technologies, making the access to the systems possible to an extent defined by the connection between the 'front-end' and the system itself.
- The users, like on the Internet, are able to manage data in the various systems in a uniform way, cutting and pasting, achieving a certain level of 'integration', on the Workstation.

The concept has the following disadvantages:

- There is no way to ensure the coherence of the total system. It consists of a number of autonomous subsystems, which from the point of view of data and functionality remain disintegrated.
- Dataintegrity is not ensured.
- In view of the complexity in the organisation of hospitals, and the complex handling of information related to the single patient, the lack of overall coherence, integration and appropriate complementarity between subsystems, makes a continued, advanced development in Healthcare IT difficult.
- Consistency of terms is not ensured.

5. Integration based on HANSA/DHE

The DHE is based on the coming Healthcare Information Systems Architecture pre-standard HISA, developed by CEN TC251. Each application stores data in the DHE database, which is common to all the applications, similar to the 'Sharing of Database' concept. The 'box' (diagram on next page) between the applications and the database, consists of synchronous services, Application Programming Interfaces, providing functional separation between the applications and the database itself, since all communication with the database is handled exclusively through the API's.

These API's and the services of DHE are functionally grouped into 5 'Healthcare Common Components', the Patient, Act, Health Data, Resource, User & Authorisations Manager. The Common Components, and the API's, are based on the DHE datamodel, which is specified and organised to form the general basis for a Hospital Information System.

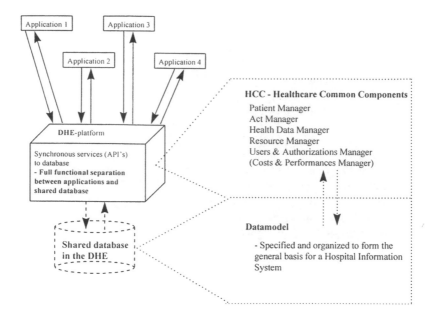

The flexibility and configurability of the datamodel provides:
- A potent HIS kernel
- Support for the applications, making the storage of healthcare related common data items possible.

    The applications will not need to know anything about the database itself, only how to invoke the relevant API's. The API's will become public, and the documentation will provide any application vendor with the specification of each of the API's.

HANSA/DHE has the following advantages:
- Similar to the traditional integration strategy based on database sharing:
  - ☞ Unambiguous non-redundant data
  - ☞ Synchronous, fast data access
  - ☞ Direct access to all data
- Without the direct coupling of the applications to the database, since all database communication is handled exclusively by the API's.
- The DHE handles a large part of the shared functionality, which the applications otherwise would have had to provide themselves.
- The possibilities in the development of applications based on such standard platform.
- The possibilities to develop advanced, specialised applications dedicated for a specific userdefined purpose, by using the common functionality in the DHE, combined with its configurability.
- Standardisation

HANSA/DHE has the following disadvantages:
- There are not yet services for asynchronous communication, message management and 'data interchange'.
- Already developed systems cannot be used directly with the DHE, but will have to be migrated or 'replicated' to some extent to the DHE.

6. The DHE from an IT and user requirements point of view

The organisation of hospitals are complex, and the handling of information related to the patient is complex. The wide perspectives in the use of IT to both support organisational, work-flow related issues as well as the handling of medical information, makes the need for integrated systems and overall system coherence in Healthcare obvious.

The DHE, which has been developed in complete conformance with HISA, the CEN TC251 Hospital Information Systems Architecture coming pre-standard, under the research and technological development programme 'Health Telematics Applications', provides a strong concept in this regard:

* Integration through the sharing of database, with non-redundant data and fast data access, through an open API, which makes the applications independent of the database itself, and which together with the datamodel provides a flexible, open and modular structure.

* This structure, based on the Healthcare Common Components 'managers' such as the 'Act Manager' which organises the various hospital activities, provides a set of services and constitute a back-bone HIS-kernel, thus ensuring the coherence in the total IT system, from a datatechnical as well as an organisational point of view.

References

[1] HISA   CEU CEN Draft European Pre-standard
                                                                         under the Red Cover Procedure
[2] HANSA [HC 1019]   CEU DGXIII
[3] UseDHE   CEU DGXIII
[4] Riche Reference Architecture   Groupe Riche
[5] Health Level Seven, Ver. 2.3, 1996   Health Level Seven
[6] The Middleware-Based Architectural Approach for
     Opening and Evolving Healthcare Information Systems   MIE96 Book, Fabrizio Massimo Ferrara,
[7] European Distributed Information Technology for
     Healthcare, Real Open Healthcare Information Systems:
     Now a Reality in Europe   MIE96 Book, A. van der Werff, F.M.
                                                                         Ferrara and G. Mobilia

Medical Informatics Europe '97
C. Pappas et al. (Eds.)
IOS Press, 1997

Post-integration of a tumor documentation system into a HIS via middleware

Schweiger R[1], Bürkle T[1], Dudeck J[1]

[1]*Department of Medical Informatics, University of Gießen, Heinrich-Buff-Ring 44, 35392 Gießen, Germany*

Abstract. Integrating autonomous applications is a difficult task since they usually represent similar informations in different data schemes. Any communication requires an agreement of sender and receiver on a common data representation. The number of interfaces to convert one data representation into another is minimized if all participants of an information system agree on one data representation such as Health Level Seven (HL7) or Edifact. Even more convenient is the use of a middleware solution like the Distributed Healthcare Environment (DHE) that keeps message transfer completely transparent to the integration process. This paper discusses a project that aims at the integration of a cancer registry system into a DHE based Hospital Information System (HIS). The project is a cooperation between the universities of Gießen and Magdeburg within the framework of the European Communities Telematics Research Project HC 1019 HANSA (Healthcare Advanced Networked System Architecture). The concept of a so called 'DHE-Adapter' to integrate existing legacy systems is explained. This adapter converts a data or message format of a legacy system into calls of the DHE programming interface. To develop a DHE-Adapter for our cancer registry system we intend to design a DHE-Adapter-Generator which would be able to produce DHE-Adapters for different systems and export formats, e.g. HL7 or Edifact. That would allow a variety of software vendors to integrate their products into the DHE without entering deeply into the DHE's programming interface.

1. The Gießen/Magdeburg project

Efforts are done to improve follow up of cancer patients by integrating informations from different suppliers such as cancer registries, laboratories, radiology departments, pathology departments or general practitioners. In Gießen a cancer registry documentation system called GTDS (Gießener TumorDokumentationsSystem) has been developed within the last years [1, 2, 3, 4], which is now sold as product and applied by 29 German cancer registry centers, among them the Magdeburg Cancer Center. GTDS is a UNIX based documentation system to support data collection about cancer patients for regular follow up care, to enhance therapy by offering therapeutic advice and to perform disease specific statistical analysis. Our approach aims at integrating this GTDS system within the DHE.

At Magdeburg Cancer Registry GTDS is not only used by registry staff for documentation but its functionalities regarding therapy support are also used by physicians. However the current front end, a UNIX terminal emulation, is awkward to use and not designed for use by medical doctors. Therefore Magdeburg intends to develop a Front End that provides a physician on demand in a convenient way with the GTDS data and functionalities. This Front End will be pre-integrated, that means it will be implemented directly on top of DHE. In this way it can be assured that each time a new supplier (e.g. laboratory, ...) is plugged into the DHE the informations will be immediately available for the user of this front end application.

The university hospitals in Gießen and Magdeburg are both participating in the European Communities Telematics Research Project HC 1019 HANSA (Healthcare Advanced Networked System Architecture). Within this cooperation we will use the Distributed Healthcare Environment as a middleware to connect GTDS with a clinician front end system. The following figure depicts the software architecture for this cooperation:

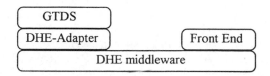

Figure 1: Software architecture of the Gießen/Magdeburg project

The two components 'DHE' and 'DHE-Adapter' are now discussed in deeper detail.

2. DHE: Distributed Healthcare Environment

The DHE is designed as an integration platform of common services to provide components of healthcare information systems with healthcare specific functionalities. In this context hospital information systems are considered as open federations of autonomous but collaborating systems, which provide an optimized support to the specific needs of the individual medical centers and functional units. To get an idea what informations are represented by DHE, an example is given: Let assume we want to integrate a laboratory departmental system. In this case front end applications would need to know which laboratory tests they can order and would like to enter such orders and retrieve the appropriate results for individual patients. The DHE divides such information in descriptive information like services offered (the different lab tests which can be ordered) and in 'live' information like requests and results for individual patients. All such informations can be accessed with a well defined DHE Application Programmers Interface (DHE-API) which can be regarded as a set of functions. A DHE user operates only with semantic entities such as patients, service points, health data items etc and does not worry about technical issue such as message passing or data management. Therefore the DHE can be regarded as an integration platform at a symbolic level that covers all areas of a HIS like resource allocation, user authorization, patient data management and others.

3. The DHE-Adapter: An Interface between legacy applications and the DHE

The DHE [5, 6, 7, 8] offers possibilities to integrate even legacy systems. In this case it is not necessary to restructure the existing applications in their overall architecture but the applications have to be equipped with a set of functionalities to support the interaction with the DHE-API. The legacy application is then encapsulated within the DHE. In this case however some kind of mapping between information models of the legacy system and the DHE is necessary. GTDS for example is an application developed independently from DHE. Here a mapping is required for the tumor data like location, histology or staging. Having completed this mapping at conceptual level one has now to translate the actual data from the legacy system, which might either derive directly from the legacy systems data base or from a defined data export scheme of the legacy system, into API calls of the DHE and vice versa. Exactly this translation is performed for the GTDS system by means of the DHE-Adapter. GTDS provides a data export format called BDT ('BehandlungsDatenTräger') that has established as a German standard for communication of health data . The DHE-Adapter will be constructed as a generic BDT-DHE-converter, therefore ensuring a connectability of many BDT based applications into a DHE-based HIS.

Our approach to build the DHE-Adapter will be even more generic. We intend to construct a DHE-Adapter-Generator which is fed only with the mapping of the information models as well from the legacy system as well from the DHE and which internally contains knowledge about the API design of the DHE. Such a general module will then deliver a set of functions which exactly perform the translation of actual data from and to the DHE. Figure 2 demonstrates this approach: The DHE Adapter Generator is fed with information models of legacy system and DHE and delivers as a result the DHE-Adapter for connection of the legacy system and the DHE API.

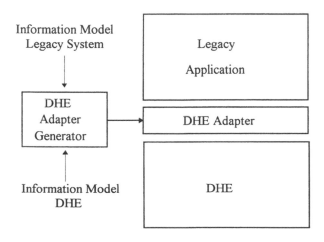

Figure 2: The DHE-Adapter-Generator

4. Discussion

The DHE is meant to establish a future European standard for internetworked healthcare information systems. The generic design ideas have been incorporated into the prestandard 'Standard Architecture for Healthcare Information Systems' of the Projectteam 13 of CEN TC251 [9]. To achieve adherence to any standard providers of healthcare information systems have to be stimulated to make their applications standard-compatible. The DHE has good chances to succeed in this undertaking since it does already support connection and interoperability with legacy systems inside the hospital. Nevertheless we consider it essential to avoid the necessity for each supplier to implement his own DHE-Adapter. A first step would be the availability of generic DHE-Adapters for specified protocols like BDT, HL7 or Edifact. The HANSA partners university of Gießen and Magdeburg will interface the cancer registry system GTDS to the DHE using a DHE-Adapter for the BDT format. To construct this adapter we will build a generator module which should then be reusable also for the construction of other DHE-Adapters e.g. for the HL7 format. If we succeed in this task other vendors of hospital information systems or components could then use the generator to connect their own systems easily to the DHE, not bothering about data models inside the DHE but only feeding their information model into the generator. This would accelerate post-integration tremendously and could give the DHE a great push from a quasi standard to a real standard.

References

[1]   Dudeck J et al. Qualitätssicherung in der Onkologie. 8. Informationstagung Tumordokumentation 1994, 111-118.

[2]   Altmann U et al. Concepts of GTDS: An Oncology Workstation. MEDINFO 95 Proceedings, 759-762.

[3]   Altmann U et al. Entwicklung und Bedeutung eines Data Dictionaries für Funktionalität und Integration eines Anwendungssystems am Beispiel des Gießener Tumordokumentationssystems (GTDS). GMDS 1995, 413-416.

[4]   Altmann U et al. Aspects of Integrating a Disease Specific System into a Hospital Information System. MIE 96, 291-295.

[5]   Ferrara F M. The middleware-based architectural approach for opening and evolving healthcare information systems. MIE 96, 264-270.

[6]   Ferrara F M. The DHE middleware Information view. GESI-12-114.2, Gestione Sistemi per l'Informatica, Rom.

[7]   Ferrara F M et al. DHE Functional view. GESI-12-114.3, Gestione Sistemi per l'Informatica, Rom.

[8]   Ferrara F M et al. DHE API of services. GESI-12-114.5, Gestione Sistemi per l'Informatica, Rom.

[9]   CEN/TC251/PT013 draft standard on 'Standard Architecture for Healthcare Information Systems'

Medical Informatics Europe '97
C. Pappas et al. (Eds.)
IOS Press, 1997

Security of Healthcare Information Systems Based on the CORBA Middleware

Bernd BLOBEL and Martin HOLENA
Otto-von-Guericke University Magdeburg, Faculty of Medicine, Institute of Biometrics and Medical Informatics, Leipziger Straße 44, D-39120 Magdeburg, Germany

Abstract. The development of healthcare systems in accordance to the "Shared Care" paradigm results in co-operative health information systems across the boundaries of organisational, technological, and policy domains. Increasingly, these distributed and heterogeneous systems are based on middleware approaches, such as CORBA. Regarding the sensitivity of personal and medical data, such open, distributed, and heterogeneous health information systems demand a high level of data protection and data security, both with respect to patient information and with respect to users. The security concepts and measures available and additionally needed in health information systems based on CORBA architecture are described in this paper. The proposed security solution is also open to other middleware approaches, such as DHE or HL7.

1. Introduction

Under the constraints of changed basic conditions of care and of increasing demands for health services, all developed countries are modifying their healthcare systems structure to a shared caring concept, extended communication and co-operation between direct as well as indirect care providers, and at least a minimum of competitiveness.

These objectives must be supported by adequate, i.e. distributed and really co-operative health information systems. Meeting these requirements, the newly developed or legacy components of information systems must realise Leguit's integration type "Integration" [3]. Only strictly object-oriented approaches, providing services comprising data *and* methods applicable to the data, are capable of such co-operation. Regarding domain specific affiliation, the achieved integration level, and platform or provider dependencies, different approaches to the middleware layer below end-user applications attempt to tackle the isolation and not-openness of legacy health information systems. Including the healthcare domain specific vertical common facilities envisaged by the CORBAmed group, the present paper is restricted to CORBA (Common Object Request Broker Architecture) as the approach probably best fulfilling the above requirements. However, the proposed security solution is also applicable to the other middleware approaches using CORBA services. A comparative study of middleware approaches for healthcare (HL7, DHE, CORBA) can be found in [1].

2. Overview of the CORBA Middleware Approach

Based on the popular object-oriented paradigm, the CORBA approach is being elaborated by the Object Management Group (OMG), created in 1989 to promote the theory and practice of object technology in distributed computing systems. An object, in general, can represent anything that is unambiguously identifiable and capable to provide one or more services that can be requested by some kind of client. Associated with each object is a set of methods and a set of attributes. The former represent the provided services, the latter represent the state of the object and the information passed during the request or produced when services are provided. Each implementation of an object consists of three parts:

- Operations, implementing the services represented by the object's methods;
- Data, which implement the object state and information represented by the attributes;
- Interface, implementing the ability to accept requests and to return information. It is specified by a special Interface Definition Language (IDL) defining passed parameters, return mode, as well as links to a request context and to exception handling methods.

The basic structure of the CORBA architecture is the Object Request Broker (ORB), which is responsible for locating an object implementation, preparing it to receive the request and communicating the data making up the request. Hence, it plays the role of an active object interconnection bus. It consists of the ORB core, which provides the basic representation of objects and communication of requests, and various client- and/or server-side interfaces. Though the ORB can be implemented in various ways, its interfaces are standardised and implementation-independent. They provide CORBA with a high degree of portability, scalability and flexibility.

Between the ORB and the application objects, implementing end-user applications, the CORBA architecture situates two layers of widely used objects. The lower layer of Common Object Services provides basic functionality for using and maintaining objects. Examples of common object services include Transaction Services, Object Lifecycle Management, Event Notification, or Concurrency Control. The higher level of Common Facilities provides general purpose capabilities useful in many applications. The facilities may be horizontal, pertaining to different application areas, or vertical, within a particular application area like healthcare. Available horizontal facilities include User Interface, Information Management, System Management, and Task Management.

The version 2.0 of CORBA includes an interoperability standard enabling one ORB to pass requests to a different ORB. It comprises bridging mechanisms, translating requests between ORBs, and communication protocols such as the General Inter-ORB Protocol (GIOP) and Internet Inter-ORB Protocol (IIOP).

To promote the importance of CORBA for the healthcare, within the OMG in 1995 the healthcare domain task force CORBAmed was created, which explicitly states as its mission „to improve the quality of care and reduce costs by CORBA technologies". It has already initiated the technology adoption process to standardise interfaces for healthcare domain vertical facilities. The authors are actively involved in these activities.

3. Security features available in CORBA

Security protects information systems from unauthorised attempts to access information or to interfere with their operation. Though the need for incorporating security services into CORBA has been recognised rather early, a comprehensive specification of the proposed security solutions has been available only at the end of 1995. Simplicity, consistency across the distributed co-operating systems, scalability and usability (transparency), flexibility of security policies, independence of security technology, application portability, interoperability, and sufficient performance were defined as goals for an object-oriented security architecture within CORBA. Fulfilling these goals, CORBA provides to users and applications transparently the required security at least on the level of their own environment. In addition, the CORBA security services are also available to security unaware applications.

CORBA provides all important security services, such as identification and authentication, authorisation and access control, security auditing, security of communication including mutual authentication of clients and targets, integrity protection and confidentiality protection, non-repudiation, and administration of security. Security is defined for domains differing from the point of view of organisational or legal conditions (security policy domains), institutional boundaries (security environment domains), or the technology platforms (security technology domains). Security pertains to various components of the CORBA architecture. A considerable part of security functions is implemented directly through the ORBs or through their bridging mechanisms. Others are confined to transaction services or to additional security services, implemented through specific security-related objects. Finally, security services are also provided by the underlying operation systems and communication services.

Each object service is ultimately requested on behalf of a principal, i.e. an end-user known to the system and separately accountable for the requests it initiates. Unless the principal has been already trustworthy authenticated outside the system (see next section), its authentication is performed by the Principal Authenticator object, associated to each ORB providing a higher level of security. The Principal Authenticator creates for each principal a Credentials object, containing the Principal's privilege attributes, e.g. the access identity, groups to which the principal belongs, roles, security clearance, and capabilities concerning various groups of objects. A security aware target application may obtain attributes of the principal responsible for the incoming request, to make its own authentication-depending access decisions. The information contained in Credentials can be obtained either directly or through the Current, an interface of the Transaction Services, which holds reference to the current execution context at both client and target objects.

The privilege attributes are first needed for making a secure invocation, which is mediated by the ORB. Whether the invocation can take place, as well as the way in which it is mediated, depends on the client and target security policies. Security policies concern such issues as access control, establishing trust in client/target, protection of messages for integrity/confidentiality, time restrictions, or delegation of privileges. If a request initiates a chain of invocations, then the security policies of all objects in the chain are taken into consideration by delegation mechanisms, including all intermediate objects.

As far as access control is concerned, applications can enforce their own access policies. Typically, details of access control are isolated from the application itself, and are implemented through an Access Decision Object, specific to the access policy. In addition, there is an Access Decision Object associated with the ORB and used for the invocation access policy, which is enforced internally by the ORB. The decision whether to allow access to a given function or data depends on the privilege attributes of the initiator of the request, control attributes of the target, and on the execution context. Access policy can be actually shared by a whole domain of objects with similar security requirements. In that case, reference to the corresponding Access Decision Object is available via the Current interface.

Similarly, applications can also enforce their own audit policies, which can be again managed via a domain structure. Each application writes its audit records to an Audit Channel object. One such object is created at ORB initialisation time and is used for all system auditing. Application can use different Audit channel objects.

Finally, CORBA supports optional Non-repudiation services, providing generation and later verification of evidence concerning performed actions and data associated with those actions. The evidence can be generated using either symmetric cryptographic algorithms requiring a trusted third party as the evidence generating authority, or asymmetric cryptographic algorithms assured by public key certificates issued by a certification authority. Keys or other information needed for generating or checking the evidence are available via Credentials.

4. CORBA Security Solutions in the Context of Healthcare Information Systems

Shared care means communication and co-operation between directly or indirectly involved care providers. In this context, in general, a client requests a service from a server. Client and/or server could be a user and/or an application. The guarantee of data security and the reliability and obligation of certain activities are basic conditions for health information systems supporting trustworthiness between physicians and patients, but also between different care providers. Legislation, rules, roles, duties, rights, conditions, and penalties are defined by the security policy. Security threats and risks have to be analysed and assessed. Counter-measures must be evaluated and implemented. These steps must be regularly repeated. Additionally to the availability of information and functions, two kinds of security are needed for the secure invocation of a service or the secure use of an application:

- the communication security, ensuring integrity, reliability (accountability), and confidentiality of communication between authenticated partners, and
- the application security, controlling access rights to the application (functional and data access rights) as well as the reliability of the application functions and data (accountability as non-repudiation).

The access rights depend on the organisational structure within the healthcare institution (mandatory access rights), on the role of the principal within the care process (e.g. caring doctor, therapeutic team, consulting doctor, nurse, administrative clerk), and finally, on the patient's consent. The case of emergency care where the roles of particular principals are not known in advance can be essentially covered using the CORBA identity domain, a special case of security environment domains.

To ensure integrity, reliability, and authentication, strong authentication mechanisms must be used, relying on user-specific knowledge (password, PIN), ownership (electronic identity cards with keys and certificates), or physical properties (such as fingerprint, voice analysis, retina analysis, face analysis). Confidentiality can be provided using symmetric and/or public key cryptographic algorithms. Nowadays, availability, feasibility and cost-benefit relation are promoting chip-cards for security mechanisms in healthcare. Those cards will contain the user's identity, private keys for digital signatures (ensuring integrity and non-repudiation of origin), as well as, if necessary, class keys for group authentication. The latter function could also be provided using the individual authentication, together with directories of group members, their roles and rights. Finally, a trust authority (trusted third party) is needed, to ensure the correctness and validity of keys by certificates, and to provide directory services (public keys for encryption and proof of digital signatures), as well as notary functions.

Functions related to the communication security can be globally organised, whereas the application security related to detailed access rights concerning a particular application can be controlled only locally, by the owner of the data or by the application administrator. In this context, the delegation mechanisms available in CORBA support the above described authentication procedures of security aware healthcare environment. The highly dynamic access rights underlying the access decisions are, in general, enforced by the application via access decision objects and additional services (like time services, account management). Using the various delegation options (simple delegation for end-to-end interactions, composite, combined and/or traced delegation) the middleware can adapt to requirements of different users and establishments. We intend to use this functionality of CORBA for our own environment. Within a project called German Model Trial, aiming at the implementation of health professional cards (HPCs), we are introducing HPCs to improve data security in a regional clinical cancer registry. Our contribution to the project includes also a sophisticated access management.

In distributed co-operating information systems, the underlying middleware provides also some integrative functions. For example, the envisaged CORBA vertical facilities Master

Patient Index, harmonising the patient identification in different applications, and Lexicon Services, supporting and managing terminology and semantics between different systems, provide functionalities supporting the intraorganisational or interorganisational interoperability of different information system components. Since those facilities will support such essential medical functions as electronic health records, archiving systems, clinical or epidemiological registries, they must ensure an adequate level of security.

In current security models, the service providers, including middleware services, are viewed as untrusted, following the basic concept to trust nobody and to organise security mainly by the communicating and co-operating partners. Especially for distributed middleware architectures involving a number of hosts, Varadharajan proposed to install, on each of them, security functions (e.g., encryption/decryption, signatures), a security information base, secure factory objects (objects responsible for creation and deletion of other objects), and secure interfaces [4]. Most of these services can also be provided by functionalities specified in CORBA.

5. Conclusions

The CORBA middleware architecture, as it has been specified so far, provides advanced security services that allow the integration of both security unaware and security aware applications typical for the healthcare area. Special conditions defined in security policies of departments, institutions, organisations, regions, countries, or even the European Union can be specified, to control the middleware security services. The CORBA security solutions are suitable to integrate external security services in healthcare proposed the within TRUSTHEALTH project funded by the Telematics Programme of the EU. Moreover, the integration of such external security services is also possible in coexistence with other middleware approaches, such as DHE and HL7 [2].

6. Acknowledgement

This work was supported within the "Telematics Applications Programme" framework of the European Union, and by the Ministry of Education and Science of the German Federal State Saxony-Anhalt.

References

[1] BLOBEL, B., and HOLENA, M., Advanced Healthcare System Architecture Using Middleware Concepts - A Comparative Study. Deliverable of the HC 1019 Telematics Project HANSA, July 1996.
[2] BLOBEL, B., and Holena, M., Security Aspects of Health Information Systems Based on Middleware Architectures. Submitted to the Int. Journal of Bio-Medical Computing, March 1997.
[3] LEGUIT, F. Interfacing Integration. In Bakker, A.R., et al., Eds., Hospital Information Systems, pp. 141-148. North-Holland, Amsterdam, 1992.
[4] VARADHARAJAN, V., and HARDJONO, T. Security Model for Distributed Object Framework and its Applicability to CORBA. In Katsikas, S.K., and Gritzalis, D., Eds., Information Systems Security, Chapman & Hall, London, 1996, pp. 452-463.

Regarding the included architectural groups, additional references can be obtained from the authors.

Medical Informatics Europe '97
C. Pappas et al. (Eds.)
IOS Press, 1997

Functional and Control Integration of an ICU, LIS and PACS Information System

D. KATEHAKIS[1], M. TSIKNAKIS[1], A. ARMAGANIDIS[2], S. ORPHANOUDAKIS[1,3]
[1]Institute of Computer Science, FORTH, PO Box 1385, GR 711 10, Heraklion, Greece
[2]Evangelismos Hospital, Ypsilantou 45-47, GR 106 75, Athens, Greece
[3]Dept. of Computer Science, University of Crete, GR 714 09, Heraklion, Greece

Abstract. The need for collaboration and data sharing among systems dedicated to individual functional areas and user groups has initiated major efforts towards the development of an integrated hospital information system. Major issues in the development of any integrated architecture that incorporates autonomous departmental systems include the development of commonly accepted interaction mechanisms, standardisation, the structure of the computerised patient record, its extensibility, as well as limitations multimedia data impose. This paper presents work done within project IHIS, a nationally funded project for the development of an integrated hospital information system that provides ICU staff with access to both the ICU assisting laboratory information system's data as well as radiological multimedia data.

1. Introduction

Hospital organisation diversity, complexity of clinical protocols and procedures, as well as the different preferences of various user groups make it extremely difficult for a single monolithic information system to effectively serve the needs of an entire health care organisation. Thus, information and telecommunications systems must primarily provide the infrastructure to permit the effective integration of distributed and heterogeneous components, ensuring overall integrity in terms of functional collaboration and information sharing.

The physically distributed resources of the health care sector and the diverse requirements of different medical facilities and clinical departments require that specialised autonomous information systems are used to support different needs, while they interact transparently to the user as a federation of autonomous systems. This approach ensures the transfer and integration of consistent information throughout a network of health care facilities, without imposing constraints on the operation of individual units.

This paper's objective is to elaborate on the architectural framework that has already been presented in [1] and to present an integrated environment, that can collect, validate, record, recall, process and communicate multimedia information related to the patient under medical observation and recovery in the ICU. This approach supports data sharing among several departments, while at the same time individual domain-specific information systems sustain their autonomy.

2. Integration Types

The logic, as well as the data structures used in clinical information systems are not only complex but also incompatible. The institutional patient meta-record (PMR) concept [2] permits the seamless integration of distributed computerised patient record (CPR) segments. The different types of integration required are *data, functional, presentation* and *control*.

The distributed architecture presented here, consists of individual clinical information systems, each of them dedicated to its particular clinical requirements and having the ability to function independently from the others. As a part of the integrated architecture each of the clinical information systems can communicate with all the other, transparently from users, and exchange information when this is necessary. This approach supports information retrieval and propagation that can be accomplished:

- by allowing direct access on the servicing department's data base server,
- by having information systems exchanging work-lists and reports either event-driven or on on-demand, and
- by allowing users to request information on particular examinations

3. Workflow Management

Workflows are activities involving the co-ordinated execution of multiple tasks performed by different processing entities [3]. In the health care domain, activities correspond to work lists, task correspond to diagnostic service requests and processing entities are the servicing information systems.

Important requirements for the efficient and reliable operation of applications supporting workflow management include deep understanding of the process to model, as well as workflow implementation and automation. Separation of work activities into well-defined tasks with certain roles, well-defined rules and procedures allows for the modelling of health care processes in a rigorous and comprehensive way. This is a prerequisite for the development of an integrated hospital information system to support automation of processes.

The Center for Medical Informatics and Health Telematics Applications (CMI-HTA) of the Institute of Computer Science (ICS), Foundation for Research and Technology - Hellas (FORTH) has designed and implemented a Work Flow Manager (WFM) agent that acts as a co-ordinator among hospital-wide spread work list managers. This agent maintains information on available services provided in the integrated hospital environment and acts as a mediator among heterogeneous information systems. In addition the WFM supports a set of services capable of providing distribution of available services in the integrated hospital environment, work list decomposition and routing, appointment reservation as well as report composition. The WFM also keeps a record of all the intra-hospital examination request and report traffic.

4. Work List Management

The outcome of a diagnostic service request is the receipt of all or some of the examination(s) results, as well as the related reports by qualified recipients. To service a diagnostic request, the requester, as well as his authorisation, should be identified. The validity of the requested procedure types, as well as their steps should be also verified. Important factors affecting the scheduled procedure steps are the availability of the attending physicians, the technical personnel, the required equipment, and of course the patient. As a result the service request procedure produces a series of instructions for the patient, the requester, and the performer, concerning each of the scheduled procedure steps.

The CMI-HTA has designed and implemented a Work List Manager (WLM) that can support patient admission to the requesting department and give the opportunity to authorised personnel to place a diagnostic service request (i.e. to schedule patient examinations to the appropriate assisting clinical information systems).

When the requesting WLM communicates with the performing WLM it has to provide information like requester identification patient related data (like demographics, patient location and mobility, etc.), requested date and time, urgency, clinical data, as well as the destination for the supplied results. Upon completion of the exam(s) that correspond(s) to the procedure step(s) that compose the requested procedure, the final report is constructed and transmitted to all pre-requested recipients. After the receipt of the report by the last recipient, the diagnostic service request is considered to be complete.

5. ICU Information System

The ICU consists of a ward, with a limited number of patients and a small group of users [4]. Under *normal conditions* the ICU monitoring devices function properly, the patient's state is steady and the medical personnel's responsibility is to watch the patient and treat him/her accordingly.

When one or more monitoring device alarms are active, then there is an *emergency situation*. Immediately after such a situation it is very important to have the patient's record updated about the injected drugs, the medical acts, as well as the acceptance or rejection of certain data recordings during the alarm period.

Another critical point for the proper health care delivery in an ICU is the seemly *shift change*. The major issue here is the critical patient information that has to be passed along, which is associated to special treatment needs. What is important here is not what has to be done, rather than what has preceded.

With the above information in mind the requirements that any ICU-oriented information system should fulfil are:

- **On-line data acquisition from various sources:** This, combined with the ability to compose new information can lead to new data presentation methods, and can provide the practitioners with new possibilities for efficient treatment.
- **Automatic data validation:** This way human errors can be minimised, and equipment malfunctions can be isolated.
- **Integrated data presentation centred around the different data modalities:** This can reduce significantly the time spent by hospital personnel moving to and from various assisting laboratories, and thus improve the productivity of the ICU.
- **Fast data manipulation:** The amount of real-time data should not cause bottlenecks.
- **Reporting, and charting:** This way documentation quality can be improved significantly.
- **Adherence to international standards:** This is the only viable solution to the problem of integration. Functional interfaces among the different systems/components of the IHIS require significant effort towards standardisation.
- **Scalability:** It should be easy for the architecture to be expanded with the addition of more clinical information systems. It should be also easily incorporated in a wide-area network of integrated hospital information systems.

The IHIS project ICU monitoring system implementation consists of three autonomous components, each of which is responsible for managing different data types. Patient data, vital sign display of both simple measurements (SM) and continuous recordings (CR) provide an integrated bedside display for ICU practitioners. Support for several viewing modes (real-time data display, daily overview, charting mode and the patient record import/export functionality) is also provided.

6. Laboratory Information System

Laboratory data can be of different type and they can be transformed to useful information only after they reach a physician. The clinical personnel's most critical actions are mainly data analysis and reporting. The procedure begins with the receipt of the physician's request and ends with the delivery of the laboratory procedure report to the receiving physicians. The intermediate steps which the procedure has to undergo are, issuing of the order request, specimen collection and processing, data acquisition and analysis, results verification and reporting.

Data acquisition is performed through the standard serial interface most of the instruments provide. After the necessary two-phase validation procedure, for eliminating transmission and data errors, data are transferred into the patient's record. For devices supporting manual data entry, only data validation is performed.

In addition the LIS, developed within the IHIS project, supports automatic patient demographic data, as well as examination schedule insertion, initiated by the local WLM, eliminating thus valuable time for data re-entry. This makes the LIS an active information system, in the sense that it is capable of responding to other information systems requests.

7. Picture Archiving and Communications System

Medical images are very important sources of diagnostic information. The Picture Archiving and Communications System (PACS) is the information system that allows for the collection of diagnostic quality images, their efficient management, the fast and reliable access to them, as well as for the intra-hospital communications of medical images [5].

Figure 1 shows the architecture of the PACS system developed by CMI-HTA, ICS-FORTH as part of the IHIS project. The architecture consists of several components that function as an integrated information system over the distributed application environment.

The Medical Multimedia Archive Server manages the permanent storage of images, while the WLM Archive Server stores the records of ordered work lists. The User Interface Component allows for browsing through the PACS PRS, the Acquisition Component is responsible for the acquisition of diagnostic images, and the Clipboard is an intermediate buffer between acquisition and the PACS PRS. The Medical Mail Client is used for the exchange of multimedia medical images for remote consultation, while the Medical Mail Server acts as a filter for medical-content email. The WLM, as has already been described, facili-

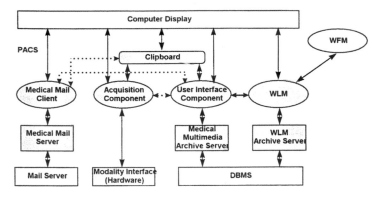

Figure 1. The PACS Architecture.

tates both the referral and the reporting process, automating medical acts by means of the WFM.

8. Teleconsultation Services

Bearing in mind that health care is an important telematics application domain, the CMI-HTA of ICS-FORTH is developing a scaleable architecture and reusable tools for the integration of domain-specific autonomous information systems. As part of this effort a simple multimedia communication component through electronic mail, for remote opinion request, has been developed. Asynchronous teleconsultation is achieved through the exchange of medical content Messaging Application Programming Interface (MIME) attachments over the Simple Mail Transfer Protocol (SMTP). This service has already been integrated with the PACS application, as shown in Figure 1.

Synchronous consultation between the radiology department and the ICU is supported by the CoMed application [6], also developed by CMI-HTA, ICS-FORTH. CoMed is a desktop medical conferencing application that allows for interactive real-time co-operation among two or more conference participants.

9. Discussion

An architectural framework for the development of an integrated hospital information system is being evaluated with the IHIS project. Although a single hospital is autonomous and devoted to the delivery of a particular set of services, the desirable continuity of care requires that different medical centres, offering complementary services and different levels of expertise, exchange relevant patient data and operate in a co-operative working environment. The sharing of information resources is generally accepted as the key to substantial improvements in productivity and to better quality of service.

References

[1]   M. Tsiknakis *et al.*, Intelligent Image Management in a Distributed PACS and Telemedicine Environment, *IEEE Communications Magazine*, vol. 34, no. 7, July 1996, pp. 36-45.
[2]   E. Leisch *et al.*, An Architectural Framework for the Integration of Geographically Distributed Heterogeneous Autonomous Medical Information Systems, *EuroPACS '96 Proceedings*, Heraklion, Greece, 1996, pp.73-77.
[3]   D. Georgakopoulos *et al.*, An Overview of Workflow Management: From Process Modeling to Workflow Automation Infrastructure, *Distributed and Parallel Databases*, vol. 3, no 2, April 1995, pp. 119-153.
[4]   P. G. H. Metnitz, K. Lenz, Patient data management systems in intensive care - the situation in Europe, *Intensive Care Med.*, vol. 2, Springer-Verlag 1995, pp. 703-710.
[5]   S. T. C. Wong, H. K. Huang, A Hospital Integrated Framework for Multimodality Image Base Management, *IEEE Transactions on Systems, Man, and Cybernetics - Part A: Systems and Humans*, vol. 26, no. 4, July 1996, pp. 455-469.
[6]   M. Zikos *et al.*, CoMed: Cooperation in Medicine, *EuroPACS '96 Proceedings*, Heraklion, Greece, 1996, pp.88-92.

Medical Informatics Europe '97
C. Pappas et al. (Eds.)
© IOS Press, 1997

Migration towards a component based HIS architecture

P. J. Toussaint, H. Lodder,
HISCOM, Schipholweg 97, 2316 XA Leiden, The Netherlands

Abstract: Changing requirements for health care information systems force the development of an open, modular architecture in which components can be integrated. This offers a flexible means for integrating different (heterogeneous) systems used by different users. Migration towards such an open, modular architecture is a difficult task. It consists of breaking down existing systems in components and integrating these components. Many authors on migration strategies focus attention on the ordering of the steps to be taken without detailing how these steps were arrived at. This paper presents a more rigorous approach for deriving a migration strategy.

1. Introduction

Allowing integration and the consistent interworking of different (heterogeneous) applications is a major need of current HealthCare systems. The distributed and highly co-operative nature of the health care service necessitates an open modular architecture in which applications can be embedded. Many technological solutions are available, ranging from health care specific (DHE [1], CorbaMed [2]) to generic (CORBA [3]). Migrating towards an open, modular architecture based on DHE middleware or on distributed object technology such as CORBA poses a number of difficult questions.

A migration strategy transforms a current information system infrastructure (the As-Is situation) into a wanted information system infrastructure (the To-Be situation). In our view the specification of a migration strategy has three parts:

1. A specification of components or business objects to integrate in our open, modular architecture, and their relations
2. A specification of the way these components and their relations can be derived or constructed from existing systems (applications and middleware solutions)
3. A specification of the order in which components and their relations are realised

The third part is very often taken as the sole part of the migration strategy [4,5]. Orderings of steps are presented without discussing how the steps were arrived at.

The components found in the first step are derived from an analysis of the business process to be supported. So, in the words of ODP [6] we assume that a component must be linked to the enterprise view of the application domain. This observation is also elaborated by Orfali et al. [7] in discussing the rise of the distributed objects or distributed components paradigm. Business Objects or Components to be embedded in a CORBA or COM/OLE environment offer a distinguished end-user functionality. This paper presents a methodology for doing that.

In section 2 we specify an As-Is and a To-Be situation that will be used for illustrating our approach for defining a migration strategy. As an example we take the business process of conducting studies at a Nuclear Medicine department. In the sections 3, 4 and 5 we elaborate the three parts of the migration strategy for our example.

2. The example case

2.1 As-Is situation

The characterisation of the current situation has two parts:
- The information systems currently in use
- The relations established between these information systems.

Our example will be a Nuclear Medicine department. There are three information systems for supporting the workflow on this department:
- **Scheduling System:** This system offers four services:
    - s_1 - using this service a visit can be registered, the visit is associated with a unique study identifier, s_2 - using this service the registered visit is scheduled, s_3 - view registered visit, s_4 - view schedule
- **Hospital Information System:** A small number of services offered by the HIS are relevant in this example:
    - s_5 - this service registers patient and assigns a unique id, s_6 - retrieve patient data/patient id, s_7 - make list of studies to be reported, s_8 - view list of studies to be reported, s_9 - report study, s_{10} - view report text
- **Image system for Nuclear Medicine:** This system offers services for approving, reporting and viewing nuclear medicine images. For this example we highlight the following services:
    - s_{11} - associate images with HIS-patient data, s_{12} - make list of studies to be approved, s_{13} - view list of studies to be approved, s_{14} - approve study, s_{15} - view images belonging to a specific study

There are currently no relations between the Scheduling System and the two other information systems. The Image System imports s_6 when it associates images with HIS-patient data (s_{11}). The HIS imports s_{14} both for the report study (s_9) and the viewing of report texts (s_{10}).

2.2 To-Be situation

The end situation is closely related to a model of the business process to be supported. This model of the business process is described in terms of: agents, their tasks, the co-operation relations between agents and the way agents restrict each other's behaviour. These concepts are related to the concepts included in the enterprise viewpoint language [see 6].

The process of conducting studies at a Nuclear Medicine department involves four actors, each able to perform several tasks:
- The Nuclear Medicine physician. Tasks: *prepare study, check diagnostic quality images, report study*
- The Nuclear Medicine assistant. Tasks: *make images, request for image quality approval*
- The Requesting physician. Tasks: *request study, review study results (report and images)*
- Administrator. Tasks: *make appointment*

The collaboration relations we take into account are as follow:
- The Nuclear Medicine physician requests the Nuclear Medicine assistant to make images after the study is prepared.
- The Nuclear Medicine assistant requests the Nuclear Medicine physician to check the diagnostic quality of the images when they are made.

The performance of a task by an agent can restrict the performance of one or more tasks by another agent. We list two of these restrictions:
- The Nuclear medicine physician must have prepared the study before images can be made by the assistant

- Study results can only be reviewed by the requesting physician when they are reported by the Nuclear medicine physician

Given this characterisation of the business process to be supported, the To-Be situation is constructed based on the following assumptions:

- Every agent wants an information system for supporting his information processing needs arising in the conduction of his tasks;
- Each task is supported by a (possibly empty) set of services.
- An information system is conceived as a set of services;
- If a set of tasks is included in a collaboration relation between two agents A_1 and A_2 (this is the set of tasks of A_2 that can be used by A_1), the information system for A_1 includes the services supporting these tasks;
- If the performance of a task by agent A_1 is restricted by the performance of a task by agent A_2, the information system for A_1 includes a service providing information on the state of the performance of the task by A_2 (is it finished, is it already started, etc.).

We will now list the optimally integrated information systems from the standpoint of our four agents.

- A_1 - **Nuclear Medicine Physician:** $IS_1 = \{s_3, s_4, s_8, s_9, s_{10}, s_{13}, s_{14}, s_{15}\}$;
- A_2 - **Nuclear Medicine assistant:** $IS_2 = \{s_3, s_{12}, s_{13}, s_{14}, s_{15}, state(t)\}$, where t is the task of preparing a study as performed by the Nuclear medicine physician;
- A_3 - **The Requesting physician:** $IS_3 = \{s_{10}, s_{15}, s_1, s_2, state(t)\}$, where t is the task of reporting a study as performed by the Nuclear medicine physician;
- A_4 - **Administrator:** $IS_4 = S_4 = \{s_1, s_2\}$

3. Migration Strategy Part 1: finding Components and their relations

The information systems in the To-Be situation do overlap in that they share services. The process of decomposing these systems aims at isolating shared services as much as possible. So, only services shared by the same systems are grouped into the same component. If two services are shared by two information systems, and there are no other services shared by these information systems, we group these two services in the same component. Middleware components are components shared by two or more information services. Components only used by one information system are called application components.

- $c_1 = \{s_1, s_2\}$, a middleware component shared by IS_3 and IS_4
- $c_2 = \{s_3, s_{13}, s_{14}\}$, a middleware component shared by IS_1 and IS_2
- $c_3 = \{s_4, s_8, s_9, state(b_{21}), state(b_{22})\}$, an application component used in IS_1
- $c_4 = \{s_{12}, state(b_{11})\}$, an application component used in IS_2
- $c_5 = \{s_{15}\}$, a middleware component shared by IS_1, IS_2 and IS_3
- $c_6 = \{s_{10}\}$, a middleware component used in IS_1 and IS_3

4. Migration Strategy part 2: realising components and their relations using existing systems

Now that we have identified the application and middleware components to be realised in our open, modular environment, we will investigate how these can be realised using the existing applications and the middleware technology we have adopted, i.e. CORBA or DHE. First thing we have to do is to associate the services offered by our components with services offered by the information systems identified in the As-Is situation. A component is mapped onto an information system currently used, when either a service offered by that component is implemented in the information system or a service in the component provides information on the state of a task, and the information system offers a service supporting that task.

In table 1 we present the mapping of the components found onto the information systems in use at the Nuclear medicine department.

Table 1: Mapping worked out for our example

	c_1	c_2	c_3	c_4	c_5	c_6
Scheduling	+	+	+	+		
HIS			+			+
Image Sys		+	+	+	+	

Note that it is possible that components derived from the To-Be situation are not supported by any of the information systems currently in use. In this case the methodology has identified new components needed to support the business process.

Given our mapping onto the systems in use, we have to take the following steps:

1. In case of an **application component**
   - if the component is supported by only one information system, the functionality of the system should be adjusted by either restricting or extending it in order to make it compliant with the specification of the component;
   - if the component is supported by two or more information systems these should be integrated in order to offer the functionality required by the component. In principle there would be no need for the use of highly advanced integration technology in achieving this goal.
2. In case of a **middleware component**
   - if the component is supported by only one information system, the function(s) supporting it should be removed (or disabled). Then the component services (including the data managed) should be implemented using the middleware technology selected.
   - if the component is supported by two or more information systems, the function(s) supporting it should be removed (or disabled) from all these information systems. In the same way as above, the component services arc to realised using the selected middleware technology.

The construction of the 6 components derived in our example using DHE middleware and the three information systems, requires the following steps:

1. c_1 is a middleware component supported by only one information system. Registering and scheduling a visit should be handled by the ACT-management module of DHE and not by the POING application.
2. c_2 is also a middleware component, but it is supported by two information systems. All the information handled in this component is information related to the image stored in the database. This information should be stored in the DHE database.
3. c_3 is an application component (within the context of the business process analysed). This component should be realised by coupling the three information systems. Actually, this is exactly what was done at HISCOM.
4. c_4 is also an application component. It can be realised by coupling POING and the Image System. Main function is the construction of a list of studies to be approved.
5. c_5 is a middleware component supported by only one information system. The service offered by this component is viewing the images associated with a study. As with c_2 this service handles information stored in the DHE database.
6. c_6 is a middleware component supported by the HIS. As with c_2 and c_5 it handles the study information stored in the DHE database.

Finally, we investigate which integration steps are needed for constructing the information systems derived in the To-Be situation. These are realised by integrating the components. For each of the information systems in the To-Be situation we indicate out of which components it is constructed.

- $IS_1 = \{c_2, c_3, c_5, c_6\}$
- $IS_2 = \{c_2, c_4, c_5\}$
- $IS_3 = \{c_1, c_5, c_6\}$
- $IS_4 = \{c_1\}$

Note that only IS_1 and IS_2 use application components. The other information systems are based solely on middelware components.

5. Migration Strategy part 3: ordering the steps to be taken

We have now provided a method for deriving the parts 1 and 2 of our migration strategy. For all components we indicated how they could be realised using the existing systems and the middleware technology adopted. The last step to be taken is ordering the construction of components. A very simple strategy could be to order the construction based on the level of genericity. In our example this strategy would lead to the following order:

1. In the first step c_5 is constructed, because it is used by three information systems identified within the To-Be situation;
2. In the next step c_2, c_6 and c_1 are constructed. These are all used by two information systems;
3. Finally, the application components c_3 and c_4 are constructed. These are used by only one information system.

This ordering could be further refined by taking organisational, technological and financial considerations into account. This aspects are not dealt with in our account.

6. Conclusion

A migration strategy for transforming a non-open architecture into an open, modular architecture consists of three parts: specification of the components and their relations that will operate within this architecture, specification of the way how these components and their relations can be realised by integrating exiting information systems and a middleware technology, and a schedule for the construction of these components. The first two parts are often taken for granted. This is unfortunate because the quality of part 3 highly depends on the availability of parts 1 and 2.

7. References

1. Friers, T, F. Ferrara, *Migration towards common middleware solutions for an open HIS architecture*, MIC'96 proceedings, Sevens et al. (eds.), 1996
2. CORBAmed RFI, Object Management Group, January 1996, (http://www.omg.org/corbamed.home.htm)
3. Mowbray, T.J., R. Zahavi, *Essential CORBA*, Wiley & Sons, 1995
4. Scherrer, J.R., R. Baud, D. de Roulet, *Moving towards the future design of HIS: a view from the seventies to the end of the nineties, the DIOGENE paradigm*, in *Hospital Information Systems: design and development characteristics; impact and future architecture*, Elsevier, 1995
5. Vaughn, L.T., *Client/Server System Design & Implementation*, McGraw-Hill, 1994
6. ISO/IEC JTC 1/SC 21, Information retrieval, transfer and management for OSI - Basic reference model of open distributed processing - Part 1 Overview and guide to use, 1992

Medical Informatics Europe '97
C. Pappas et al. (Eds.)
IOS Press, 1997

Program package for paramedical investigations (EEG, EKG, radiography, biochemical investigations, pathological anatomy, nuclear medicine)

Smaranda Constantinescu[1] , Adina Raclariu[1] , Tania Butufei[2] and Mariana Purice[3]

[1] Software ITC S.A., [2] Hospital "Gr. Alexandrescu", [3] Institute of Endocrinology, Bucharest

Abstract. The purpose of this program package is to provide computer-based assistance for the work performed in paramedical investigation laboratories: functional investigations, radiology, biochemical investigations, pathological anatomy, nuclear medicine, in hospitals, polyclinics, medical practices. The common characteristics regarding the management of the work done in such laboratories has made a global approach of the problem possible. The modular design of the program package has allowed its stagewise development, thus offering the possibility of integration with the medical information management in each laboratory.

The program package for paramedical investigations has a two level structure

• programs and data bases pertaining to the main program;

• programs and data bases specific to each type of computerised laboratory.

The **SCALAB** application is aimed at optimising laboratory work with a view to assisting the specialist in most of the activities performed in the biochemical investigation laboratory. Among the facilities provided we mention: *data input facilities* (screen formats, vertical menus for assisting the user, explanatory message windows, "on-line" validation of input data, detected errors are sanctioned immediately by error messages and possibly sound sequences, supplementary facilities of the Windows environment are used, dialogue and editing boxes, push buttons), *data display/listing facilities* ("browse" type display, display/listing in tabular form, display as "push buttons", display within windows).

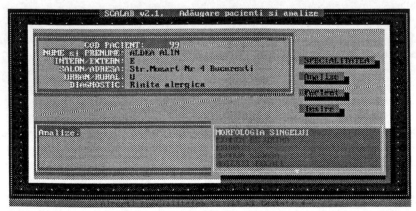

Patient data input screen

The working data of the application are grouped into two streams:

Input data:

• data contained within the patient records: name, forename, date of birth, date of the biochemical investigation, the department or clinic which sent the patient, diagnoses;

• one or more biochemical investigations.

The output data are organised as reports and statistics as follows:

• report containing data about the patients for which certain biochemical investigations have been performed;

• report containing data about the patients for whom the full set of biochemical investigations has been performed;

• report regarding the investigations for a certain patient;

• statistic containing the investigations performed during a trimester, semester or year;

• statistic of the investigations by the medium of origin of the patients (urban or rural) [2].

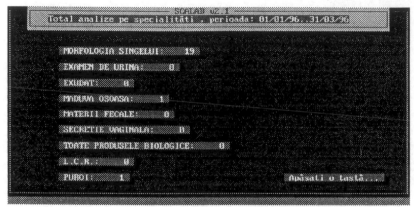

Screen displaying the statistic total of the investigations

The **EXFUNC** application is an application whose function is to collect the data displayed in functional investigation records, to store them in an appropriate manner and to process them in order to obtain, at a given moment, reports and statistics. The following types of investigation are performed in the functional investigation laboratory [5]:

Electroencephalogram - described according to the ICD-10 standard by the following types of diagnoses: slower wave activity in the theta band, increased activity of the slow waves, 8-13 cps alpha rhythm, very slow toward flat Eeg, delta rhythms of 1-4 cps.

Electrocardiogram - described according to the ICD-10 standard by the following types of diagnoses: P wave absent, widened QRS complex, lengthened QT interval, two-phase QRS-T route, abnormally low or high ST segment, increased, decreased or flattened T wave amplitude, U wave present, atrial tachycardia, arhythmia-brachycardia, arhythmia-tachycardia, atrioventricular block of the first degree, ventricular non-polarisation disturbances, ventricular tachycardia, atrial or ventricular fibrillation, atrial, nodal or ventricular extrasystoles, heart stop.

The evoked potentials are of the following types: visual, auditive, somato-sensorial.

All these investigations and diagnoses require a strict record of them to be kept, both quantitative and qualitative. In the functional investigation laboratory a ledger is kept in which the following information is recorded: record number, patient name and forename, age, clinical diagnosis, result interpretation, who performed the investigation. The investigations to which the patients are subjected as well as the results of these investigations are very important, because they help to decide whether surgery is to be performed or not in the given case.

The **RADIOLOG** application is an application whose function is to collect the data displayed in radiographic records, to store them in an appropriate manner and to process them in order to obtain, at a given moment, reports and statistics.

The types of radiographs performed in the radiography rooms, because they are of a wide variety, such as: standard (simple) radiographs, radiographs using contrast substances; tomographs.

In each radiography room a ledger is kept in which the following information is recorded: record number, date when the radiograph has been made, patient name, age, address, the department that referred the patient, the type of investigation, the room where it was performed, the number of incidences, the result of the radiographic investigation.

The result of the investigation is recorded in a radiographic examination bulletin, which is of great importance because it also constitutes a forensic medical document. The investigations performed upon the patients are the object of a statistic [1], [4]:

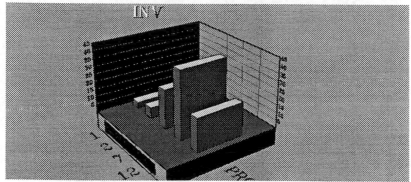

Screen presenting the 3D plot attached to the statistic by investigations.

NUCLEAR is an application whose function is to collect the data from the nuclear unit records, to store them and process them with a view to producing, at a given moment, certain reports and statistics.

Within the nuclear medicine laboratory, the radioisotopic investigations are grouped into two large categories: "in vitro" and "in vivo", the latter category being further subdivided into three groups: RIC, LIN scintigraphy and gamma camera scintigraphy.

• The nuclear medicine laboratory ledger contains the following information: record number, date, patient name and forename, age, sex, referring department or hospital, method of performing the investigation, kind of investigation, number of radioisotopic pictures, result of the investigation, remarks.

• The types of investigations and the types of isotopic substances corresponding to each type of investigation are in a large number.

• The isotopic investigation bulletin with the final result contains the following information: bulletin number, date of the investigation bulletin, patient name and forename, age, department, date when the investigation was carried out, the substance used, the mode of use, the name of the person who controlled the dose, the batch from which the radioactive substance was taken, the producer of the radioactive substance (usually the Atomic Physics Institute), delivery number, date of delivery, result of the investigation, recommendations, number of hours of surveillance, number of days of surveillance in hospital after the investigation.

Screen presenting the results from the investigation bulletin.

The statistic reports produced by the laboratory are:
• monthly consumption of consumable materials (films, radioactive substances)
• number of patients/month for whom radioisotopic investigations have been performed
• number of radioisotopic investigations

The **AP** application helps to establish the clinical diagnosis and to decide whether the given case is a surgical one or not. The histopathological examination is useful only in situations where during surgery it is not possible to decide about the nature of the tumour. In this case tumour samples are processed and sent to the pathological anatomy laboratory.

The importance of the anatomo-pathological diagnosis within the patient's file:

• From the point of view of the current medical activity in the clinic, the pathological anatomy laboratory plays an especially important role by the implications regarding the modification of the therapeutic conduct toward the patient, the moment when the precise anatomo-pathological diagnosis is established being crucial for the patient. The laboratory provides the medical information on the basis of which the patient's chances of survival are estimated.

• The pathological anatomy (histopathological) laboratory adds details to the clinical diagnosis made on hospitalisation. The respective domains of the two diagnoses (clinical and histopathological) are different: the clinical diagnosis describes the disease generally, while the anatomo-pathological (histological) one is a microscopic diagnosis.

The histopathological diagnosis correlated with the localisation of the pathological process and the possibility of a radical surgical intervention achieve a prognostic indication of the future evolution of the patient.

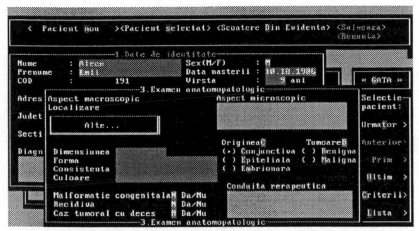

Patient selection screen.

The main objectives pursued by the informatisation of the nuclear medicine, functional investigations, radiography, biochemical investigations and pathological a anatomy laboratories are the timely, accurate and complete delivery of the results of the investigations requested by the physicians, the elimination of double record keeping in the laboratories involved, the optimisation of information transmission between the laboratory and the departments served, the delivery of the specific statistic reports to management and the statistics department.

The use of laboratory informatic applications in medical research facilitates information management, fast and high-quality processing of information, and information exchange between similar laboratories.

References:

[1] Petru Muresan, Book for mathematical methods in health status analysis, Medical Publishing House, Bucharest 1989.

[2] Daniel Schwartz Statistycal analysis of the surviving data, Flammarion Publishing Press, Medicine-Sciences, 1990.

[3] OMS, International classification of maladies, Medical Publishing Press, Bucharest, 1993.

[4] Ilie Vasilescu, Computer-based Statistic for human scientes, Military Publishing Press, Bucharest, 1992.

[5] Popescu Ovidiu: Medical Informatics, Medical Publishing House, Bucharest, 1988.

[6] Francois Gremy avec la colaboration de A. Aurengo, B. Auvert, P. Degoulet, B. Giusiano, M. Goldberg, H. Tevernier: Informatique medicale. Introduction a la methodologie on medicine et sante publique.

Medical Informatics Europe '97
C. Pappas et al. (Eds.)
IOS Press, 1997

A database on pesticides in Italy: a progress report

Petrelli G *, Mariotti S *, Siepi G *, Carrani E °, Roazzi P°, Tropeano R *, Mucci N⁺

*Istituto Superiore di Sanità -Epidemiology & Biostatistics Lab
°Istituto Superiore di Sanità -EDP, Rome- Italy
⁺ISPESL-Occupational Medicine Dept., Rome - Italy

Summary

An existing database on pesticides, running in the DOS/Windows environment, is operative at the National Institute of Health and has yielded useful informations for several published researches. The database is currently being restructured for the purpose of making it available on the Web. An HTML interface, allowing to formulate queries on the database from the Web is presently under development, and it will be made available, once the problems related to confidentiality of certain parts of the database are solved. The database in its present form is presented and necessary changes foreseen in the Web edition are discussed.

Introduction

Occupational handling and spraying of pesticides involves exposure to the active ingredients, but also to several different chemicals, which are used as solvents. The presence of active ingredients and organic solvents in pesticides is highly relevant to cancer risk (1) and to male infertility (2, 3). Spreading of information on the substances used in the pesticides is essential for assessing the risk and for preventive purposes.

The National Registry of Pesticides, a database containing information on the technical formulation of pesticides and their single active ingredients and solvents used, has been operative at the National Institute of Health since 1984 (4). As an example of using the archive for monitoring the risk associated to pesticides, a research trying to relate the decline in the past 50 years of male fertility on one side, and chemical agents with experimental evidence of male reproductive toxicity on the other side, was conducted using the data of the Register (5). The results indicate that several pesticide products notified to the Italian Registry contain active ingredients and/or solvents severely affecting testicular function and sperm morphology in laboratory animals.

While the present form of the database has already proved to be very helpful for the Local Health Units of the National Health System, which requested it to get information useful for their health control activities on agricultural products, an implementation of the same database on the Web, would make it more easily reachable and most important of all, easily upgradable with new substances being introduced every day. A new formulation of the database, constisting mainly in the implementation of an HTML interface between the database itself and the Web protocol would yield several important advantages.

Organization of the database

According to the Italian law, the marketing of a pesticide must be authorized by the Ministy of Health. Information about new pesticides notified to the ministry of Health are organized in a Register, which contains up to date thousands of technical formulation proposed for use in Italy between 1971 and 1996. For each registered product the following items are stored:1) Name of industry;2) Name of product; 3)Number of registration; 4) Date of registration; 5) Toxicological class; 6) Active ingredients (name and concentration); 7) Solvents; 8) Name of factory; 9) Factory address; 10) Type of factory. The database includes 8500 products of pesticides (20.000 records, one record for each registration, consequentely the number of records is different from the number of products because each product can be authorized many times). The inquiries can be performed by using built-in facilities with every combination of items as selection keys. Specific programs are being developed in order to simplify the inquiries most frequently performed.

Some of the information of the register was made available to the Regional Health Authorities, by means of floppy disks containing a subset of the database implementation. The withdrawn products (those products which are considered dangerous by the Health Authorities and therefore revoked) are stored in a separate file.

The conversion of the database in a form suitable to accept queries from the Web is currently being implemented. Every researcher in the Public Health field with access on the Internet, subject to the condition that the user is registered and a password for the use of the archive has been assigned by the maintenance staff, will be able to get information about the substances registered in the database. A simple HTML interface is being developed, to translate queries in a form suitable to be understood by the DB vista SQL method used. The heart of the interface, the Common Gateway Interface (CGI) is written in ANSI C. Problems of confidentiality of certain parts of the information contained in the archive will be solved by restraining access to these parts.

Conclusion

Public Health is one of the areas where worldwide exchange of information is of especially high priority for many reasons, among whom the fact that spread of epidemics and environmental pollution does not stop at the national borders. For this reason, the easy access and transmission of up-to-date information will promote quick decision-making. At the same time the World Wide Web is becoming quickly the major way of acquiring information in all scientific disciplines, for its suitability to fast distribution of information. The Web version of the Pesticides Register will yield wider access possibility, along with a much easier upgradability.

References
1. Petrelli G., Siepi G., Miligi L. and Vineis P. Solvents in pesticides. Scand J Work Environ Health, 1993; 19: 63-65.
2. Traina M. E., Ade P., Siepi G. , Urbani E. and Petrelli G. A review of the effect of pesticide formulations on male fertility. Int. J. Environ. Health Res, 1994; 4: 38-47
3. Petrelli G., Traina M. E. Glycol ethers in pesticide products: a possible reproductive risk? Rep. Tox.; 1995; 9: 401-402
4. Petrelli G. Archivio dei fitofarmaci. Potenzialità e sviluppo. Igiene dell' Ambiente e del Territorio, C. G. Ed. Med. Scient, Torino, 1989: 489-510.
5. Petrelli G., Mucci N., Siepi G., Pace F. Antiparassitari agricoli valutati per potenziali effetti cancerogeni, mutageni e tossico-riproduttivi. Med. Lav., 1996; 87: 110-121.

Acknowledgements

Part of this work was made possible by a grant of ISS Project "Prevenzione dei fattori di rischio della salute materno-infantile" (Art 12 D leg.vo 502/92).

Medical Informatics Europe '97
C. Pappas et al. (Eds.)
IOS Press, 1997

Pre-hospital Health Emergency Management as an Integrated Service of the Regional Health Telematics Network of Crete

Erich LEISCH[1], Manolis TSIKNAKIS[1], and Stelios C. ORPHANOUDAKIS[1,2]

[1] *Institute of Computer Science, FORTH, PO Box 1385, GR 71110 Heraklion, Greece*
[2] *Dept. of Computer Science, University of Crete, GR 71409 Heraklion, Greece*
{erich,tsiknaki,orphanou}@ics.forth.gr

Abstract. In this paper, a Pre-hospital Health Emergency Management System (PHEMS) is presented, which is being developed on the basis of a common reference architecture that has been defined at a European level by partners from ten EU member states in the course of the ongoing HECTOR project. The PHEMS, which is implemented as an autonomous system, will be integrated as an added-value service into the Regional Health Telematics Network of Crete. The PHEMS architecture is based on a 'perception-cognition-action' paradigm.

1. Introduction

The health emergency management domain and the information systems used in it can be characterised in the following way: Health emergency management services are usually not supported by a single information system, but by a number of task-specific Heterogeneous Autonomous Distributed Systems (HADS). Quite often, those systems are not co-operative by themselves, which leads to the necessity for redundant user input and sometimes to co-ordination problems or inefficiency. Another characteristic is the requirement for those systems to show a 'soft real-time' behaviour in response to emergency service requests and to continuously incoming information about a dynamically changing emergency situation. Parts of an emergency management system can be implemented as autonomous agents [1]. Such agents are being discussed and used in the context of a new approach to Artificial Intelligence [2].

The presented system is mainly based on existing technology and incorporates new multimedia and telecommunications capabilities. It is designed to cover a well-defined spectrum of scenarios and situations in the health emergency management domain.

The Regional Health Telematics Network of Crete will provide a set of services, in order to support the different tasks that contribute to high-quality healthcare provision for the inhabitants and the visitors of Crete. The Pre-hospital Health Emergency Management System (PHEMS), although designed as an autonomous system, will provide its services in the context of that Health Telematics Network. This is possible, because integration and interoperability issues played an important role in the design of the PHEMS and of the Regional Health Telematics Network of Crete.

2. Scenarios

The scenarios described in this chapter imply the involvement of four actors, namely the Health Emergency Co-ordination Centre (HECC), its Mobile Units (MU), and the partners at the co-operating hospitals and Primary Care Centres (PCC).

2.1 Trauma Transportation Telematics (TTT)

Crete, a highly populated tourist island, faces an increased number of emergency calls, mainly trauma from road accidents, especially during summer. It is planned to test the efficiency and applicability of emergency teleconsultation with the mobile unit and of preparing the receiving hospital to manage the patient, by transmission of vital signs such as ECG, blood pressure measurements, etc., and of real-time camera pictures of the accident scene and of the patients that are sent to the HECC.

2.2 Real-Time Teleconsultation (RTT)

Doctors in remote primary care centres quite frequently face difficult cases (trauma, cardiac arrests, drug intoxication, etc.) without the appropriate experience or expertise to manage them successfully. In this scenario, teleconsultation and telediagnosis based on previously transmitted vital signs and medical pictures are used in combination with formalised medical protocols aiming at improving the morbidity and mortality statistics of rural emergency cases.

2.3 Inter-Hospital Transportation Teleconsultation (ITT)

The transportation of critically ill patients is a difficult task and their supervision through telematics services seems to be of invaluable help. As ICUs are sparse in the island, transportation of such patients between hospitals is frequently required at a regional, national, or trans-national level. In this scenario, joint teleconsultation and telediagnosis of the sending as well as the receiving hospitals and the mobile unit are tested.

3. Approach

In order to establish a sound basis for an architecture design and a detailed functional specification of the services to be implemented at the pilot site of Crete, a formal requirements analysis was conducted. This formal analysis, which served also as a means to communicate with the domain specialists about the REQUIRED applications and services, was done by means of a CASE tool, which supports system development methodologies that cover the analysis and design stages. Using that CASE tool, mainly the process of responding to emergency service requests has been described. The primary actors (e.g., health emergency co-ordination centre, hospitals, mobile units, etc.), the data stores (e.g. knowledge bases) and the data processes with their associated data flows (e.g., communication messages) were identified and described. That process model, which was successfully verified in co-operation with the local partners (mainly EKAB), was also used for the description of the HECTOR reference architecture.

The HECTOR reference architecture, which is based on the *perception-cognition-action* paradigm [6], defines the conceptual model, the services, the user interface guidelines, the message formats, and the levels of interoperability for a HECTOR-compliant PHEMS.

4. Patient Record and Emergency Episode Folder

At the hospitals (or other healthcare providers), clinical multimedia data are organised in a *patient-centred* manner in so-called 'patient record segments'. They are mainly accessed via the patient identification (patient card, name, date of birth, passport number, etc.).

In contrast to that, at the HECC and its associated mobile units, clinical multimedia data created during an emergency episode are organised in an *episode-centred* manner in emergency episode folders. The patients involved in an emergency episode are assigned a 'preliminary patient identification number' that is composed of the 'episode identification number' and a patient counter. After identifying a patient, his/her emergency episode folder contents become a patient record segment of his/her 'virtual patient record'.

In addition to the primary central emergency episode archive at the HECC, there are decentralised secondary emergency episode archives at the mobile units, the hospitals, and the primary care centres. Those secondary archives are used to keep data temporarily, until they are transferred (via batch mode) to the HECC's archive, thus reducing the need for online communication.

5. Architecture

As already mentioned, the HECTOR architecture uses a *perception-cognition-action* paradigm. That paradigm is illustrated in the figure below.

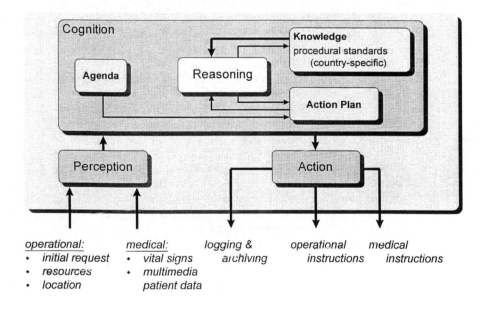

Figure 1 : The HECTOR paradigm

The *perception* part of the HECTOR architecture is responsible for taking or sensing information from the environment. This information may be of operational or medical nature. Operational perception data may be incoming calls, i.e. emergency service requests, but also information about available resources or data describing the current location of mobile units, patients, etc. Medical perception covers the acquisition of vital signs, the retrieval and exchange of clinical multimedia data (e.g. patient record segments), and the annotations that are exchanged during telediagnosis or teleconsultation sessions.

The most challenging component of the architecture is the *cognition* subsystem. It is supposed to give instructions and recommendations that are based on the perceived information (see above) and on knowledge about operational and medical procedures, that are stored in simple rule databases or in more sophisticated knowledge bases. Decisions are made by co-operating autonomous agents. Typical problems that are to be solved by the cognition component are the effective and efficient management of resources under dynamically changing conditions or the determination of the adequate set of therapeutic or life-saving actions, triggered by continuously acquired vital signs from a patient.

Operational *actions* are, for instance, the allocation of resources such as mobile units, the exchange of operational instructions between the HECC and the mobile units, and the maintenance of the emergency episode archive. Besides that, medical instructions and therapeutic protocols are exchanged and applied.

6. Services

6.1 Medical Services

The medical services provided by the PHEMS comprise access to clinical multimedia data stored in patient record segments, telediagnosis and teleconsultation on such data, the acquisition of vital signs, and the determination and application of predefined medical procedures.

By means of these services, clinical multimedia data from the patient record archive as well as currently acquired vital signs and real-time pictures from the accident scene can be exchanged between the HECC, the hospitals, the primary care centres, and the mobile units. Vital signs include ECG, non-invasive and invasive blood pressure measurements, oxygen saturation, capnometry traces, and temperature.

Based on the exchanged clinical multimedia data, telediagnosis and teleconsultation sessions with multiple participants at different sites can be established, thus making medical expertise available at remote locations.

Another way of providing medical decision support is through the use of locally stored predefined standard medical procedures that may be triggered automatically by vital signs at the assistance site or remotely by a doctor at the HECC.

6.2 Operational Services

The HECC-based resource management is the most important operational service. It implies the gathering of resource and status information from the involved actors (perception), the optimal use of the available resources under dynamically changing situations (cognition), and the issuing of resource assignments and other operational instructions (action). In order to achieve an optimal management of resources, an approach was chosen that is based on the concept of co-operating autonomous agents, each of them taking care of a small manageable subset of optimisation goals of different importance, thus resulting in the desired overall system behaviour [1, 2].

Resources are mobile units, medical personnel, beds in hospitals, equipment, etc. At the mobile units, hospitals, and primary care centres, incoming resource requirements are compared with available local resources. Information about available resources as well as status information about them is sent to the HECC on demand or on a regular basis. Resource assignments made at the HECC are presented and registered.

The tracking of mobile units, the location of assistance sites or patients could be seen as part of the resource management. They are mentioned here separately because of the specific GPS/GIS technology used in this context. Location, however, is only partly based on GPS data; also traditional location information (city, address, etc.) is exchanged and used at the HECC to keep spatial information up to date.

A series of online tutorials covering the operational and medical procedures that have to do with pre-hospital health emergency management will be provided. It will be used not only for the education and the training of the HECC staff, but also for the involved partners at the hospitals and primary care centres.

7. Interoperability Issues

A satisfactory level of interoperability has to be achieved in three areas. First, the components of the HECTOR system have to use a common model and common standards. Second, it must be possible to integrate the HECTOR system with the Regional Health Telematics Network of Crete. Third, it should be possible that a HECTOR system can co-operate with another Emergency Co-ordination Centre (ECC) through the exchange of a minimum set of standard message classes, in order to forward an emergency request or to co-ordinate a co-operative response, e.g. by utilising foreign resources.

Acknowledgement

This work has been funded in part by the HECTOR project under the Telematics Applications Programme of the European Commission.

References

[1]   P. Maes, Modeling Adaptive Autonomous Agents. *Artificial Life Journal*, vol. 1 (1&2), 1994.

[2]   R. A. Brooks, Intelligence Without Reason, MIT Media Lab, MIT, MA, USA, AI Memo 1293, 1991.

[3]   S. C. Orphanoudakis *et al.*, Development of an Integrated Image Management and Communication System on Crete, *Computer Assisted Radiology - CAR '95 Proceedings*, Berlin, 1995, pp. 481-487.

[4]   M. Tsiknakis *et al.*, Intelligent Image Management in a Distributed PACS and Telemedicine Environment, *IEEE Communications Magazine*, vol. 34, no. 7, July 1996, pp. 36-45.

[5]   E. Leisch *et al.*, An Architectural Framework for the Integration of Geographically Distributed Heterogeneous Autonomous Medical Information Systems, *EuroPACS'96 Proceedings*, Heraklion, Greece, 1996, pp. 73-77.

[6]   B. Hayes-Roth, Architectural Foundations for Real-Time Performance in Intelligent Agents, *Real-Time Systems* (May 1990).

Medical Informatics Europe '97
C. Pappas et al (Eds.)
IOS Press. 1997

W.W.W. Cooperative Multimedia Interface in Medicine

Courtin C. [a], Séka L.-P. [a], Cléran L. [a] and Le Beux P [a].

[a] *Laboratoire d'Informatique Médicale, Faculté de Médecine, Université de Rennes 1, avenue du Pr. Léon Bernard 35043 Rennes Cédex, FRANCE*

Abstract. The World Wide Web is now the most used multimedia information system on Internet allowing, by means of Web browsers such as Netscape Navigator or Mosaic, distribution or consultation of hypermedia documents. Although the Web has appeared only recently, the growth of its use has generated the emergence of numerous information and knowledge bases in the medical field. We suggest to investigate extended functionalities in order to introduce cooperative activities in our medical information system. These new activities allow asynchronous exchange of records and synchronous cooperation for a better coordination of the work within and between hospitals.

1. Introduction

Our first purpose is to offer to a large public a multimedia man/machine interface on Internet allowing exploration of our medical information and knowledge bases. Multimedia items (texts, images, and sounds) of about 3,500 clinical cases, which are stored in the images database ICONOWEB in the Medical Information Department of Rennes, may be shared simultaneously by several Web users.

Our second purpose is to present feasability results of adding cooperative functionalities to the existing multimedia interface in order to carry out a cooperative system on Internet. This investigation is aimed at the use of our medical information system for establishing co-diagnosis by several physicians. Such activities define telediagnosis which is a part of telemedicine.

Finally, we present a prototype W.W.W. multimedia interface we have developped in the Medical Information Department of Rennes.

2. Materials and Methods

2.1 W.W.W. in the medical field

Taking charge of patients in a hospital generates a huge volume of medical and clerical information which is shared by multidisciplinary staff (physicians, radiologists, nurses, secretaries, etc.). Sometimes, completion of a patient's record involves medical examination in another medical department. It follows therefrom that patient's record has to be carried wholly or partly between different places either by the patient himself, by post, or by hospital mail. Computerizing medical records would avoid scattering of included data and allow rapid and secure transmission of it by a telecommunication network [1]. The quality of patients' care depends directly on the quality, security, rapidity, and low cost of transmission devices. Development of new technologies involved the emergence of numerous software applications providing physicians with facilities to access and explore medical databases. In our Medical Information Department, we put our existing medical database at the public's disposal as soon as the Web appeared [2]. Indeed, most of current Web browsers, such as Netscape Navigator or Mosaic, support multimedia information. The official definition of World Wide

Web (W.W.W. or Web) is : wide-area hypermedia information retrieval initiative aiming to give universal access to a large universe of documents [3]. A medical record is intrinsically multimedia as it mixes various types of data : texts, still images, video, vocal or sound items, and spreadsheets. Thus, the Web is suitable for supporting medical information.

3. C.S.C.W. in the medical field

3.1 Groupware activities

Connection to a telecommunication network allows a rapid and secure transfer of medical information between physicians. Also, Internet access permits computerized medical records to be available everywhere and at any time. Thus, a physician would be able to get a patient's record in the case of an emergency admission in any hospital by requesting authorization directly, via the network, to the original hospital. Such a practice would avoid redundant medical examinations which are time consuming and costly.

   Groupware and new technologies of telecommunication allow remote physicians to work together. Such activities, called C.S.C.W. (Computer Supported Cooperative Work), involve communication, coordination, cooperation, and collaboration facilities. The use of transmission devices in the medical field defines telemedicine which encompasses mainly teleradiology, telediagnosis, and teleassistance.

3.2 Network technology

Networks are characterized by the nature of the communication support (telephone, coaxial cable, radio relay system, optical fiber), and especially by the communication protocols used [3] which are software providing several users with dialog boxes, data exchange facilities through the network. C.S.C.W. systems conception requires consideration of three types of criteria [4] : hardware, software, and network. Hardware criteria refer to the target machines and the input/output devices. Software criteria are related to the operating system, the window system, and the graphical user interface. Network criteria encompass various types of networks : L.A.N. (Local Area Network), M.A.N. (Metropolitan Area Network), W.A.N. (Wide Area Network), and various communication protocols. W.A.N. are networks allowing interconnection between computers wherever they are in the world.

   Performances of teleradiology systems depend on the technology of the network. The development of new technologies has instigated the creation of new types of network : I.S.D.N. (Integrated Services Digital Network) [5], the A.T.M. (Asynchronous Transfer Mode) technology allows improved data compression and then fast transfer of still images, video, voice or sounds. It is worth noting that I.S.D.N. technology offers reasonably fast Internet access.

3.3 C.S.C.W. systems

As shown above, existing C.S.C.W. systems are dependent on hardware (the target machines and the input/output devices), software (the operating system, the window system, and the graphical user interface) and network technology (L.A.N., M.A.N., W.A.N., and communication protocols). With the purpose of casting off these constraints, we have chosen to use well-known Internet browsers, such as Netscape Navigator, to carry out our man/machine interfaces. Nowadays, all types of network (L.A.N., M.A.N., W.A.N.) can be connected to each other. In other words, the international network consists of interconnection between local and national networks. Internet is the most famous international network which is spread all over the world. Every network client program uses different protocols for establishing communication : H.T.T.P. (HyperText Transfer Protocol) for W.W.W. (World Wide Web), Gopher protocol, Wais protocol, or F.T.P. (File Transfer Protocol). There is a lower protocol behind all of these programs called I.P. (Internet Protocol) and supported by most of the networks, especially by Internet.

   Locally, our medical information system is settled on intranet allowing interconnection between various types of machines (Macintosh, P.C., UNIX) using Ethernet protocol. Until now, Internet was well-suited for interactive activities between a client and a server. However, dynamic activities are quite limited in H.T.M.L. pages, and then cooperative activities can not be supported with current Web browsers[1]. This issue conveys us to use the Java language supplying cooperation facilities in H.T.M.L. pages. In the next subsections, we attempt to present detailed features of the Java language allowing activities in a C.S.C.W. system via a H.T.M.L. interface.

4. Java language, the Solution !

4.1 Features of the Java language

The Java language, a new object-oriented computing language related to C++ [6], is designed to be machine independent and platform independent. In other words, the aim of this language is that all compilers accept the same programs and that all Java programs compute the same result on all machines.

The Java language may be integrated into H.T.M.L. pages as programs doing specific tasks. Java is object-oriented (well-adapted to the management of medical records included items), simple (for instance : memories' issues have been solved by means of integrated garbage-collector), robust, secure (a full control mechanism is integrated for checking imported code and then protects the local station against viruses or infiltration ; Java supplies confidentiality facilities which are indispensable in medicine), independent of architecture (Java does not produce specific micro-instructions but byte-code program, by means of a javac compiler, which can be interpreted by a virtual Java processor), portable (use of standard in terms of network and internal data types), efficient (a Java interpreter runs a compiled program, already optimised), distributed (Internet protocols such as H.T.T.P., F.T.P. Telnet, are integrated ; client/server architecture can be easily implemented), multi-thread (simultaneous processes) and dynamic (dynamic loading of various classes).

4.2 Java in H.T.M.L. pages

As far as the H.T.M.L. page is concerned, the Java program « x » (or applet) appears in a specified area defined in the H.T.M.L. program as following [7] :

    <APPLET code=« x » width=20 height=20></APPLET>

The included Java applet is an objet which may be a video, or a vocal item (for instance : comment of radiograph), or any other program.

4.3 Java communication mechanisms

The next two subsections deal with R.M.I. (Remote Method Invocation). The sockets are the basic communication mechanism provided by Java. This mechanism is simple and flexible enough for making general communication tasks. It implies implementation of application level protocols in order to exchange messages between client and server.

Unlike the sockets, the R.P.C. (Remote Procedure Call) mechanism is placed at procedure call level. Procedure calls are transparent whether they are local or remote. This mechanism hits a snag when communication between objects placed on various remote machines is necessary, it is therefore not suitable for distributed objects systems. Remote object calls are managed by proxies[2] on distributed object systems.

Java is a third generation language (3G.L.) entirely portable which uses internal libraries supplying high-performance multimedia functionalities (AudioClip, java.awt.image), graphic interface objects and events management such as cursor movement (A.W.T. : Advanced Windows Toolkit), network management functionalities (java.net), and some other facilities. All of the systems supporting the Java interpreter allow A.W.T. graphic objects to be manipulated.

---

[1] Netscape 4.x should allow some cooperative activities.

[2] A network proxy is a conduit between the computer and the Internet used to access to the latter.

Java threads run in the same space and they can share the access to the same attributes and methods of an object. Therefore, attributes and methods may be characterized as being synchronized, and a monitor may be associated to every instance of the object. In this case, the thread has to be dedicated to a monitor in order to know whether the instance is already used or not.

5. Results

Today, our multimedia information system contains hypermedia documents describing more than 10,000 diseases on A.D.M. database [2], and about 3,500 clinical cases (i.e. : anomynous patient records) stored on ICONOWEB database. The man/machine interfaces which explore existing medical data and knowledge of our system have been carried out thanks to H.T.M.L. forms providing interaction with users. Thus, physicians can use any Internet client program (browser) to access our interfaces on any platform (Macintosh, P.C., UNIX).

5.1 ICONOWEB multimedia system

The ICONOWEB project is aimed at medical students or physicians who want to see similar clinical cases or merely want to train for medical diagnosis. The ICONOWEB multimedia system comprises various types of medical information which is set up on a relational database management system (ORACLE), programs for indexing texts, creating new multimedia documents, and multimedia man/machine interfaces.

The medical data and knowledge consist of books referencing medical images (EDICERF), the clinical cases or reports (ICONOCERF), and the description of deseases (A.D.M. dictionary). ADM-INDEX program uses the latter for indexing texts in the first two kinds of documents : the books and the clinical cases.

ADM-INDEX program makes links between clinical reports (or cases) and the A.D.M. dictionary, EDICERF books and the A.D.M. dictionary, clinical reports and EDICERF books. After determining the corresponding links, the query process analyses conceptualy the user's request in order to display (by means of a matching process) all clinical cases (by chapter : Diagnosis, Context), EDICERF books (by chapter : Pediatry ...) and A.D.M. deseases which contain the query concepts. Thus, the user can get the related information on navigating easily, via a H.T.M.L. multimedia interface, on the server.

The system presents cases as questions if a concept is present in the chapter Context, displays the report without diagnosis and commentaries, and allows the user to suggest diagnosis. In this case, ADM-INDEX plays an important role as it draws a parallel between the user's answer and the concepts in the diagnosis and then gives an answer and a correction.

5.2 Cooperative activities

The foremost concern of extending the capabilities of our system comes from the need for real time cooperation between physicians and medical students. Our feasability results are based on a detailed survey of Java possibilities, and on the cooperative Java applet « Cafet.class » developped by Mr. Lapointe on the « PauseJava » site [8]. The Java applet, included in a H.T.M.L. page and automatically loaded as soon as the latter is consulted, allows real-time discussion between several users. An identification facility allows new comers to join the current discussion. A dialog area displays textual exchanges in a comprehensive way : various colours, icons (see figure 1).

Using the same communication protocol, cursor location of connected users can be transfered (as easily as characters) and then displayed in a shared area. Analogously to the mechanism of the « Cafet.class » applet, several physicians can discuss through a similar dialog area and show specific regions of interest on a X-ray by means of telecursor ; both the applet Java display areas (text and image) may be inserted in the same H.T.M.L. page. It is worth noting that an applet can communicate with other programs in three ways :

- by invoking public methods of other applets on the same H.T.M.L. page (subject to security restrictions).
- by using the A.P.I.[3] defined in the java.applet package viewer that contains it.
- by using the A.P.I. defined in the java.net package to communicate over the network with other programs. The other programs must be running on the host that the applet originated from.

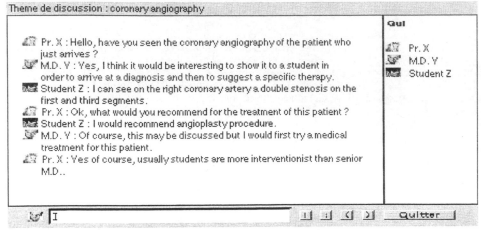

figure 1 : cooperative Java applet

6. Conclusion

The opened system W.W.W. can be used either to enhance and to standardize existing multimedia medical information. Hence, the emergence of the Java language and the choice of the Web for supporting our medical multimedia information system offer large perspectives of development for new facilities. Besides, unlike stand alone applications, the use of Web browsers allows easy and continuous maintenance of both medical data and multimedia interfaces. We are working on a prototype using the Java language to extend the functionalities of our medical information system in order to permit cooperative activities beween remote physicians and medical students.

References

[1]   Beuscart R., Debaecker C., Foucher C., Dufresne E. « Multimedia et médecine : un outil pour améliorer la communication médicale » Informatique et Santé La Revue No. 16 (1st trimester 1994) pp. 25-30
[2]   Pouliquen B., Riou C., Denier P., Fresnel A., Delamarre D., and Le Beux P. « Using World Wide Web Multimedia in Medecine » Medinfo 95 Proceedings, Ed. R.A. Greenes and al. (1995) pp. 1519-1523.
[3]   Le Beux P., Denier P., Burgun A. « Le Multimédia : C.D./R.O.M. et/ou clients serveurs Hypermédia » Ed. Informatique et Santé (1994) pp. 223-242.
[4]   Reinhard W., Schweitzer J., Völksen G. « C.S.C.W. Tools : Concepts and Architectures » I.E.E.E. (may 1994) pp. 28-36.
[5]   Arpège « Gestion de réseaux : concepts et outils » Ed. Masson (1992)
[6]   Rodgers R.P.C., M.D. « Java and Its Future Biomedical Computing » Journal of the American Medical Informatics Association, Vol. 3, No. 5 (Sep./Oct. 1996) pp. 303-307
[7]   Wiley John & Sons, Inc. « JAVA Sourcebook. A Complete Guide to Creating Java Applets for the Web » Ed. Anuff, of HotWired (1996)
[8]   Lapointe P.-N. « le bar » http://www.u-strasbg.fr/reseau_osiris/doc_tech/java/bar/

---

[3] Application Programming Interface

Medical Informatics Europe '97
C. Pappas et al. (Eds.)
IOS Press, 1997

PRONET Services for Distance Learning in Mammographic Image Processing

L. Costaridou[1], G. Panayiotakis[1*], C. Efstratiou[1], P. Sakellaropoulos[1], D. Cavouras[3],
C. Kalogeropoulou[2], K. Varaki[2], L. Giannakou[2], J. Dimopoulos[2]

[1] *Department of Medical Physics, School of Medicine, University of Patras, Greece*
[2] *Department of Radiology, School of Medicine, University of Patras, Greece*
[3] *Department of Medical Instrumentation Technology, TEI Athens, Greece*

Abstract. The potential of telematics services is investigated with respect to learning needs of medical physicists and biomedical engineers. Telematics services are integrated into a system, the PRONET, which evolves around multimedia computer based courses and distance tutoring support. In addition, information database access and special interest group support are offered. System architecture is based on a component integration approach. The services are delivered in three modes: LAN, ISDN and Internet. Mammographic image processing is selected as an example content area.

1. Introduction

Due to the rapid evolution in methods and technological innovations in medical imaging and the poor representation of medical image processing in clinical routine [1], the need for medical physicist's and biomedical engineer's training is increasing. The advantages of computer based learning methods have been exploited in stand alone learning systems in medicine [2-4]. The evolution of these systems to distance learning systems with the use of telematics technology constitutes a current methodological trend in learning [5-7].

PRONET involves the development and demonstration of an integrated training and support service for professionals, using innovative technologies, as telematics.

In this paper PRONET services relative to medical physicists and biomedical engineers and to some extend radiologists distance learning need are presented, in the domain of mammographic image processing.

2. Materials and Methods

2.1. User Needs

One of the first phases of PRONET was the collection of user requirements concerning services that will best meet user needs. Figure 1 summarises the medical physics and biomedical engineering user group preferences.

---

* Corresponding author

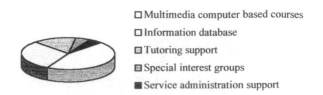

☐ Multimedia computer based courses

☐ Information database

▨ Tutoring support

▨ Special interest groups

■ Service administration support

Figure 1: Top ranking of services clearly indicate an increased need for multimedia computer based courses, followed by access to an information database.

2.2. Architecture

To meet the above stated user requirements PRONET provides a series of training sessions. The sessions are implemented using multimedia technologies over the Internet. These sessions are based on interactive multimedia courses and on-line tutoring support through video/audio conferencing, white-board and electronic e-mail facilities. This functionality is based on a four-level architecture presented in figure 2.

The PRONET system architecture is based on an integration and customisation approach of components. These components are developed using commercial products, that are market proven. The main benefits of this design are: (i) reduced development time, (ii) system modularity which allows easy system modification to satisfy future needs and (iii) compliance with existing standards.

2.3. The PRONET Services

The PRONET service is being released on the World Wide Web, using HTML, CGI, Perl and Java facilities, as well as multimedia authoring tools and relational databases for the courseware creation. The user environment consists of a PC, an Internet connection, a Windows environment and a Netscape browser.

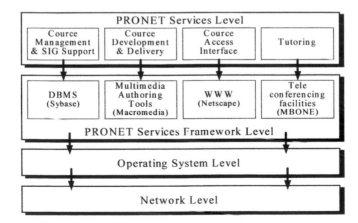

Figure 2: The functionality of the system is presented as a four-level architecture, the PRONET service, the PRONET service framework, the operating system and the network.

PRONET forms a network which is currently composed of three nodes. These nodes are named Access Service Points (ASPs) and contain all the necessary hardware, software and networking infrastructure to support the service. Such a network offers improved effectiveness of information access, since ASP nodes function as 'one stop' information shops for PRONET users.

PRONET services are adapted with respect to the available bandwidth of the end user. The access modes provided are: LAN (high speed access), ISDN (via local ISDN connections) and Internet access.

Users may use personal workstations (appropriately equipped) and basic Internet services in order to access the PRONET service.

2.4. Multimedia Course Structure

Three courses (10 hours in total duration) addressing different medical physics and biomedical engineering subjects are developed. The course structure is hierarchical, composed of units and chapters, schematically presented in figure 3.

2.5. The Database Contents

The PRONET service includes access to an information database supporting medical physics and biomedical engineering scientific/professional needs. This information base provides access to resources such as: scientific/professional organisations, european universities offering courses and programs, european organisations responsible for directives and recommendations, planned conferences and events in Europe and technical reports.

3. Results and Discussion

Mammographic image processing has been selected as it represents a functionality directly supporting image information extraction, which is related to diagnosis.

Content is organised to reflect both theoretical and case-oriented approaches. The theoretical approach consists of image enhancement concept definition and methods description such as wavelet based contrast enhancement, Difference Of Gaussians (DOG) and Gabor filtering [8-10].

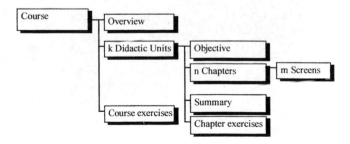

Figure 3: The structure of a multimedia course. The course structure allows the definition of general description templates, that are of generic character and are used for course development.

In describing the methods, emphasis is given to the presentation of the effects of key input parameters to processed images, which is offered as an additional functionality enriching the interactive character of the course.

Clinical images originated from the department of radiology of the university hospital of Patras and digitised (ScanJet II cx/T, HP). Images have been off-line processed using scripts (MATLAB v4.2) or original C++ code. Public domain routines have also been used (Wavelab Toolkit and Wave 2).

As an example two characteristic screens are presented in figures 4 and 5. In the first screen the structure and the key steps of a dyadic wavelet based algorithm is presented. In the second screen, an example of the application of the same algorithm on a mammogram is presented. The case is designed to visually convey the effect of different input parameters of the algorithm on the reconstructed image.

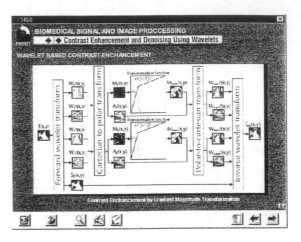

Figure 4: Wavelet based contrast enhancement. The effect of the algorithm is presented by means of an artificial object (phantom). The icons correspond to full scale grey level images at intermediate «key» steps of the algorithm.

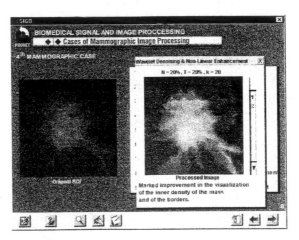

Figure 5: The effect of a selected wavelet enhancement method and its N, k, T parameters on a mammogram. Contrast enhancement is qualitatively assessed by radiologists.

The distance learning scenario of PRONET is based on exploratory learning, offered by the interactive multimedia courses, complemented by distance tutoring services following course attendance. Tutoring support services rely on real or differed time tutor-learner communication, depending on available bandwidth. Thus for LAN or ISDN accessed ASPs, the tutoring scenario relies on video-conferencing, where as for Internet access ASPs wide board technologies and e-mail are used.

Both interactive multimedia courses and tutoring services are accessed through an integrated uniform client environment, currently under development. This environment also incorporates access to the information database and special interest groups.

Finally, the effectiveness of the distance learning services offered, with respect to mammographic image processing, will be evaluated in a designed and planed evaluation phase, following the full scale implementation of PRONET.

Acknowledgement

The PRONET project (Multimedia Computer Based On-line Training and Support Service for Professionals) is funded by the Commission of the European Communities in the framework of the Telematics Education & Training programme (contract E1017). The authors would like to thank all project partners for their contribution to the project.

References

[1] H-P. Meinzer and U. Engelmann, Medical Images in Integrated Health Care Workstations. In: J. van Bemmel, A. McCray (Eds.), Yearbook of Medical Informatics 96. ISBN: 3-7945-1759-8. IMIA-Schattauer, 1996, pp. 87-94.

[2] E. Hoffer and O. Barnett, Computers in Medical Education. In: E. Shortliffe and L. Perrault (Eds.) L. Fagan and Wiederhold (Assoc. eds.), Medical Informatics: Computer Applications in Health Care. ISBN: 0-201-06741-2. Addisson-Wesley, New York, 1990, pp. 535-561.

[3] L. Costaridou, K. Hatzis, G. Panayiotakis, B. Proimos and N. Pallikarakis, A learning tool in medical imaging: using procedure graphs in radiographic process simulation, *Medical Informatics* **20** (1996) 251-263.

[4] L. Costaridou, C. Papanikolaou, C. Efstratiou, K. Hatzis, N. Pallikarakis and G. Panayiotakis, Modeling X-ray imaging procedures: A tool for generating learning tasks. In: J. Brender, J.P. Christensen, J.-R. Scherrer, P. McNair (Eds.), Proceedings of MIE '96. ISBN: 90-5199-278-5. IOS Press, Amsterdam, Ohmsha, 1996, pp. 1047-1051.

[5] M. Muehlhauser and J. Schaper, Project NESTOR: New approaches to cooperative multimedia authoring/learning. In: I. Tomek (Ed.), Computer Assisted Learning, Lecture Notes in Computer Science 602. ISBN: 3-540-55578-1. Springer-Verlag, Berlin-Heidelberg, 1992, pp. 453-465.

[6] J. Greenberg Integrated Multimedia in Distance Education. In: H. Maurer (Ed.), Proceedings of ED-MEDIA '95, World Conference on Educational Multimedia and Hypermedia. ISBN: 1-889094-15-0, Graz, Austria, pp. 13-16.

[7] U. Hübner, FJ. Schuier and J. Newell, SAMMIE A2032 - Software Applied to Multimodal Images and Education, *Computer Methods and Programs in Biomedicine* **45** (1995) 149-152.

[8] S. Mallat and S. Zhong, Characterization of signals from multiscale edges, *IEEE Transactions on Pattern Analysis and Machine Intelligence* **14** (1992) 710-732.

[9] A. Laine, J. Fan and W. Yang, Wavelets for Contrast Enhancement of Digital Mammography, *IEEE Engineering in Medicine and Biology* **14** (1995) 536-549.

[10] P. Sakellaropoulos, L. Costaridou, D. Cavouras, A. Bezerianos, G. Panayiotakis and B. Proimos, A tool implementing DOG and Gabor filtering on mammographic images, In: Proceedings of VII Mediterranean Conference on Medical & Biological Engineering, MEDICON '95, Jerusalem, 1995, p. 75.

Medical Informatics Europe '97
C. Pappas et al. (Eds.)
IOS Press, 1997

Telemedicine:
Evaluation or Stagnation

Michael O'Rourke; Stephen Gallivan
Clinical Operational Research Unit, University College London
London WC1E 6BT

Abstract: Telemedicine is attracting attention as a new means of delivery health care, but research indicates a low level of useful analysis of projects This paper reviews the potential of telemedicine and suggests the use of appropriate evaluation techniques can enable that potential to be realised. The importance of quantifying benefits and introduction of wider perspectives is discussed and advocated.

Introduction

There is considerable interest in telemedicine globally, in both developed and emerging countries. An appropriate definition for telemedicine is. [1] "The delivery of healthcare and the exchange of healthcare information across distances using telecommunications technology"

The attractions of the concept are readily apparent. Medical expertise is an expensive resource, which generally benefits from a concentration of expertise, and the associated supporting disciplines and facilities. In remote areas or third world countries, access to such expertise will be limited by geography or a lack of availability or both. But even in developed countries, there is a desire to maximise the best expertise available, and to benefit from the technical improvements, particularly in respect of very high speed communications, which are changing the way in which most businesses are conducted.

Known projects include a proposal to link all 80 primary care centres in Iceland to a common EPR system, and to hospital laboratories, emerging departments and pharmacies. A telemedicine network is planned for India with centres of expertise serving as hubs for the 90 most populous cities. Visions such as these could transform the way in which health services are delivered, with impacts on cost, culture and effectiveness. More modest, but equally interesting applications are under way in the UK, including remote clinics for antenatal care, image transfer from a remote hospital and interactive education in diabetes.[2]

In spite of this enthusiasm very little appears to have been done to assess the impact of telemedicine projects in quantitative terms. A preliminary literature search conducted by the authors revealed virtually no material which would assist in determining the success or failure (however defined) of such projects. In fact, there is evidence to suggest that proper analyses are absent. A useful paper by Bashur [3] discusses this amongst other things. It seems that the time is ripe for raising the profile of evaluation as integral part of telemedicine projects, so that they can demonstrate in objective terms their potential beneficial impact.

The Scope of Telemedicine Projects

Telemedicine can include transfer of patient information over networks, movement of images such as CT scans, MRI's, radiographics and pathology images, and video recording of patient interviews and examinations for clinical or educational purposes. A recent survey[1] revealed telemedicine applications in use in Australia, Canada, Finland, France, Germany, Italy, Japan, Netherlands, Norway, Switzerland, Sweden, the UAE and the UK. International organisations and their interests were also noted including EFMI.

The scope of such projects can transform all aspects of healthcare delivery. Healthcare workers have the opportunity to use powerful technology linked through world networks in a manner which would have been considered infeasible just over a decade ago. Applications can permit the remote scanning of pregnant women, eliminating the need for unnecessary travel and maximising the use of expensive equipment. Educational programmes offer better prospects for medical awareness and healthier lifestyles. The availability of appropriate medical expertise is no longer dependent on the physical co-location of patient and doctor. Towards the end of life, telemedicine home care systems offer a humane and cost-effective alternative to hospital care. But is telemedicine anything more than the evolutionary development of medicine using current technology, in the same way that the internal combustion engine has transformed transport. Why should it receive any special attention?

There are several consequences of telemedicine which can impact on the health care policies of nations and organisations. In part, this is due to the spread of technology to world citizens which increases its use and familiarity: it cannot be ignored or "uninvented". One observer [3] has noted impacts of cost, quality and access, which would enable a more considered view to be taken of telemedicine. Cost is always likely to be a significant factor. As governments and agencies are under continuous pressure to contain the costs of healthcare, rising expectations from increasing populations create a tension in service delivery. Proponents of technology will suggest that its use will deliver the benefits and realise expectations in the most effective fashion. But technology which is innovative can also be expensive, and healthcare providers are reluctant to make investments without the prospect of real return.

The quality in the delivery of solutions may be most debatable. The struggle to deliver the "best" or the "most appropriate health" care is a continuous challenge to all professionals. Adding in a dose of new and different technology is not a guarantee of improvement. Access to the facilities available through telemedicine raises many questions. Rather than the raft of current projects, with many individual applications, it is possible to consider instead a planned introduction of facilities, consistent with equivalent national infrastructure, which would match carefully the needs of areas and populations, and deliver appropriate nodes and contacts within a structured healthcare system, smoothing out current inconsistencies and gaps.

In order to begin to address such questions, there is need for a much greater awareness of the actual impact of telemedicine, and the way in which it might be developed, to bring about commensurate improvements in health care. Whilst there may exist questions of definition, acceptance or utility, it seems clear that there is a dearth of evaluation methods or material which could assist in the impartial assessment of telemedicine applications.

The need for evaluation

The pressures upon Governments and agencies to deliver appropriate healthcare to increasing numbers has caused attention to be paid to technologically based solutions, most notably in relation to clinical care where increased sophistication is the norm. But greater use of computer technology appears to have had relatively little impact on the management and organisation process supporting healthcare delivery. The work of Lock [4] in England highlighted the low priority accorded to the evaluation of computer projects in NHS hospitals. A recent editorial the BMJ [5] bemoaned the poor quality of published information of IT and expressed a willingness for the journal to consider submissions in the field. [6] [7] There is currently a somewhat one-sided debate taking place, indicating that few, if any, NHS hospital computer projects justify their (often significant) costs. The recent studies of the UK Audit Commission and National Audit Office [8] indicate the pitfalls which occur, and show the interest taken by Government in examining such developments.

If improvements through telemedicine are to be made in healthcare delivery, then it is vital that worthwhile initiatives are not constrained by a late 20th century version of Luddism. The use of a dispassionate and comprehensive evaluation method would seem to be a prerequisite. A preliminary review of evaluation topics which would be relevant to telemedicine applications included: Objectives (necessity, corporate policy, competitive advantage, efficiency); Technology (reliability, security, appropriateness, standards); Costs (start up, revenue, hidden, re-chargeable); and Social/Ethical (patient needs, professional acceptance, confidentiality, socio- economic acceptance, effect on healthcare structure and operation). These issues can be amplified and used to inform the debate on evaluation. But this paper suggests that there are two areas which would provide a central focus and offer the opportunity for a greater synthesis of the outcome of telemedicine projects; the quantification of benefits and wide scale introduction.

The importance of quantifying benefits

Benefits are normally claimed for any pilot. The benefits should be clearly identified and measured, to reduce or eliminate ambiguity of results. It is important to ensure that claimed benefits can be realised, and that underpinning costs and returns have been properly calculated. The benign acceptance of parties affected by change should not be assumed. It is valid to claim for expected benefits (as opposed to those actually achieved), where the project is capable of easy replication or can obtain synergistic benefits through links to other systems. It should be possible to express at least the majority of claimed benefits in cash terms.

An analytical approach to the evaluation of a telemedicine system would start with a simple examination of a series of questions, gradually building up a structure that could be used to estimate, in quantifiable terms, the beneficial aspects . Such a sequence of questions might be: What is it that the systems is trying to achieve? What is currently being done because this system isn't in place? If the system were in place, how many people would use it? For each person that uses it, is there a way of estimating the benefits? This dialogue, as it were, is the Devil's disciple aiming to cut through enthusiastic froth and focus onto the true costs and benefits.

The precise sequence of questions depends on the telemedicine application envisaged. An inherent difficulty associated with evaluation of telemedicine, is that there does not appear to be a universal evaluation methodology and it is unlikely that such an ideal is realistic. The grounds for judging telemedicine for dermatology are quite different from those appropriate for organ transplant. Consider the case of a telemedicine system whereby fetal ultrasound images are transferred from remote areas to a tertiary referral centre for expert interpretation. Here the sequence of questions might be summarised as shown in

Table 1. An analytical evaluation framework can be developed from such a structure in a fairly routine fashion. This relies on obtaining estimates of factors affecting the process many of which are available from existing data sources (for example, what percentage of pregnancies have an ultrasound abnormality, what proportion of the population live beyond easy travelling distance from a expert referral centre, etc). Combining such estimates to give an analytical estimate of the annual net benefits of a particular telemedicine project is likely to be a useful evaluation technique. The key is to ask the right questions and to avoid focusing on topics amenable to quantification.

The two principal features of telemedicine are firstly, the geographic aspects whereby information can be made accessible over huge areas and secondly, that information can be transferred quickly. These are perhaps the cornerstones on which to base the questioning dialogue that leads to a successful analytical evaluation. Is a telemedicine system proposed in order to broaden accessibility, to speed up communication or both. If the system weren't present, could patients travel or could the postal services or FAX be used for communication?. How many patients need increased accessibility? How important is speedy communication for a particular application (for a transplant, crucial - for most dermatology, not important at all).

Table 1. Dialogue indicating the evolution of an analytical evaluation framework.

Question	Comment
What is the system to achieve?	Improving the access to expert advice Detecting problems early Reducing the need for widespread specialist fetal medicine services
What currently happens without the system?	Ultrasound is done at present site Suspicious cases are dealt with by post or patient referral to tertiary centre. X tertiary centres are available
If the system were in place, how often would it be used?	Most pregnancies are routine Y% need expert opinion (derivable from public health records) Z% have no ready access to expert opinion (derivable from demographic/geographic sources)
For each person who uses the system, what are the benefits?	Reducing probability of adverse pregnancy outcome (estimable) Reduced travel costs. (estimable) Reassurance (difficult to quantify)
What are the longer consequences	Restructuring of tertiary referral system Changing role of specialist consultation

Widescale introduction

It is rare for consideration to be given to the full implications of a widespread application of a specific project, despite pressure from research sponsors to do so. There may be a vision, but many initiatives fall into the deep gulf which seems to exist between vision and reality.[9] Yet the chances of a successful implementation could be considerably improved, by the introduction of wider perspectives, say, related to the delivery of national targets. What may be absent from the formal evaluation process is a recognition of success factors, against which a small project could match its expectations of wider acceptance. It would be valuable to explore the factors affecting success or failure of a project when being deployed as a multiple, not a single, application. For example, a telemedicine application might service local towns A-J from city X, a reflection of current local practice. But with distance costs a negligible factor, the same towns (plus many more) might be just as conveniently be supported from city Y, 500 km distant, with city X becoming a satellite too.

Such an approach requires a radical and well informed policy to the provision of healthcare facilities. Where such policies are determined for a discrete area - county, province, city - the administrative boundaries provide definition of area, population and service measures. Where policies have a reliance on competing or market arrangements, decisions on the methods of service delivery are likely to be more dynamic.

There could be scope for more broadly based pilot schemes, capable of providing a better perspective on regional or national service delivery. Such pilots would be more costly, but their success or failure - correctly measured - would be evident.. A balance would have to be drawn between the duration of a pilot scheme, and assessment of its impact, given the pace of changing technology and variations in the service delivery organisations themselves. Effective funding, project control and dissemination of results is axiomatic.

Summary

The potential value of telemedicine applications, with the possibilities of changing the way in which types of healthcare can be delivered suggests that a formal means of evaluation would be welcome. A specific literature search on evaluation in telemedicine has revealed little of value. The time would appear right to consider an appropriate means of evaluating telemedicine projects. A range of factors are present, but this paper suggest that a focus on two - quantifiable benefits and widescale use - would generate the most useful information.

Evaluating benefits depends on the nature of the telemedicine application. An interrogative structure has been proposed which could lead to the development of analytical methods to assist evaluation. Key questions would include the benefits of improved accessibility, and the advantages of improved speed of communication between patient and the medical expert. The value of such techniques would assist in determing the best means of wider introduction. More comprehensive, but tightly defined pilots are suggested to provide realistic information on actual implementation over a representative population set.

REFERENCES:

[1] Ferguson EW, Doarn CR, Scott JC, Survey of Global Telemedicine, Journal of Medical Systems Vol 19 No.1,pp 35-46, 1995. [2] Images of Healthcare technology, Department of Trade & Industry 1996 [3] Bashur RL, Telemedicine Effects: Cost, quality and access. Journal of Medical Systems Vol 19 No2, pp 81-91, 1995 [4] What value do computers provide to NHS hospitals BMJ 312,1407-1410,1996. [5] Tonks A, Smith R; Information in Practice BMJ Vol 313 p 438, 28.08.96 [6] Audit Commission. For your information HMSO 1995 [7] Audit Commission. Setting the record straight. HMSO 1995. [8] NHS Executive: The Hospital Information Support Systems Initiative:HC 332 session 1995-96; 17.04.96 [9] O'Rourke CM, Theory and practice: extremes of IT strategy; current perspectives in Health Computing ED: Bryant, Roberts, Windsor 1987.

Medical Informatics Europe '97
C. Pappas et al. (Eds.)
IOS Press, 1997

Health Telematics in Ukraine:
Problems and Prospects

Oleg Yu.Mayorov M.D., Ph.D., Dr.Sc.[1],
Victor M.Ponomarenko M.D., Ph.D., Dr.Sc.[2], Valentin V.Kalnish Ph.D.[2]
Igor V.Charin[3], Vladimir V. Sergienko[3], Dmitrij V.Sleduk[1]
[1]Dept. of Medical Informatics, Kharkiv State Advanced Training Institute for Physicians,
[2]Ukrainian R&D Institute of Public Health,
[3]Ukrainian Association of Computer Medicine
UACM, P.O.BOX 7313, Kharkiv 310002, Ukraine
e-mail: uacm@uacm.kharkov.ua

Abstract: The state of medical telecommunication networks in Ukraine is described. The concepts of creating and architecture of the National Direct Access Computer Network 'UkrMedNet' are given.

1. A Summary of the National strategy of the informatisation for health and social care

In August 1996 Ukraine celebrated the 5th Anniversary of its Independence. Nowadays preparations are in full swing for a radical reform of the entire system of health care.

The directions of high priority of the health care reform in Ukraine are the introduction of insurance medicine and institution of family doctor.

It must be underlined that the health care is going to be reformed in the country suffered from the ecological disaster of the global scale - the Chernobyl disaster. It influenced and still influences the health of hundreds of thousands of people. Also note that Ukraine occupies 607,7 thousands of sq. km and has the population of about 52 million.

Under these conditions the key roles begin to play the state-of-the-art information technologies which make it possible to solve all the above problems quickly, effectively and least expensively.

The basis of the comprehensive infrastructure of medical informatics is the creation of the National Direct Access Computer Network 'UkrMedNet'. The 'UkrMedNet' project has been developed according to the Concept of the State Policy in informatising the health care in Ukraine [1] (adopted in June, 1995), Order of the President of Ukraine No. 186/93 from 31.05.1993 'On the State Policy of informatisation in Ukraine', decision of the Cabinet of Ministers of Ukraine No. 605 from 31.07.1994 'Problems of Informatisation'.

The project has been studied and approved at the meeting of the Working group of the Ministry of Health of Ukraine on 19.02.1996.

The goal of the project is to organise a system of medical and ecological information exchange in Ukraine, as well as outside, based on the state-of-the-art communication technologies.

Ukraine already has an experience in the creation of national medical networks and databases which are to be integrated into 'UkrMedNet'. First of all there are two most developed medical networks operating within the framework of the acting national computer network of the first generation 'HealthNet'. For this the latter will be transformed into 'UkrMedNet'.

The most sophisticated of these two is the National register of the persons suffered from the Chernobyl disaster. This Register monitors the health of nearly 600,000 persons. A computer network has been created in order to maintain this Register, covering 25 districts and cities under direct central administration - Kiyv and Sebastopol.

The second most sophisticated network is the net of the Sanitary and Epidemiological Service of the Ministry of Health of Ukraine based on the computer centres of the district health care administrations (ca. 70 computer centres) which transmits operative information on the current sanitary, epidemiological and ecological situation to the Ministry of Health of Ukraine. These nets are integrated in a common net called 'HealthNet'.

At present the National Open Direct Access Medical Net-work is under creation on the basis of existing HealthNet and some other autonomous medical networks. This project also envisages the integration of all existing separate medical nets, medical universities and medical R&D institutes of Ukraine into one 'UkrMedNet', as well as the creation of a common informational space and its integration into the European one.

2. The main objectives are aimed to:

1. Update the National medical computer network to the state-of-the-art level using advanced computer technologies, communication lines and telemetry technologies, integrate it into the Internet.

2. Integrate the medical universities and R&D institutes of Ukraine into the Internet.

3. Create and maintain WWW servers supporting both Ukrainian and Russian and English languages, support references to these WWW-servers; integrate the Chernobyl Register net into 'UkrMedNet' and create a WWW server containing the Chernobyl Register information. Provide the 'UkrMedNet' users with the access to the created WWW servers, and provide this access via European partners (providers), to all countries (in Europe, both Americas, Asia and Africa).

4. Hospital information systems (HIS) of various levels (district hospital, regional hospital, specialised institute) equipped with up-to-date telecommunication facilities for transmitting biological signals and pictures (EEG, ECG, Ro-grammes etc.), texts, graphics, audio and visual information according to the telemedecine concepts; integrate these systems into the 'UkrMedNet' and provide an access to the Internet therefrom.

5. Create and maintain the data banks on the patients requiring organ transplantation and unite them with the existing cell and tissue banks within the information-and-co-ordination nucleus of the 'Ukrtransplant' system; connect the State information system of organ, tissue and cell transplantation in Ukraine to the similar European 'Eurotransplant' system via the Internet.

6. Train medical specialists to work with the telematics applications, advocate the utilisation of up-to-date communication technologies in health care. The project envisages the creation of a Republican or International Training Centre based on the Department of Medical Informatics and IT in Health Care Management of the Kharkiv State Advanced Training Institute for Physicians, and preparing and conducting a course of lectures and workshops on the theoretical aspects and implementation of the telematic applications in the health care of Ukraine.

7. Load the servers with the information on the following sections:

- Strategically important information on radiological, epidemiological and toxicological monitoring;

- Data bases with quick access information and instructions on urgent measures in emergency situations;

- Information on the branches of medicine;

- Medical information for general public, including: diabetes, epilepsy, pregnancy, cardiovascular diseases, healthy way of life and rational nutrition, toxicology and pharmacology, data on prohibited food products, current pharmacological advises, other relevant information for general public.

- Information from other fields of knowledge necessary for health care (biology, physics, chemistry, etc.);
- Some data on industry and agriculture;
- Other information of economical, geographical and demo-graphic nature;
- Information specially selected and prepared for medical students;
- It is planned to create a data base related to business activity, first of all medical insurance, paid medical service and products of health care.

The information will be organised on the net in the form of hypertext distributed data bases with multimedia components (graphical, photo, audio and video illustrations) located in the WWW servers of the National (central) telecommunication node, inter-regional nodes and WWW servers of the specialised institutes (i.e. institutes of oncology, neurology and psychiatry, children and adolescents health protection, maternity health care, AIDS institute).

This will make accessible to the general public the vast amount of information accumulated by the concerned leading R&D and other organisations in Ukraine. We suppose that this work will compose a part of the programme of development of telecommunication means in Ukraine.

3. Organisational basis of the project

The project is co-ordinated by the Ukrainian Association of 'Computer Medicine' (UACM), which is an amalgamation of 56 R&D institutes, universities, scientific societies, hospitals and enterprises located in various districts of Ukraine, dealing with the development and utilisation of informational technologies in health care. The UACM has a Scientific Council consisting of 68 leading scientific experts in the fields of medical informatics, medicine, radioelectronics from Ukraine, N.I.S., USA, Japan, Great Britain, France and Poland. Such an association makes it possible to reach in the best way the project goal and objectives and co-ordinate the efforts of the participants of the project.

Within the framework of the National Network of Ukraine we will support all district and regional subject information projects.

4. 'UkrMedNet' architecture

'UkrMedNet' is a three-level structure.

The first level of the Net consists of the National and four Interregional nodes. All the nodes of this level have a similar structure and service 5 or 6 districts (district nodes). It will be connected to the National node in Kiyv.

The Ukrainian National node performs also the functions of the interregional node for Kiyv and adjacent districts.

All Interregional nodes are directly connected to:

a) national node; b) one of interregional ones; c) one of Internet nodes which is not a part of the Net of the Ministry of Health care of Ukraine. Such connection layout ensures doubling of the connections of the first level nodes, i.e. ensures virtually 100%-proof data transmission. This enables us to consider the proposed architecture to be highly reliable.

The National and Interregional nodes ensure connection to the Net of the second-level nodes, as well as direct connection of large scientific, medical organisations and universities. The second level of the Net is formed on the basis of the district health care departments. The second-level nodes are connected to the nearest inter-regional node. They ensure connection to the net of medical organisations located in the district, preferably connection to the Internet which is not a part of the net of the Ministry of Healthcare.

The third level are regional nodes and end users. They are connected to the nodes of the district health care departments. Within the scope of this project this level is built on the basis of organisations - members of UACM, as well as all health-care organisations willing to join the project at their own expense or at the expense of the Ministry of Healthcare of Ukraine within the scope of the programme of development of telecommunications in Ukraine.

5. Benefits

Due to the development of the Ukrainian National Medical Network will obtain the possibility to exchange medical, ecological and scientific information.

Physicians, scientists in R&D institutes and universities will obtain access to the necessary information, receive electronic copies of scientific journals and articles, be able to run programmes unavailable on their equipment.

A unique regional computer network for calculating and analysing sanitary-and-epidemiological situation will be created as a component of the integrated network of the Ministry of Healthcare of Ukraine.

The Ukrainian national systems on transplantation of organs, tissues and cells, connected at present with 'Eurotransplant' will be incorporated in the unified European computer system of organ trainsplantation, thus giving Ukraine a real opportunity to join the progress in this field. The information technology adapter to the national conditions will be created for supporting organ, tissue and cell trainsplantation operations on the national and regional levels.

Basing on the international experience a technical project with standardised patterns of data bases and solutions will be created, as well as standard programme modules with standard input and output files to be used in central and regional information and analytical systems in order to ensure the functioning of all data bases of the higher level.

Due to the network development the EU countries will obtain the possibility to carry out many joint projects together with medical specialists in Ukraine. Thus, the R&D potential will be stabilised.

Using up-to-date information technologies, many scientists in Ukraine can fruitfully and effectively co-operate with colleagues from other European countries literally staying at home.

For the country occupying a vast territory, which has found itself in a dramatic economical situation, very important will be the creation of consultative telemedical centres. This will make it possible to provide at low cost the population, first of all in remote rural regions, with qualified consultative and diagnostic medical aid.

Thus, the creation of the National Direct Access Computer Network 'UkrMedNet' has a tremendous medical and social significance for Ukraine and will accelerate the integration of the country into the world informational space.

References

[1] V.M.Ponomarenko, O.Yu.Mayorov, The Concept of State Policy in Informatising the Healthcare in Ukraine. *Ukrainian Radiological Journal* 1996, 4(2): 115-118.

Medical Informatics Europe '97
C. Pappas et al. (Eds.)
IOS Press, 1997

Collection of Data in Clinical Studies via Internet

E. Keim, H. Sippel, H.-P. Eich, C. Ohmann

Theoretical Surgery Unit, Department of General and Trauma Surgery,
Heinrich-Heine-University, Düsseldorf, Germany
theochir@www.uni-duesseldorf.de

Abstract. This paper describes a system enabling data collection in multi-center clinical trials via WWW and Internet. The form-based data entry is based on HTML documents with JavaScript linked to a relational database (mSQL) via a cgi program (w3-msql). The design has been applied to a multi-national study in acute abdominal pain, for which eight clinical forms have been developed. The system is now in test use and experiences with this approach are presented.

1. Introduction

Data collection in multi-center controlled clinical trials is a major problem. A lot of effort has to be put into the quality assurance of the data. Normally data collection in this type of trials is performed via a clinical form or computer programs distributed to the individual centers. Several problems arise, such as formal errors and implausible data if a documentation form is used. If computer programs are applied for data collection, the necessary assumptions concerning hardware and system software have to be fulfilled in order to allow installation, and the programs including updates have to be distributed. Data collection in multi-center clinical studies can be considerably simplified if this is done via Internet. Provided that adequate measures of data protection and data security are undertaken, a data collection via Internet would give consistent and complete clinical data tested for errors and implausibilities without the restriction to specific hardware and software. Therefore we have developed a system enabling data collection via Internet in controlled clinical trials.

2. Description of the System

The basic component of the system is a SUN Sparc-20 web server and the Apache 1.2 server software. Using HTML editors the necessary documents for the system were created as HTML documents and stored on the server. As the underlying relational database *mSQL Version 1* was used, which provides the system with a subset of the ISO standard SQL which was sufficient for the purpose of the study [1]. The connection to the server software was established by the cgi program *w3-msql*, which interprets SQL statements included in HTML forms and performs the necessary operations on the database.

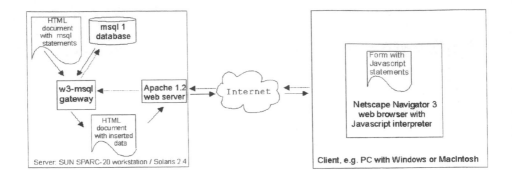

Figure 1: Flow of data in the documentation system

The new Internet programming language *JavaScript* (an HTML extension by Netscape) was used to perform plausibility checks before the data are sent to the server and entered into the database. By this procedure unnecessary data traffic is avoided because the server only receives quality-assured data. Fig. 1 shows the flow of data in our system.

In order to fulfil the rules for data protection and security, only anonymous data are transferred to the database. In addition all users receive an individual login name and password with access only to their hospital's data, controlled by the server software and the database.

3. Clinical application

The conception has been applied to a world wide clinical trial in acute abdominal pain. This trial is supported by the World Organisation of Gastroenterology (OMGE). In this trial acute abdominal pain will be studied with respect to the distribution and presentation of diseases, the spectrum of diagnostic procedures, the diagnostic accuracy of clinicians and management and outcome of disease. Data collection will be performed according to international standards. For documentation of the clinical data eight data entry forms have been developed: history, clinical examination, X-ray, ultrasound, laboratory, diagnosis, operation and outcome. The design of these forms has been based on similar forms, used in a C++ program for IBM compatible PC's [2].

The documentation is organised according to the entities „patient", „hospital stay" and „clinical document". In fig. 2 an example of a document is presented. Error controls and plausibility checks are incorporated. Clinical documents can be entered, edited, printed or deleted. A participating center has only access to the data of its own hospital. The complete system is installed and a test phase started on Feb 1st 1997, after which data collection in this multi-center trial will be started.

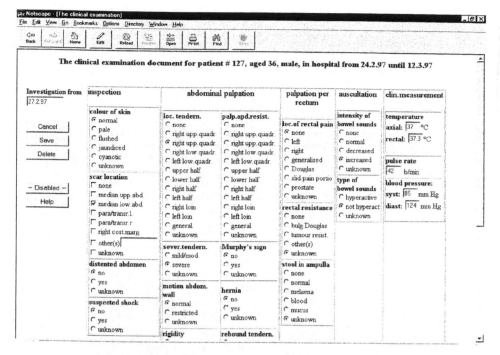

**Figure 2: Documentation form for a clinical examination (HTML-document,
including JavaScript for error and plausibility checks)**

4. Discussion

The integration of data collection forms and databases via Internet and WWW could be
achieved according to the given conception. However certain restrictions had to be
considered due to the limits of the mSQL database. It is hoped that with future versions of
this database system the problems can be solved. If not, alternative models and approaches
have to be taken into consideration. Another problem is the performance of the Internet in
general and the response time using the database. The size of the documents cause delays
because they have to be transmitted over and over again through the Internet. However,
Internet database technology has just begun to evolve and all major companies (e.g. Oracle,
SUN) are working to overcome these problems. A new concept for database access (JDBC)
via WWW has already be defined.

Little experience is available with respect to controlled clinical trials and data collection
via Internet. More information is expected from our multi-national trial. Not only data
collection can be supported by WWW and Internet, but also other aspects of multi-center
clinical trials, like randomisation and evaluation of inclusion and exclusion criteria [3].

A lot more work has to be put into the aspects of data security and data protection.
Different laws in the participating countries have to be taken into consideration (e.g.
necessity for the encryption of data). It is planned to expand the clinical application to a
general system for the support of documentation in multi-center clinical trials.

5. Acknowledgements

This work was supported by grant of the Deutsche Forschungsgemeinschaft (DFG Oh 39/3–2).

6. References

[1] D.J. Hughes: Mini SQL „A Lightweight Database Engine", available from http://hughes.com.au
[2] C. Ohmann C *et al.*: Integration of a data dictionary and a clinical database in an expert system for acute abdominal pain. In: R.A. Greenes *et al.*: MEDINFO 95 Proceedings. North-Holland, Amsterdam, 1995, pp 943 - 946.
[3] T. Kiuchi *et al.*, A World Wide Web-based User Interface for a Data Management System for Use in Multi-institutional Clinical Trials - Development and Experimental Operation of an Automated Patient Registration and Random Allocation System, *Controlled Clinical Trials* **17** (1995) 476-493.

Medical Informatics Europe '97
C. Pappas et al. (Eds.)
IOS Press, 1997

Survey among Physicians by means of Dynamic Access to an Internet Information Server Database

S. Hölzer, H. Kraft, A.G. Tafazzoli, J. Dudeck, Institute of Medical Informatics
Justus-Liebig-University Gießen, Heinrich-Buff-Ring 44, D-35392 Gießen, Germany

Abstract. Current database management systems, client-server architecture and the internet infrastructure are simplifying the exchange of information. Large and widespread electronic medical record systems are accessible via platform-independent browsing applications. The following brief summary shows one of the manifold conceivable applications of these technologies in medicine. It describes a survey among physicians with the scope of quality assurance in medicine. The dynamic, platform-independent, world-wide access to databases offers interesting aspects in medical informatics.

1. Introduction

Biomedical information systems are primarily designed to support medical patient care, to facilitate cooperation in research and to promote continuing education of medical staff. Due to progress in science medical knowledge is increasing very fast and the standards in diagnostic procedures and treatments in all disciplines are changing rapidly. Therefore there is a strong need for facilities to spread the new findings and to implement these results into medical practice in a fast way. The premise in medicine and other science is to get up-to-date information throughout the world. Client-server architecture, relational or object-oriented database management systems and internet technologies as well as the increasing infrastructure are improving the information access, representation and retrieval over the past years. Large and widespread electronic medical record systems are simply accessible via platform-independent browsing applications (1,2). Physicians are able to get local or internal information about their patients as well as general information from external servers. The internet environment and its tools are offering an easy-to-use, consistent, multimedia data transfer and information-retrieval which can be used both on physicians desktop and at home (3,4). In the past, these facilities have primarily been used to access electronic medical libraries (5-9). The direct individual access to databases by means of dynamic generated queries seems to be more interesting (10-13).

2. Methods and results

An Internet Information Server (IIS) is a tool for internet connectivity that serves Web pages and FTP clients. Via Internet Database Connectors (IDCs) one can connect any Structured Query Language (SQL)- or Open Database Connectivity (ODBC)-compliant database to an Internet Information Server. The Internet Information Server uses two files. The IDC file defines a protocol that the server needs to connect to the database. It describes the database portion of the connection. The Hypertext Markup Language (HTML) Extension file (HTX file) describes the HTML portion of the connection. The server merges the HTX file with the database and sends it to the client. The figure below illustrates this process.

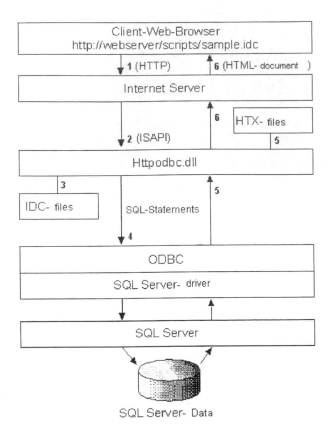

SQL Server- Data

We are using these possibilities to start a nation-wide survey among physicians to obtain information about the utilization and demands of further medical training in the Federal Republic of Germany. In the corresponding electronic data form which is a HTML document, physicians are asked about the frequency of use of textbooks, journals, hospital-internal training, internet offers and participation in national and international congresses. We allow the user to name references that were found to be especially helpful for their clinical routine. In order to sort and evaluate the data in detail, we also record the medical discipline, year of approbation and the actual medical status of the participants.

This way a pool of relevant and up-to-date medical literature is built up. We expect sufficient and representative data of the most important disciplines such as internal medicine, surgery and pediatrics within one half to one year depending on the acceptance and the frequency of access by German physicians. We will spread the received data sorted by discipline and training mode in order to allow users to get required information by dynamic queries.

3. Conclusion

In spite of its great significance with respect to the quality assurance in medicine, there are no exact data concerning the utilization of medical training facilities among physicians in the Federal Republic of Germany. The outlined concept is a practicable way to perform such a survey. We establish a possibility to get an easily accessible overview of current standards and the State of the Art of treatment in each medical discipline. This gives physicians a picture of both current research issues and practical clinical trends from a pool of relevant and topical medical literature as well as recommendations for their further training. The physician will be able to improve his training by consulting the top ranked medical references.

The dynamic access to medical databases seems to be advantageous in various fields. In addition, the presented way of using an internet information server and a SQL-compliant database permits to test the performances of the applied hardware and software under practical conditions. One of the future objectives is the establishment of an interactive database for drug side effects.

References

1. Hahn H, Stout R. The internet complete reference. Berkeley, Calif: McGraw Hill 1994;

2. Kehoe BP. ZEN and the art of internet. Englewood Cliffs, NJ: PTR Prentice Hall 1994;

3. Prokosch HU. Hospital Information systems: A pragmatic definition. Elsevier, Amsterdam 1995;

4. Willard KE, Hallgren JH, Sielaff B, Connelly DP. The deployment of a World Wide Web (W3) based medical information system. Proc Annu Symp Comput Appl Med Care 1995;771-775.

5. Kahn RM, Molholt P, Zucker J. CPMCnet: an integrated information and internet resource. Proc Annu Symp Comput Appl Med Care 1994;98-102.

6. Kleeberg P. Medical uses of the Internet. J Med Syst 1993;17:363-366.

7. McKinney WP, Wagner JM, Bunton G, Kirk LM. A guide to Mosaic and the World Wide Web for physicians. MD Comput 1995;12:109-14,141.

8. McKinney WP, Barnas GP, Golub RM. The medical applications of the internet: informational resources for research, education, and patient care. J Gen Intern Med 1994;9:627-634.

9. Frisse ME, Braude RM, Florance V, Fuller S. Informatics and medical libraries: changing needs and changing roles. Acad Med 1995;70:30-35.

10. Cimino JJ, Socratous SA, Clayton PD. Internet as clinical information system: application development using the World Wide Web [see comments]. J Am Med Inform Assoc 1995;2:273-284.

11. Cimino JJ, Socratous SA, Grewal R. The informatics superhighway: prototyping on the World Wide Web. Proc Annu Symp Comput Appl Med Care 1995;111-115.

12. Kassirer JP. The next transformation in the delivery of health care [editorial] [see comments]. N Engl J Med 1995;332:52-54.

13. Sittig DF, Kuperman G, Teich JM. WWW-based Interfaces to Clinical Information Systems: The State of the Art. AMIA 1996;694-698.

Medical Informatics Europe '97
C. Pappas et al. (Eds.)
IOS Press, 1997

Application of Telematics
for Improving Multiple Schedules

Johan H. OLDENKAMP[1], Constantijn HEESEN[2] & John L. SIMONS[3]

Telematics Research Centre, PO Box 589, 7500 AN Enschede, The Netherlands

Abstract. Nurse scheduling is an important, but also a very complicated management task. Performing this task results in a nursing schedule. These nursing schedules strongly influence the performance of a nursing ward. This paper describes research results on the application of several knowledge acquisition techniques for the development of a decision support system. This system informs the nurse scheduler about the quality of an arranged schedule. This paper next shows how this system can be used to improve multiple schedules in combination with the application of telematics. This improvement is based on the communication between schedulers who have a shortage or a surplus of nurses at certain days of the schedule. By means of internal reallocation of nurses for a short period of time, the total schedule quality of all nursing schedules can be improved.

1. Introduction: Quality Factors of Nursing Schedules

Providing health care in hospitals and other health care organisations is a continuous process. This means that health care organisations are required to operate on a twenty-four hour a day, seven days a week basis. In order to provide this care the nursing staff need to be scheduled.

Nurse scheduling, like staffing and employee scheduling in general, is an important management task [1]. The outcome of nurse scheduling — which is the nursing schedule — strongly influences the continuity in nursing care, the amount of absenteeism, and the total personnel costs (*e.g.* [2], [3], [4], [5]).

Because of these consequences, it is important to have an insight in those features of nursing schedules that positively influence the performance of health care organisations. The totality of these features will be called the 'nursing schedule quality'.

In order to investigate this nursing schedule quality, the QUINS project was started. The main objective of this research project is to facilitate, if possible, an improvement of nursing schedules in practice. The approach is based on the assumption that informing schedulers about several quality factors will result in a higher nursing schedule quality. This approach has been called Quality Indication Scheduling, of which QUINS is an acronym.

The next section summarises the main results of this QUINS project. The paper then describes a follow-up research that applies telematics in order to adjust multiple schedules. This

---

[1] Dr. Johan H. Oldenkamp is a member of scientific staff at the Telematics Research Centre, PO Box 589, NL-7500 AN Enschede, The Netherlands.

[2] Constantijn Heesen is an associate member of scientific staff of the Department of Management Informatics of the Faculty of Management and Organisation of the University of Groningen, PO Box 800, N:-9700 AV Groningen, The Netherlands.

[3] Prof. John L. Simons is the scientific director of the Department of Management Informatics of the Faculty of Management and Organisation of the University of Groningen, PO Box 800, NL-9700 AV Groningen, The Netherlands.

paper ends with conclusions about useful applications that could result from the suggested future research.

2. Results of the QUINS Project

The QUINS project consisted of four research phases. After the first phase, the QUINS project had resulted in a conceptual model of nursing schedule quality consisting of five independent quality factors. These five factors are completeness, optimality, proportionality, healthiness, and continuity. The *completeness* factor represents the degree in which the quantitative demands for occupation per shift are met. The *optimality* factor represents the degree in which nursing expertise is distributed over the different shifts. The *proportionality* factor represents the degree in which each nurse has been given about the same amount of night shifts, evening shifts and weekends off. The *healthiness* factor represents the degree in which has been taken care off the welfare and health of the nursing staff. And finally, the *continuity* factor represents the degree in which there is continuity in the nursing crew during different shifts. These first results of the QUINS project were presented at the 1995 Amsterdam Medical Informatics Conference [6].

In the second phase of the QUINS project, a ranking experiment was conducted. The objective of this experiment was to operationalise each of the five factors of nursing schedule quality. This was done by asking nurse schedulers to rank several alternative patterns of shifts according tot their own view on high quality. The results of the ranking experiment showed that the nurse schedulers ranked most patterns of shifts in the same way. These results were presented at the 1996 Medical Informatics Europe Conference [7].

An auditing experiment was conducted in the third research phase. Five nurse schedulers were asked to give each of fifteen nursing schedules a quality mark on a scale from one to ten. The results of a least-squares analysis showed that nearly 80 percent of the given quality marks can be explained on the basis of a weighted sum of factor values. In this explanation, the factor values are generic (*i.e.* are the same for all nurse schedulers), while the summation weights are specific (*i.e.* vary per nurse scheduler) [8].

In the fourth and last phase of the QUINS project, a scheduling experiment was conducted. In this experiment eight nurse schedulers were asked to arrange a nursing schedule. This experiment showed that informing nurse schedulers about the factor values of the arranged schedule results in an average increase of nursing schedule quality of thirty percent [8].

3. Using the QUINS model for further improvement

In the previous section we described the quality concept of nursing schedules. Each ward has its own schedule and therefore in a hospital several nursing schedules are made. Informing each scheduler about the quality factor values improves the nursing schedule quality. In this section we investigate a possibility to further improve the quality of nursing schedules. We will use the quality factors in two additional ways: as *process indicators*, when to start an information exchange, and as *content indicators*, to determine which information has to be communicated.

A way to improve the quality of a schedule is by exchanging nurses between wards. For example, the schedule of ward A has a low optimality factor. This could be improved if a nurse from ward B, having the right expertise, would work for some time at ward A. The quality of schedule B will decrease by this action, but as long as the quality does not drop below some minimum value, the actions is allowed. What is needed to initiate an exchange of nurses between two wards is an adjustment of the particular nursing schedules by a communication process. There is little indication that the adjustment of nursing schedules is happening on a large scale in current nurse scheduling practice, but we expect that this will happen in the future. The improvement of the schedule quality is important because it enables better nursing and lower costs. A second reason to believe that there will be more co-ordination of schedules is the fact that using decision support tools for nurse scheduling reduces the workload of the scheduler. There will be more time to take factors, such as the adjustment of a schedule to another schedule, into account.

The coordination of schedules is a problem that has been dealt with before, although not in the domain of nurse scheduling. In group calendaring and scheduling (C&S), the adjustment of schedules is of utmost importance. C&S is the planning of meetings between persons in an organisation and the scheduling of a room for a meeting. It is only possible to plan a meeting if the agendas of the individual persons indicate free time. In other words, the agendas need to be adjusted. This scheduling problem has some of the characteristics of the adjustment of nurse schedules: each ward scheduler has his/her own schedule (agenda) and this schedule has to be co-ordinated with another schedule.

There are some important differences between C&S and nurse scheduling. In the first place in C&S it is clear when a communication between schedules should start, that is when a new meeting has to be planned. In nurse scheduling it is more difficult to determine the circumstances that initiate a new conversation. Another difference is that in C&S it is clear which person is needed for a meeting, in nurse scheduling a type of person is needed, usually not a specific person. A third difference is that in nurse scheduling it is not directly clear if the exchange of a person that seems available will result in a better overall quality of schedules. The result of an exchange of a nurse can be that the decrease of the quality of the delivering ward is larger than the increase of the quality of the receiving ward.

The quality factors can support schedulers with the adjustment of their schedules, although it is not required to use quality factors. The basic conversation for adjusting nurse schedules, without using quality factors, consists of the following:

1. The scheduler examines the schedule and finds a part of the schedule that needs improvement.
2. The scheduler requests another scheduler for a specific nurse on a specific time.
3. The other scheduler examines his/her schedule to see if the request fits into the schedule.
4. The scheduler gives an answer to the request.

It is difficult to determine when a scheduler should start a conversation with another scheduler. We can use the quality factors to do this. If a schedule scores low on a quality factor, the scheduler should try to improve the schedule by repairing part of the schedule [9]. If that is not possible the scheduler can start a conversation with another scheduler. To do that the scheduler has to decide which type of nurse is needed at what time to improve the schedule. Than the scheduler can request the other scheduler for a particular nurse. The receiving scheduler also uses the quality factors to determine if the request can be fulfilled. The conversation steps are:

1. The scheduler examines the schedule and tries to improve the schedule on the basis of quality factors. If a quality factor is still below some minimum value then a nurse from another ward is needed
2. The scheduler requests another scheduler for a specific nurse on a specific time
3. The other scheduler uses the quality factors to see what will happen should the request be accepted.
4. The scheduler gives an answer to the request (accept of decline).

The conversation described here follows the conversation rules of Winograd and Flores [10], *i.e.* a request is followed by an acceptance or a reject. The quality factor has two roles. The first is a process indicator role. The scheduler determines when a quality factor is below some minimum, at that time a conversation should start. The second role is a role as content indicator. The scheduler decides which type of nurse is needed and at what time on the basis of the quality factors. A telecommunication network may facilitate the communication between schedulers. Communication can also be done by phone, but then the two schedulers need to be present at the same time. An electronic mail program or another message sending facility, such as a groupware application, is a better option. Calendaring systems use special mailing protocols based on MIME[1] or IMAP 4, to structure the communication process. This is essential when more than two wards are involved in the communication process.

The conversation as described above can directly be implemented by using an e-mail program. A disadvantage is that the user has to use two separate applications, a scheduling support system and an e-mail program. Our current research focuses on the integration of communication facilities and scheduling support systems.

4. Conclusions

This paper described how telematics could be used for adjusting multiple schedules. By informing nurse schedulers of other wards about the quality factors of an arranged nursing schedule together with additional information, these nurse schedulers can decide how to borrow nurses from other wards or to lend nurses to other wards. In this way, the total of nursing schedule quality of all nursing schedules of a health care organisation can be increased. In future research, the described application of telematics for improving multiple schedules will be evaluated in practice.

We only looked at the situation where two nurse schedules are adjusted. To support the situation where several nurse schedules need to be adjusted, agent technology can be used [11, 12, 13]. Also ideas can be used from Calendaring, but the adjustment of nurse schedules is more complicated.

References

[1] Chen, J.-G. & Yeung, T.W. (1992). Development of a Hybrid Expert System for Nurse Shift Scheduling. *International Journal of Industrial Ergonomics*, vol. 9, no. 4, pp. 315-328.
[2] Okada, M. (1992). An Approach to the Generalized Nurse Scheduling Problem; Generation of a Declarative Program to Represent Institution-Specific Knowledge. *Computers and Biomedical Research: an international journal*, vol. 25, no. 5, pp. 417-434.
[3] Randhawa, S.U. & Sitompul, D. (1993). A Heuristic-Based Computerized Nurse Scheduling System. *Computers & Operations Research and their Application to Problems of World Concern: an international journal*, vol. 20, no. 8, pp. 837-844.

[4]   Weil, G., Heus, K., Francois, P. & Poujade, M. (1995). Constraint Programming for Nurse Scheduling. *IEEE Engineering in Medicine and Biology Magazine: the quarterly magazine of the Engineering in Medicine & Biology Society*, vol. 14, no. 4, pp. 417-422.

[5]   Weil, G., Heus, K., Francois, P., Jacques, P. & Poujade, M. (1996). GYMNASTE, a Solver for Nurse Scheduling using Constraint Programming: a Technical and Sciological Challenge. In: J. Brender, J.P. Christensen, J.-R. Scherrer & P. McNair (Eds.), *Medical Informatics Europe '96*. Amsterdam, The Netherlands: IOS Press. pp. 1032-1036.

[6]   Oldenkamp, J.H. & Simons, J.L. (1995). Quality Factors in Nursing Schedules. In: J. van der Lei & W.P.A. Beckers (Eds.), *Strategic Alliances between Patient Documentation and Medical Informatics*, the proceedings of AMICE 95, Amsterdam, The Netherlands, November, 27 till 29, 1995. Meppel, The Netherlands: Krips Repro. pp. 69-74.

[7]   Oldenkamp, J.H., Lettenga, M.S. & Simons, J.L. (1996). Nursing Schedule Quality in Theory and Practice. In: J. Brender, J.P. Christensen, J.-R. Scherrer & P. McNair (Eds.), *Medical Informatics Europe '96*. Amsterdam, The Netherlands: IOS Press. pp. 863-866.

[8]   Oldenkamp, J.H. (1996). *Quality in Fives: On the Analysis, Operationalization and Application of Nursing Schedule Quality*. Dissertation, Faculty of Management and Organisation, University of Groningen, The Netherlands. Capelle aan de IJssel, The Netherlands: Labyrint Publication.

[9]   Zweben, M., Davis, E., Daun, B. & Deale, M. (1993) Scheduling and Rescheduling with Iterative Repair. *IEEE Systems, Man, and Cybernetics*, vol 23, no 6, pp. 1588-1596.

[10] Winograd, T. & Flores, F.M. (1986). *Understanding Computers and Cognition*. New Jersey: Ablex Publishing Corporation.

[11] Shoham, Y. (1993). Agent-oriented programming. *Artificial Intelligence*, no. 60, pp. 51-92.

[12] Davis, R. & Smith, Reid G. (1983). Negotiation as a metaphor for distributed problem solving. *Artificial Intelligence* no. 20, pp 63-109

[13] Heesen, C., Homburg, V. & Offereins, M. An Agent View on Law. *Artificial Intelligence and Law*, Accepted for publication.

Note

[1] MIME stands for Multipurpose Internet Mail Extensions, and IMAP refers to Internet Message Access Protocol.

Medical Informatics Europe '97
C. Pappas et al. (Eds.)
IOS Press, 1997

European Citizens Advisory Systems based on Telematics for Communication and Health

Dr. Jörg F. Maas, M.A. (Hannover - Germany)

Abstract: The objective of Citizens Advisory Systems for Health in Europe is to provide background information in preventive health care, to offer data-based and knowledge-based facilities and to reduce costs within the national and European wide health systems. In order to do so, easily accessible human-computer-dialogues and systems have to or have been already developed, allowing every citizen to obtain the right information at the right place at any time with any intensity which is wished. The paper will describe the already existing standards, will explain the ideal type and the technical and social implications which have to be taken into consideration for these systems.

1. Prerequisites

If one talks about European cooperation between partners from industry and academia - within telematic oriented research projects or others - one has to reflect 4 important aspects by running these projects: technology transfer, indicator for innovation and research, manageability within existing limits, and politicalization. These aspects constitute the frame of any European cooperation and project environment, they represent both the challenge and the necessity for those consortia and for the European dimension within a worldwide competition in innovative technology.

Before I will go into further detail of telematic needs, standards and wishfull thinking within such a framework, let me introduce first the specifications and prerequisites of EU-projects in general.

The first aspect of the 4 characterizes the specifics of cooperation between industrial and academic partners. Research, in this sense, is not only a general necessity for innovation according to the Greenbook of the European Commission, it also has a connotation within the cultural sense of "joy of science". There is, in other words, a complexity between partners from industry and academia in terms of how they cooperate, how they invent and how they commercialise their ideas and products: academia in this sense is mostly the theoretical inventor with vague ideas about reality and commercial interests; industry, however, represents the market orientation together with what one calls the "enterpreneurial spirit" representing a clear sense and calculation for costs, productivity, innovation and investment. Their cooperation, henceforth, originates technology transfer in its original meaning with consequences for new political orientations and streams for Europe, leading from a Greenbook to a Whitebook and further on towards another Frameworkprogramme.

This definitely reflects the development for telematics oriented research within the EU within programmes like ACTS, ESPRIT, DELTA, TELEMATICS, TEN TELECOM, INFO 2000 and INCO from the end of the 80s until today.

According to the 1994th report for scientific and technology indicators of the

European Commission, 1/3 of all participants of programmes within the 3rd Frameworkprogramme were partners from public institutions receiving 1/4 of the overall budget of the EU. 1/5 of all partners came - on the other side - from industry, but receiving more than 1/3 of the available funding. These statistical data confirm what has been found out in the so-called IMPACT-study done by the BETA-institute in Strassbourg: industry takes significant advantage of cooperations with universities in general. The advantages, however, were of more significance to companies with more than 500 employees than for those with less.

The development for telematic oriented research again is somehow different from a point of view of market shares: research is mostly done in SME´s, whereas profit orientation is to more than 50% based within big consortia, European branches of multis from all over the world or traditionally powerful European companies like Siemens, Philips, Bull and others.

The third aspect deals with the fact that not innovation is linear proportional to funding from Brussel, rather restricted by the splitting of the overall budget divided by member states and programme lines. Due to the joining of Finland, Austria, and Sweden in March 1996, the European Council has decided to increase the budget of the 4th FRP of 800 Mio. ECU up to a total sum of 13.1 Billion ECU. This money, however, went equally to the already existing programme-lines and member states and has not been used for the enforcing of already defined top-priority projects or programme-strands. Another increase was originally planned but will probably not go into action due to budget shortages in Brussels. Instead, any additional money will probably go directly into the so-called "task forces" agreed upon by the commissioners Edith Cresson, Martin Bangemann and Neil Kinnock: among others at least 3 telematics and multimedia-oriented research schemes will be designed (Railway and Alarming Systems for the Future, Intermodal Traffic Systems, Multimedia-Software Development for Education and Training).

The 4th aspect is highly undefineable, since political issue are sometimes black boxes for most of the EU-citizens and also for the EU-politicians themselves. The budget for the 5th FRP represents with about 4% a rather small and politically unimportant part of the EU budget. But, everybody expects new challenging perspectives and innovations from European research, not knowing how to share the little money among the principles being set up over the last 5 years.

The EU reflects on the principle of subsidy/subsidiarity, knowing exactly that also the national budgets are decreasing and that a national priority list will not always predetermine the European priority list for research and development.

This, however, correlates with a rapidly changing market for telematics-products, in which prices are dropping of about almost 50% within a year together with expectations rising for the labour market and its solutions by using telematics- or home-based-work places. The questions remains whether industry just ignores political discussions and expectations in Brussels for saving market shares and values. Or to put the question the other way around: is the ongoing political and scientific discussion in Brussels about future outlines and developments of new information and communication technology really up-to-date and still realistic, if one takes into consideration market and product line changes ?

For those being familiar with the new call within INFO 2000 the question arose, whether a defined maximum project budget of 100.000 ECU for the MIDAS-NET is really a stimulating factor to innovate, to transfer technology and to commercialise. Frankly speaking, I doubt it.

2. Telematics and the Frameworkprogrammes

How, now do these facts - mostly well known - affect telematic-based systems for health and prevention and to what extend might they improve or delay neccessary research?

In the late 1980s and early 1990s, many countries experienced fundamental changes in the structure and funding of their health services. The US-system failed to improve their national health system; in Britain, a fundamental review and restructuring of the NHS (National Health Service) based on internal market forces has entailed a split along commercial lines between purchasers and users on the one hand and providers of health care on the other.

These changes were information intensive and depended on the systematic collection and processing of information and data on all levels of prevention and health care.

Also in the Netherlands, reforms based on competition within the public sector have been gradually introduced with an emphasis on consumer needs and choices. This was also the premise behind major reforms in Germany and Belgium, just to name only a few European states. The increasingly competitive environment for healthcare has involved changes in customer requirements, technology, competitors, economic structure and legislation.

In Europe, the ongoing ageing and increasing diversity of minority groups as well as public awareness about health matters create an enormous demand for preventive health information. Any computer based Citizens Advisory Systems (CAS) has to deal with the following aspects:
- to offer background information in preventive health
- to offer data-based and knowledge-based facilities to make citizens aware of offers, needs and habits throughout Europe
- to give the opportunity for independent decisions for every citizen
- to give the chance to become informed about different EU-standards and structures
- to offer information about treatment and medication within existing legal boundaries

3. User Needs Analyses

European studies for the identification of user needs and expectations have been undertaken within the last months. Almost all users and in addition to the key-informants from hospitals, universities, companies, health insurances and public bodies regarded CAS´s as important and as real information suppliers. The needs ranged from a simple directory of local services in clinics etc. to multi-media information which might facilitate a decrease of personal communication between doctors and patients at any time about any issue. Multi-media information should be user-driven with an easy access for everybody, at any time at any place. Most key informants preferred a double solution: stand-alone systems in public (so-called: kiosks) and networked equipment for private use at home.

Regarding the function of a CAS, the following answers have been given:
- information system should give general health care information: 100 %
- should work as a medical encyclopedia: 68,75 %
- should contain infotainment: 31,25 %
- should educate users or groups: 18,75 %

General information is preferred compared to life-rules and informations about deseases. The information should be given anonymously, detailed according to the wishes and expectations of the user and should be easy to understand ("as simple as possible, as compex as neccessary").

87 % prefer public locations in medical contexts (in hospitals or alike)
75 % prefer libraries
62 % prefer public places like city halls etc.
50 % would like to have access from their homes
10 % would contact multi-media centers.

Some of the key-informants indicated that the best location is the privacy at home, but they thought it not be feasible under the existing technological infrastructure within Europe. Most key-informants do not have a multi-media PC at home or do find the price for modems and hardware-equipment still to high (prices vary up to 150 % between for example Portugal and the Netherlands).

Most key-informants indicated that the offered configuration has enough possibilities because it covers all the carriers of information nowadays being available. But they also indicated that the hard- and software-specifications are too technical to understand. Offering sensory or olfactorial stimuli might be original and easy to use but according to price-standards not feasible. The question what technical standards are preferred has been answered as follows:

81 % prefer usual equipment (PC etc.)
81 % prefer print-outs
56 % prefer video
12 % prefer statistics
12 % prefer touch-screen
 6 % prefer sensory
 6 % prefer olfactory

A majority of the key-informants preferred a mixture of text, pictures, video sequences, and interactive text.

Any CAS should be considered as information supplier with main attention on information, not on treatment, medication and self-diagnosis. The value of health advisory in general is primarily the prevention of illness, secondary the restriction of existing illness and tertiary the restriction of the consequences of illness (Damoiseaux, 1993).

We found out, that users and key-informants indicated that on the one hand the system can partly take over the task of doctors concerning some minor questions about health issues. This means, that people will visit a doctor less frequently. On the other hand: demand generates supply; information about health issues evokes new questions. Therefore, doctors will be visited and seen more frequently.

Users and key-informants state that two topics are important to the general public: information and entertainment. From a preventive point of view, information about health is important because there is so much information regarding health and illness already, that it is important to indicate which information might be of help for which user in which situation. Next to information a user is interested in entertainment, which especially holds true for the MTV-generation (age 10-35). For healthy people the relevancy of information is also based on easy accessible infotainment.

Another aspect is diffidence in case of a socially sensible illness. A married man who had an homosexual contact and who is afraid of being infected by AIDS will find the threshold of visiting a doctor very high. An anonymous and impersonal contact might be solution. Practical information with a high relevancy should be given priority in this context by using multimedia-information-supply.

4. CAS-specifications

In cooperation with health insurance companies in Germany and Europe standards have been defined according to user needs, providers expectations, and cost regulating issues for using telematic-based citizens advisory systems.

These standards might be divided into 10 points:

1. A reform of medical renumeration and calculation has to be taken into consideration. Costs should be calculated more on the basis of consultancy, therefore preventive medicine instead of on the use of high technology equipment. With this respect, multimedia applications might be of help, assuming that these applications are multi-valent and differentiating according to the users expextations and knowledge.

2. The family doctors model should be further developed which might lead to the fact that more resources might be saved rather than vasted. This model would improve the quality of care on a personal basis with the help of telemedicine, telediagnosis and videoconferencing-technology.

3. The principle of "as much out-patient care as possible, as little in-patient care as necessary" should be applied. Changes are already under way in some European member states towards out-patient clinics on a poli-medical clinic basis: different doctors with different expertises are sharing one clinic for the advantage of patients and citizens within the community and for reducing costs.

4. A competition in the out-patient area might increase the quality of analysis and treatment and could initiate so-called medical quality-circles towards ISO 9000 sq. standards. Analysis and treatments standards, continuing training schemes and on line information could be given by using innovative CAS´s.

5. The initiation of an effective competition in the supply area of medicine would also be of help in order to regulate prices for treatment and medication towards a positive list of drugs and therapies. In cooperation with networks of pharmacists and the pharmaceutical industry for example, those positive lists could be published, updated and commented in the CAS´s.

6. It is anachronistic that doctors define the content and quality of their services and treatments and that they also define the quality of their profession themselves. CAS might be of help to define together with insurance companies and user groups associations the content and quality of medical analyses and treatments in the near future. In the context of more and more limited budgets, TQM-measures will be recognised as appropriate tools for evaluation procedures and decision making processes.

7. An optimization of information and consultancy systems run by insurance companies and doctors together with telecom-branches and research units might also optimize national and/or European health systems. In times of shortages of public budgets for health services, a better use of the already existing resources might be of help. Whether or not this only applies to the health prevention aspects or also to the treatment and medication sector waits to be seen.

8. Socio-political strategies should be developed in order to increase the awareness for health care matters. The corporate promotion of a safe and sound body and soul should be rather a general political task than one only in the field of offering data in the right way and attractiveness.

9. Health prevention should be based on the general national risk structure. This risk structure takes into consideration ageing structure, nutrition, life style, economic structures, information infrastructure and morbidity rates within the community. These types of information should be made public and accessible to every citizen and should be taken up into curricula development schemes in schools and education.

10. Controlling systems within hospitals and health systems have to be made more effective. The planning, preplanning and the accounting of resources have to be improved according to national budgets but also with regard to european-wide comparisons.

The study we have undertaken and the project CATCH which is under development now is a multilingual and multimedia-version. In CATCH, hospitals, insurance companies, universities and research units and the telecom sector is involved to build a European version of a CAS together with partners in Portugal, the Netherlands, Germany and Great Britain. The study and the technological standards will be published soon. Earlier information might be obtained from my office.

Medical Informatics Europe '97
C. Pappas et al. (Eds.)
IOS Press, 1997

Medical Emergency Aid through Telematics: design, implementation guidelines and analysis of user requirements for the MERMAID project

G. Anogianakis[1,2], S. Maglavera[1], A. Pomportsis[3], S. Bountzioukas[2], F. Beltrame[4], G. Orsi[5]

1 BIOTRAST s.a., 111 Mitropoleos Str, GR-54622 Thessaloniki, Greece
2 Department of Physiology, Faculty of Medicine, Aristotle University, Thessaloniki
3 Department of Informatics, Aristotle University, Thessaloniki
4 DIST-University of Genoa, Italy
5 TSD-Projects, Milano, Italy

Abstract. MERMAID is an EU financed telemedicine project with global reach and 24-hour, multilingual capability. It aspires to provide a model for the provision of health care services based on the electronic transmission of medical information, via ISDN based videoconferencing. This model will not be limited to medical diagnostics but it will encompass all cases where the actual delivery of health care services involves a patient who is not located where the provider is. Its implementation requires the commissioning of an expensive telecommunications infrastructure and the exploration of a number of solutions. In fact, all categories of telemedical applications (audio and video conferencing, multimedia communications, flat file and image transfer with low, medium and high bandwidth data requirements) will be considered while the full range of network choices (Digital land lines, Cellular/Wireless, Satellite and Broadband) will be tested in terms of cost/performance tradeoffs that are inherent to them and the developmental stage each of these options occupies in their in its life cycle. Finally, out that MERMAID utilises advanced land based line transmission technologies to aid the remote patient by making available the specialist care that is best suited in the particular case.

1. Introduction

MERMAID is an EU (DGXIII) Healthcare Telematics programme (1, 2), that it was set up in response to Council Directives 92/29 and 93/103. These directives provide the basis for using "long distance medical consultation" to protect the safety and health of maritime workers. MERMAID therefore intends to provide an untegrated multilingual medical emergency service around the world and use telematics to transfer medical expertise to sea-borne vessels (3). In this respect, it has conducted a series of survey on telemedicine user requirements (4) that attempted to place maritime telemedicine within the presently emerging framework for practicing telemedicine around the world. The reasoning behind such a survey was that although MERMAID is strictly a maritime telemedicine and emergency medicine project, it can neither ignore current telemedical developments, nor grow into a trully "global 24 hour multilingual telemedicine surveillance and emergency service" by isolating itself from other facts of the field of the telemedicine[1].

2.   The MERMAID survey

To place the MERMAID surveys conclusions into perspective, one must mention that it was compiled on the basis of the replies from 1853 medium size and large (> 1000 gross tons) ocean going vessels. According to the Maritime Administration of the U.S. Department of Commerce: (5) This corresponds to 7.5% of the total world merchant marine for this class of vessels. It also corresponds to 2.5% of the world total when all ships over 100 gross tons are taken into account (6). Finally, it corresponds to appoximatelly 20% of the EU merchant marine capacity.

MERMAID has succeed to estimate for the first time the size and depth of the maritime telemedicine market. Thus:
1. The merchant marine and the sea related activities are estimated to employ 1,500,000 workers world-wide. Of these 410,000 people work aboard medium size and large ships, 140,000 being officers and the rest (270,000) as deck and engine crew. Officers come to a large extent (>40%) from OECD countries while crews from developing or underdeveloped countries (>60%).
2. Most ships have an adequate marine communications infrastructure for supporting telemedicine applications, especially those operating at high seas. However, high speed data (HSD) capability is not widely available and at present, only a small number of ships (<5%) can take advantage of the full spectrum of telemedical services that are technologically feasible (Table 1). It is noted that only 18,5% of the vessels surveyed are fitted, so far, with the Global Maritime Distress and Safety System (GMDSS) i.e. the new standard in marine safety

Type	Percentage %	Type	Percentage %
INMARSAT A	55	Fax	49
INMARSAT B	4	Radio/Telex	3,7
INMARSAT C	37,5	INMARSAT -M	0,1
Intelest	0,6	MARINET	1,8
Capability of High Speed Data	5	TOR	0,1
Modem	13,5	Mobile Telephone	0,8
Telephone	56		

Table 1: Percentage of vessels capable of operating over the different marine telecommunications systems

3. Most modern ocean going vessels have some kind of computer capability. 85% of the operators currently use personal computers on board their vessels, 76% are utilising telephones and facsimile equipment, while 48% use modems for transfering data to and from their vessels. Operating systems used are either DOS or Windows.
4. The number of marine telemedical calls is estimated between 15,000 to 20,000 per year world-wide. In general, the incidents reported are restricted to either sudden illness (37%) or accidents (63%). 9 out of the 10 cases reported as "sudden illness" are in fact "neglected" cases that suddenly deteriorated.
5. 43% of the operators expressed an interest for a 24 hour emergency, multilingual and multidisciplinary telemedicine service while 73% of these operators, who reported their interest for such a service, said they would be willing to pay a subscription for it.

---

[1] G7 Conference (Building the Information Society for the Citizens of the World), February 1995, Brussels

3.   Review of the Communications technologies of interest to MERMAID (7, 8)

Communications technologies of interest to MERMAID can be viewed from two main vantage points: that of Transmission Media and that of Networking Systems. Regarding Transmission Media the following subjects can be considered of importance:
1. Fiber Optics
2. Copper Cable (HDSL/ADSL and Coaxial Cable)
3. Satellite Communications
4. Cellular Radio Technologies
5. Wireless Data Networks
6. Radiotelephony for navigation
7. Radiotelephony on airplanes
8. Radiotelephony on trains

Similarly, regarding Networking Systems the following subjects bear on the MERMAID project and its future infrastructure development strategy:
1. Asynchronous Transfer Mode (ATM)
2. B-ISDN Protocol Reference Model for ATM or I.121 (Physical Layer, ATM Layer, ATM Networking, ATM Adaptation Layer or AAL)
3. ATM Networks and Services Introduction Scenarios
4. ATM and competitive Narrowband Services (Global Networking with N-ISDN)
5. Packet Switched Networks
6. The Internet

4.   Implications for the MERMAID implementation

Based on the current mix of marine communications capabilities that exist aboard ocean going vessels it has been decided that the MERMAID medical telecommunications software that is currently under construction be adapted to accommodate all types of maritime users, irrespective of whether they are INMARSAT A, B or C adherers. Furthermore it was decided that the Medical telecommunication software should include:

1. A medical record system that can guide the user through patient history and objective examination.
2. A multimedia HELP function with text and illustrations based on the WHO and the EU (DG V) requirements for help at sea, to guide paramedics through all the diagnostic procedures they have to perform for the teleconsultant and through all therapeutical procedures which the teleconsultant might prescribe.
3. A database with all information on the vessel's stocks of medicine and medical equipment.

The MERMAID telemedical approach itself will be a two level approach that will include:
1. A basic level at which the MERMAID medical with the INMARSAT satellite communication system in mind communications system that will include the medical record and a HELP/guidance system will be used.
2. A second level at which more enhanced and technical sophisticated features such as interactive video, sound, EKG transmissions etc. will be used, features that can only be used for ships equipped with INMARSAT A or B.

Finally, the development of programme modules for training and education of the seafarers in the use of the MERMAID medical communications system will be given top priority as such modules they constitute the firmest basis for the promotion of the proper practice of telemedicine at sea.

5. Guidlines for the implementation of the MERMAID telemedical scenario

1. MERMAID capitalises on the fact that ISDN is the first widely available public network, which is based on international standards, that can provide support for integrated services. This makes it the obvious current choice to support wide area telemedical applications.
2. Communications satellites provide a means of transmitting data between geographically remote locations. The MERMAID choice, INMARSAT, provides a telecommunications capacity which PTTs may lease to provide world-wide data communications and to use for building Virtual Private Networks.
3. The MERMAID telemedical scenario considers that the first and foremost piece of information of value to a clinician for reaching a correct diagnosis is *the first-hand contact, view and examination of the patient*. Experience suggests that in the absence of the visual prompt of the patient's presence, medical practitioners make errors in history taking which result in a number of dangerously incorrect diagnoses. MERMAID therefore, has adopted telemedicine methods and scenarios that include live images of the patient transmitted to the remote physician and offer the possibility for on-line interaction, discussion and consultation with the patient and/or those attending him.
4. Experience has shown that, with monitor resolution as low as 200 lines per picture height and 10 frames per second, clinicians are already able to diaenose much more effectively than with voice only communication. MERMAID will be using image quality considerably above that threshold.
5. Telepresence is the virtual presence of a distant person at a site, giving that person a sense of perception at the site. When added to a medical teleconsultation scenario, such as the one used by MERMAID, it gives all the benefits of image transfer and enhances the efficiency of the session. In this respect the following parameters have a significant affect on the feeling of reality: (a) Image size, (b) Image definition, (c) Personalised images, (d) Localising sound with images.
6. Locally stored but remotely controlled multimedia material will be used to make medical instructions more explicit. The subjects to be covered by this material will include, among others: (a) First aid instructions, (b) Poisoning related structured history taiing, (c) Trauma related structured history taking, (d) Infectious diseases, (e) Venereal diseases, (f) Emergency treatment of marine disaster victims, (g) Environmental vessel contr, (h) , Prevention of diseases, (k) On-board administration of pharmaceuticals, (I) Pharmaceuticals index and dosa, (m) Surgical equipment and usage
7. The three main components necessary to set up the MERMAID telemedical scenario are the following: (a) *Source of expertise*, i.e., definition of land-based stations where physicians standing by (or on call) will be able to offer their services in case of emergency, (b) *Communications channel, i.e.,* ensuring communications with open-sea vessels across the globe, (c) *Terminal equipment* for the capture and transmission of visual and audio information. This should be: operationally safe within the intended environment, able to support the intended functionality, cost justified, easy to learn, easy to use, adherent to data communication standards, in ordep to promote versatility and interoperability

8. Other issues involved in the realisation of the MERMAID scenario are: (a) *Training*. In particular, self-training applications with possibilities for distance training will be used, substituting formal person-to person interaction by simple point-of-uqe instructions, explanatory documentation, on-line multimedia ppesentation and help, (b) *Consultation protocols* for both ocean and land-based sites. Telemedical consultation will have an impact on both resource usage and work patterns at both ends, (c) *Medical Records*. The representation, content, storage, and integration of medical records to this scenario may prove to be of great importance for the suacess of the proposed scheme, (d) *Medical practitioner concerns*. While it is possible that the land-based hub will not always feature a medical practitioner with the required expertise the problem mainly concerns the qualifications of the respondent at the ocean site.

6.   Conclusions

MERMAID attempts to combine mobile satellite technologies, VSAT technologies and ISDN protocols in order to realise a Global State-of-the-Art System for the provision of health care services to the Maritime Sector. In this respect it must be pointed out that the technologies chosen guarantee:

1. reliability, since the technological platforms that were chosen have been extensively tested over the past 20 years.
2. continuity, since bandwidth is casily upgradable to at least 2Mbps over the existing technological platforms
3. seamless connectivity, since the technological platforms that were chosen have been fully integrated into the worldwide telecommunications networks
4. ease of upgrading, since the next step upwards to the technologies chosen is ATM which is the natural successor to ISDN
5. implementation at the lowest possible cost, since they utilise (and interface) existing and implemented technologies for every branch of the proposed MERMAID network
6. downward compatibility, since all the technologies chosen can accommodate smaller scale implementations. For example, besides HSD Inmarsat A can accommodate different levels of interaction, all of which can be utilised for telemedical purposes.

References

1. George Anogianakis, The New Flying Doctor, Ocean Voice April 96
2. George Anogianakis and Stavroula Maglavera, MERMAID rescues those in peril on the sea, European Hospital Management Journal, Vol. 3 Issue 1 1996
3. INMARSAT fact sheet on Telemedicine
4. MERMAID HC-1034 Deliverable D1.1: "Report on the analysis of user requirements", Healthcare Telematics, DGXIII, September 1996.
5. The Economist Pocket "World in Figures" 1993 Edition, London, UK
6. David Wright and Leonid Androuchko, Telemedicine and developing countries, Journal of Telemedicine and Telecare, Vol. 2, Number 2 1996
7. George Anogianakis and Stavroula Maglavera, Medical Emergency Aid through Telematics (MERMAID), Health Care in the Information Age, H. Sieburg, S. Weghorst and K Morgan (Eds) IOS Press and Ohmsha, 1996
8. George Anogianakis, Stavroula Maglavera and GFA Harding, Medical Emergency Aid through Telematics (MERMAID), Medical Informatics Europe '96, J Brender at al (Eds), IOS Press, 1996

Medical Informatics Europe '97
C. Pappas et al. (Eds.)
IOS Press, 1997

A Multimedia Man-Machine Interface
for the Disabled and Elderly

P. Angelidis, G. Anogianakis, S. Maglavera
BIOTRAST S.A., Thessaloniki, Greece

1. Introduction

In geographic Europe alone, where the overall population is around 800 Million, there are currently about 100 million elderly people and 50 million people with a disability (this figure includes disabled people who are also elderly). The figures for the European Union are currently about 77 million elderly people and 43 million people with a disability.

There is a growing movement in the EU to improve the rights of disabled people. The problems of providing assistance are high and they are exacerbated by the difficulty of finding professional staff to assist the disabled and elderly and by the high cost of such assistance. Specialised products can enable individual users to perform everyday tasks more easily and less expensively.

More and more companies are becoming willing to support these moves - both as an employer and service provider. Disabled organizations have been keen to point out specialist products and services that are of key importance to disabled people. One of the areas of high interest and wide research activity is *Domotics*, i.e. the design of assistance machines that replace humans in performing household activities.

The interface we are presenting in this work is part of a fully automated robot which enables severely disabled or bed-ridden users to play o more effective and active role in everyday domestic activities. The project was financed by the EU within the DGXIII TIDE programme under the name MOVAID (MOBILITY AND ACTIVITY ASSISTANCE SYSTEM FOR THE DISABLED)

2. Description

2.1 General principles

The Multimedia Man-Machine Interface (MMMI) of MOVAID is the gateway to the system. It enables able-bodied users or disabled with limited hand functionalities (enough to operate a mouse) to access the available functions in order to perform certain tasks.

The MMMI provides:

- a tool to pass instructions to the system
- an overview of system status, system responses and messages, particularly when some user reaction is required.

The main design disciplines of the MMMI are:

- ergonomically correct interface, as easy as possible to learn and use
- minimal number of steps to complete each process and task
- easily accessible interface components
- interface components accessible to the user are selected according to the user's expertise
- the system should not intimidate the user
- task execution follows the KISS (Keep It Simple and Stupid) principle, whereas interface design is distinctively intelligent.

2.2 Functional Description

The MMMI interacts in the front level directly with the user. It aims to serve the user manipulate the system, give orders and directions, watch the requested action as it evolves and in some cases configure the system.

In the back level the MMMI provides tools (in form of functions) to pass instructions to the rest of the software modules and especially the supervisory module (SM), to accept feedback from the rest of the modules particularly when some user reaction is required and an overview of system status, system responses and messages.

The primary role the MMMI fulfills is to provide the user with an easy and friendly access to the system and the system with a tool for communication with the user.

The task of the MMMI is basically twofold:

1. to receive user's requests;
2. to 'translate' the user's request into a list of Elementary Actions and sent them to the supervisory module.

Two different sub-modules, corresponding to the above mentioned tasks, could be identified within the MMMI: the 'Graphical Interface' in the front level and the 'Interpreter' in the back level.

The Graphical Interface guarantees that the user can only ask for allowed actions. For example, if the first part of action requested by the user is "GO TO THE BATHROOM", the second part cannot be "OPEN THE MICROWAVE OVEN".

The sub-module directly communicating with the supervisory module is the Interpreter. It interprets the correspondence between the user's input and a proper list of Elementary Actions, by accessing both its own local data-base and the system data-base.

In some cases, this correspondence can be dependent on the objects and/or actions involved. For example, if the user asks "OPEN" combined with "MICROWAVE OVEN", the list of actions generated by the Interpreter must be different from the one generated in case of "OPEN" "REFRIGERATOR". So, the MMMI accesses to the System Data-Base, whenever appropriate indications, associated to the objects or the movements of the system, are required.

The following picture shows the functional scheme of the modules interacting with the MMMI. The arrows highlight the interfaces between the modules and the MMMI.

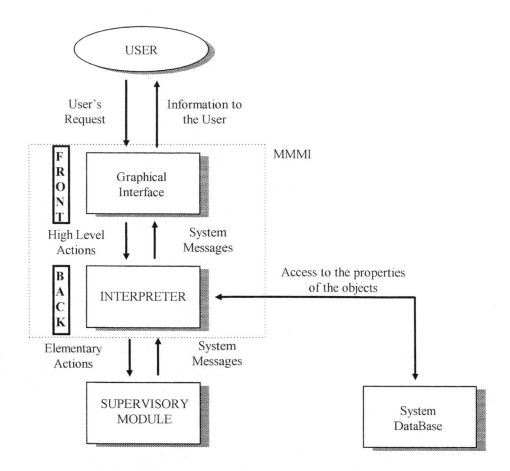

Figure 1 The functional scheme of the modules interacting with the MMMI

Functionally, the MMMI is organised in four levels. Each level allows different ways of manipulation; the higher the lever, the more advanced the user requirements, the complication of the instruction and the higher the freedom degree. The style and effort of interaction from the user point of view is different according to her/his skills and experience with the use of the MOVAID system. In fact, the following different levels of use have been defined (at any level the user is allowed to access to all the functions available at the lower levels, plus some functions typical of the current level of use):

- Beginner: training procedures, self-explanatory commands, only pre-defined macros, indication of objects on the screen;

- Standard: simplified on-line help, pre-defined macros, indication of objects on the
  screen, optional involvement in error management;

- Advanced: no on-line help, pre-defined macros, indication of objects on the screen,
  involvement in error management;

- Expert: no on-line help, pre-defined macros, indication of objects on the screen,
  involvement in error management;

Each level is designed to provide functions to fulfill the manipulation level described in the design concepts of the MOVAID system.

Another task of the multimedia MMI is to monitor the status of the mobile unit. It is able of displaying the position of the mobile unit, messages from the Supervisory module, pictures from the cameras, and other information that presents to the user the status of the mobile unit and help for its navigation in the house environment.

The multimedia MMI is also able of recording sequences of low level functions into "macros" for faster execution of tasks by the user. Macros will be used for making frequent tasks more easy, after the user has learned the system better. In this way, the user will be able to "customise" the system. Additionally, functions and pre-programmed sequences can be provided for use by a third helper.

The MMMI is designed to provide on-line guidance and help to the user through a series of multimedia objects including sound, graphics and text.

2.3 Technical specifications

MMMI's main purpose is to display the commands and actions available to the user in a user-friendly form, accept the user's response, and then pass the commands to the Global Supervisor module where the commands will be interpreted and processed.

The multimedia MMI supplies support for all low level functions of the mobile unit. The user is able of moving the mobile unit forwards or backwards, turn the mobile base clockwise or counter-clockwise, handle the arm movement and the cameras. Support for low level function is important for the adaptability of the system even though it makes handling more difficult. It also makes the system more interesting for the user to explore and find out more things that can be done with it. Low level function support is also import for critical situations, that the system cannot handle, and returns some sort of error message to the user. These are moments where the user must handle the mobile unit manually to get it out of its critical situation.

The multimedia MMI has a two-way communication with the user to accomplish. First the input to the module must provided at the lower level through the mouse. This way certain multimedia devices can be added to the system that makes access to it more human friendly. Those devices emulate mostly the mouse. Devices like that, that emulate the mouse are touch screens, joysticks, digitizer boards, head controlled devices, sound recognition equipment.

From the above it is clear that command input to the multimedia MMI had to be made as much as possible with straight commands, and not with invocation through many level menus or even typing of commands. The user have a list of actions and a list of items that must associate them with the help of the mouse (and this way with every device that emulates it). For example touching the word GO and the item KITCHEN, makes the mobile unit to start the process of moving to the kitchen.

All the commands of the system are represented with actions and items as described above, and this is the backbone on which every other way of interaction will be based on.

Video and sound makes the user interface even more friendly. Besides video windows that display the "vision" of the mobile unit, video can be used for on-line help, showing the user how to handle a certain device. All the messages from the system to the user can be made with sound. Also certain cartoon-like figures can be used for giving the user advises about certain matters. All the interaction between the MMMI and the user is displayed in figure 2 below.

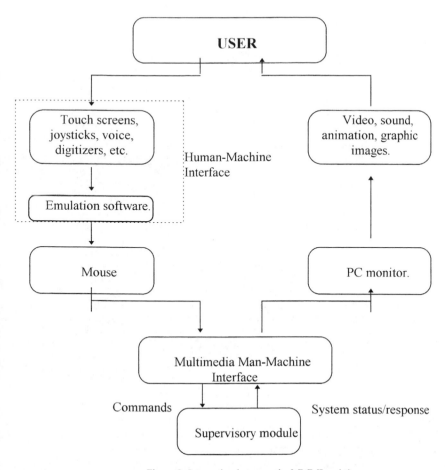

Figure 2 Interaction between the MMMI and the user

3. References

[1]   EUROSTAT, (1992). Rapid Reports, Population and Social Conditions: Disabled People - Statistics. Commission of the European Communities, Luxembourg

[2]   S. Hasino *Aiding Robots,* Advanced Robotics, vol. 7, no. 1, 1991, pp. 97-103

[3]   WS3 *Robots for Disabled and Elderly People*, International Conference on Robotics and Automation, May 27, 1995, Nagoya, Aichi, Japan.

[4]   P. Dario, Project Coordinator TIDE Project #1270 *Mobility and Activity systems for the Disabled*, Feb. 1994

[5]   C. Laschi, E. Guglielmeli, L. Leontaridis, P. Dario, TIDE Project #1270 Deliverable 5.1/6.1 *Design Specifications of the Workstations*, Apr. 1995

[6]   P. Dario, E. Guglielmeli, B. Allotta and M.C. Carozza,   *Robotics for Medical Applications*, IEEE Robotics & Automation Magazine, vol. 3, no. 3, Sep. 1996, pp. 44-56

Medical Informatics Europe '97
C. Pappas et al. (Eds.)
IOS Press, 1997

An EKG Monitor Network

Mihajlo KOMOCAR
IMTEL Computers, Bul. Lenjina 165B, 11070 Belgrade, Yugoslavia

Srecko ATANASKOVIC, Zoran SAVIC
IPME, Ustanicka 152/41, 11000 Belgrade, Yugoslavia

Dejan IGNJATIC
LTS, Dobrovoljacka 9, 11080 Zemun - Belgrade, Yugoslavia

Abstract. A networkable kardiomonitor CM-3 is described as well as the associated central monitoring device CEMON. CM-3 allows archiving as well as efficient control of all relevant measurements, alarms and trend data in the last 2 years of use of the equipment. This data is easily reviewed, printed or saved on removable media to be included in the hospital patient documentation. The network is based on standard Ethernet bus architecture and PC Ethernet adapters. This high speed medium allows efficient real time control and immediate reaction to each alarm situation. Easy integration with other parts of the hospital information system is possible. In addition, critical monitor files can be efficiently backed up and possibilities are open for hierarchical storage with high security options.

1. Kardiomonitor CM-3

Kardiomonitor CM-3 is the commercial name for a hospital monitor whose functions include EKG, oximetry, plethysmography, blood pressure measured by invasive or non-invasive means, respiration (frequency, rhythm and intensity of respiratory movement) and temperature. The intensive development of microcomputer technology has led to a fast increase in accuracy of measurement, quality of presentation and an increase in the measured and stored parameters. While in 1991 monitors could store 2 h of trend data, today the CM-3 can store an unlimited number of selected events with a pre and post history of 10 min. duration with immediate review, archiving and post review. There are over 20 firms producing monitors with very similar methods for measuring biomedical parameters but usually with different methods of presenting, archiving and indication of alarm states. That is why special recommendations have been made which besides technical characteristics define general factors of quality of monitors regarding human factor design[1]. These factors are ease of use, ease of overview of critical events, ease of instruction, recording and printing data, etc.

Two significantly different types of data for logging and archiving can be distinguished. The first type is numeric data with a low frequency of measurement which does not require large memory resources. The trend data fits into this category: pulse, temperature, blood pressure. If this data is logged once a minute, a daily log takes up about 40 kB of memory, or about 15 MB per year.

The situation with analog data like EKG is significantly different. To store them in a form where they can be easily accessed for subsequent review and analysis an analog to digital conversion of these signals must be made. The CM-3 works with a sampling rate of 500 Hz and A/D converter resolution of 12 bits so that additional processing of the signal is possible. For storing a minute of EKG data 45 kB of memory are necessary. For an average of 10 alarm situations per day and a storage of 5 min. per event, the necessary daily capacity is 2.25 MB or 820 MB per year[2].

The CM-3 has 4 MB of RAM memory for storing current data and a hard disk of 1.7 GB capacity for archiving data. This is several times larger than competitive monitors and also reflects a speedy and easy data access. The CM-3 has also the ability to issue a release diskette of a specific patient with all the characteristic and relevant data of case history, which can be used later if the patient returns to the hospital.

2. Central Monitor CEMON

Hospital monitors are by their nature and application tied to monitoring critical parameters of the state of the patient and so require the presence of hospital staff, it is useful to separate part of the monitor functions which are not directly involved in patient monitoring (administration, additional analysis, printing, archiving, monitor configuration...) and free the monitor from such tasks. In addition to these tasks, the central monitor with an EKG monitor network allows easy integration into the hospital information system, acquisition and storage of data in a way applicable to EDP, as well the application of modern methods of patient data security.

The central monitor includes the following functions:
- monitoring all state parameters of the patients connected through the network of Kardiomonitors CM-3.
- enables remote setting of some of CM-3 functions
- administrative and case history data entry for patients
- generating reports and reviews of gathered data.

3. Network Organization

Simultaneous monitoring of all the patients on the network was the demand that had a critical influence on the network design. The volume of data created in patient monitoring has been estimated above, and by taking into account that up to 16 CM-3 monitors may be connected to CEMON at a time, we can estimate the data throughput. The data has to be transferred with maximum speed, minimal latency, as monitoring of critical data requires immediate attention.[3]

A rough estimate of the average amount of data to be transferred and processed as 10 kB/s. The intensity of this data transfer varies as there can be asynchronous requests for the transfer of archived data from individual monitors, initiated at the CEMON or CM-3. In these situations the intensity of data transfer increases several times and approaches the capacity of the transfer medium. The communication base is the standard Ethernet cable (IEEE 802.3 standard) which is usually used in LAN networks. Its declared bandwidth is 10 Mb/s. Figure 1 shows the architecture of the Kardiomonitor net. The element for communicating with the hospital information system, usually a LAN, can be a device for that purpose (router, bridge). A direct connection can also be made so that the stations on the LAN share a segment of the cable with the Kardiomonitor net. This is possible as the communication protocol between the CM-3 and CEMON has been realized in such a way that it is transparent to potential existing protocols on the same cable. The protocol is realized directly using the SPX protocol service and peer-to-peer communication.

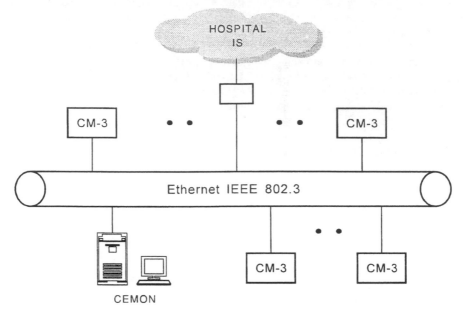

Figure 1. - The architecture of the Kardiomonitor network

4. Central Monitor Functions

The basis of the CEMON consists of a 486 personal computer with DOS operating system version 5.0 or higher. A minimum of 8 MB RAM is required and a SVGA graphics adapter with at least 1 MB of graphic memory. On this platform the application subsystem for the realization of the central monitor functions has been implemented. The "RT Kernel" library routines for a "multitasking programming system" have been used. Borland C++ is the programming environment.

The start of the application, as well as a series of security sensitive functions have been secured by a mechanism of passwords.

An addition to the programming system of the central monitor is a set of routines which are executed on the Kardiomonitor CM-3 and which realize a set of functions for connection, data transfer and disconnection for communication on the net.

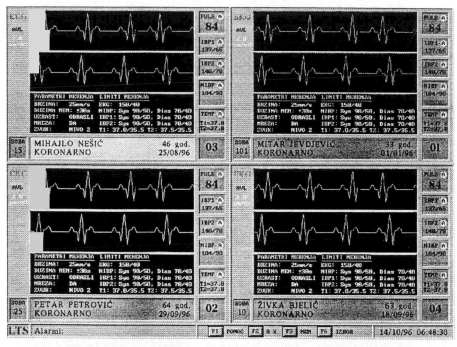

Figure 2. - 4 monitor view

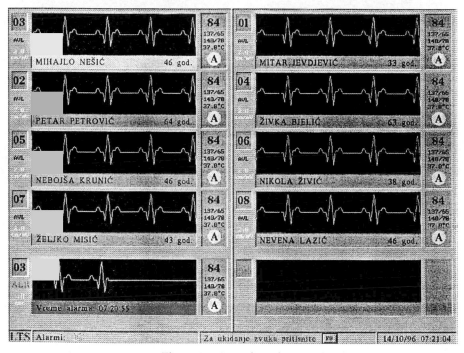

Figure 3. - 8 monitor view

The overview and control of individual Kardiomonitors has been realized through a system of windows allocated to these monitors. It is possible to view 4 monitors at once on the screen of the CEMON, displaying identical data as on the monitor,
as well as 8 monitors with a reduced data display. This is shown in figures 2 and 3. The figures show simulated data.

5. Conclusion

Kardiomonitor CM-3 has been created by careful elimination of negative characteristics of existing monitors, primarily in the access to critical and archived data. Modern microprocessor technology has enabled the realization of an economic and modern monitor for measuring, monitoring, archiving and analysis of a large number of biomedical parameters, quickly, simply, efficiently and accurately.

Of the numerous advantages of a Kardiomonitor network system the following may be highlighted:
- the system can be integrated into a perspective or existing hospital information system
- offers a series of qualitative new possibilities in the following and monitoring the status of a patient, resulting in the application of adequate and timely therapy
- enables an entry into the application of high technology solutions in this field at a lower price and higher autonomy than other products on the market.
- enables an easy application of hierarchical storage and data security options.

References

[1] Health devices, Physiologic Monitoring and the Standard of Care, Vol. 20, March-April 1991, ECRI.

[2] D. Dumeljic, D. Ignjatic, Biomedical Data Archiving in Up To Date Medical Equipment such as Kardiomonitor CM-3, 281-283, Medicinska Informatika 96, zbornik radova, 28-31 oktobar 1996.

[3] S. Atanaskovic, R. Petkovic, Z. Savic, M. Komocar , Central Monitor for Networking with Kardiomonitor CM-3, 275-280, Medicinska Informatika 96, zbornik radova, 28-31 oktobar 1996.

Medical Informatics Europe '97
C. Pappas et al. (Eds.)
IOS Press, 1997

Color Perimetry with Personal Computer

N. Accornero, M. Capozza, S. Rinalduzzi, A. De Feo *
G.C. Filligoi, L. Capitano **

*Dipartimento di Scienze Neurologiche ** Dipartimento infocom
University of Rome La Sapienza

ABSTRACT

Color visual field analysis has proven highly sensitive for early visual impairments diagnosis in M. S., yet it has never attained widespread popularity usually because the procedure is difficult to standardize, the devices are costly, and the test is fatiguing. We propose a computerized procedure running on standard PC, cost effective, clonable, and easy handled.

264 colored patches subtending 1° angle of vision, with selected hues and low saturation levels are sequentially and randomly displayed on gray equiluminous background of the PC screen subtending 24°x40° angle of vision. The subject is requested to press a switch at the perception of the stimulus. The output provides colored maps with quantitative informations.

Comparison between normals and a selected population of Patients with Multiple Sclerosis and with Glaucoma without luminance visual field defects, showed high statistical difference.

1. Introduction

Color visual field analysis has proved highly sensitive for the diagnosis of early visual impairments in multiple sclerosis and other visual diseases [1, 2, 3, 4, 5]. Yet it has never attained widespread popularity because the procedure is usually difficult to standardize, the devices used are costly, and the test is fatiguing for subjects to perform.

Our primary aim was to assemble a low cost, reliable instrument that could be handled easily by technician and patient alike, a real diagnostic tool using a commercial PC with standard peripherals.

2. Methods

A 486 PC, equipped with an SVGA card (480x640, 16.7 M of colors) generated color visual stimuli on the computer monitor, collected data from patient responses through a hand held switch (right button of the "mouse" pointing device) and displayed results in graphical and numerical form. The software, assembled in Visual Basic, runs under the Windows interface. Color perception was randomly tested for three chosen hues (red, green, and blue) with two low saturation levels within a contrasting gray equiluminous background (10 lux). The chromatic contrast was quantified considering 100% of contrast (level 2) a distance of 1 unit of the axis of the CIE (Commission Internationale de l'Eclairage) diagram from the central gray along the three red, green blue (RGB) color axes of our monitor and consequently 50% of contrast half a unit, (level 1) [6]. Each stimulus appeared as a small disk subtending a visual angle of 1° with boundaries progressively smoothing toward the gray background.

Each stimulus was displayed for 300 ms at the first level of saturation and then for a further 300 ms at the second. After a random pause lasting 800-1500 ms another stimulus (random colored) was generated in a different screen location. The new location was randomly chosen on an 88-point grid positioned to sample the inner 10° of the visual field with a spatial frequency of 3° and the outer field within 24°x40° with a resolution of 4°.

The relatively low spatial resolution of the grid proved to be a good trade off between accuracy and time of examination.

Towards the end of the examination points perceived at highly different contrast (2 levels) from at least three neighboring points were re-tested and the minimum difference in contrast was taken for that point.

For testing, the subject sat in front of the screen with the head fixed in a head-rest at a calibrated distance, so that the active display area subtended a visual angle of 40°x24° (approximately 30 cm with a 15" display monitor). With one eye covered, the subjects looked at a marker on the center of the screen and had to press a switch as soon as they perceived a local change on the screen. If necessary subjects wore glasses to correct refraction. Subjects were not asked to recognize the color of the stimulus although collaborative normal people could correctly discriminate colors almost all over the screen. When the subject pressed the switch the stimulus disappeared and the position, hue and saturation were memorized. Another stimulus was then randomly generated. The temporal window for the acceptance of the switch signal outlasted the stimulus presentation by 200 ms.

The central fixation point was checked by the operator with an infra-red TV camera pointing towards the patient's eye.

In normal subjects, the complete test required about 8 minutes per eye because not all the points perceived at the lower saturation level were tested for the higher level. In complete color blind subjects the test require 10 minutes for eye.

At the end of the examination an interpolation algorithm was executed, to fill the total matrix of 960 points. Three color maps for each eye were then displayed on the screen with a quantitative analysis of the levels of color perception

In the "setup" procedure large tiles differing in color and saturation were displayed on the screen so that their illuminance and chrominance could be measured. With a professional TV luxmeter (Minolta Chroma-meter x-y 1) that provided illuminance (in lux), chromaticity coordinates (x-y) and color temperature (k) according to CIE. Simple mouse or keyboard commands allowed illuminance, hue and saturation to be adjusted for each stimulus level and background.

3. Subjects

Ten normal subjects (both sexes 20-50 years), Ten Definite Multiple sclerosis patients, ten patients with primary open angle glaucoma have been enrolled for a pilot study.

All subjects selected had normal central visual field luminance test, and normal foved color test (Lanthony).To compress data and quantify the topographical results, we summed all the stimuli for each color perceived at the first level of saturation (weighting + 1), the stimuli perceived at level 2 (weighting 0) and stimuli not perceived at all (weighting -1). The sum total, which we termed the Color Perimetry Index (CPI), ranged from - 960 to + 960 per color and per eye. Because normality testing indicated that this variable had a normal distribution, data were analyzed with Student's t-tests. P values of <0.05 were considered significant. Analysis of variance was used to test differences between groups.

4. Results

The device we developed for clinical perimetric testing accomplished the task well and proved easy to handle. With these stimuli settings, normal subjects on average perceived the

50% contrast stimuli only within 10° of the visual field but they perceived the 100% contrast stimuli almost all over the screen, exept for the blind spot area.

No statistical differences emerged between colors, or between sexes, with the color setting used.

Repetitive testing in 8 subjects did not show statistical differences among the consecutive tests. Discriminant analysis with nine variables, three levels of perception, 50% saturation (level 1),100% saturation (level 2), and "not perceived" (level 3), for the three colors, completely separated the eyes of normal subjects from those of M.S. and glaucoma patients (Fig. 1, 2).

Principal component analysis (two components) indicated "level 1" and "level 3" for red color for MS. group and for blue for glaucoma group as the most significant.

Green color did not shows significative difference from red but wider variance.

5. Conclusions

The analysis of the results proved this computerized test procedure to be reliable for quantifying color perception in the central visual field for clinical purposes. We appear to have reached a good trade off between accuracy and rapidity. Rapidity is an important requisite since fatigue causes the test results to deteriorate to the extent that they cannot be upgraded even by a time-consuming increase in the sampling resolution of the visual field.

The utilization of standard low cost computer equipment without dedicated peripherals has some drawbacks concerning precision and stability of color setting of the monitor that requires frequent controls with a photometer but has the great advantage of availability of the instrumentation and duplication of the procedure.

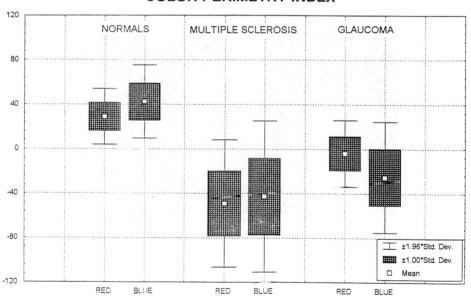

Fig. 1 Distribution of the color perimetry index for red and blue color in normal subjects, multiple sclerosis and glaucoma patients.

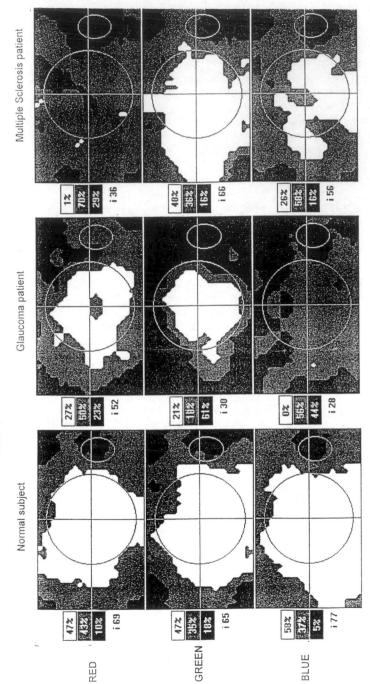

FIG. 2

Gray scale print out of computerized color perimetry:
comparison between a normal subject and two pathological ones.
White: 1 level of detection of color saturation, Gray: second level, Black: not seen

Our data on MS and glaucoma patients indicate that chromatic visual field analysis is highly sensitive, since all the patients we tested with normal luminance perimetry, normal foveal chromatic tests showed significative impairment with Chromatic perimetry.

The comparison between colors confirm that detection of long wave-lengths (RED) is particularly impaired in MS patients and correlates with the severity of the visual system involvement. While detection of short wavelenght (blue) is particularly impaired in glaucoma patients and correlate with the increase of the intraocular pressure.

References

[1] L. Fallowfield, J. Krauskopt. Selective Loss of Chromatic Sensitivity in Demyelinating Disease. *Investigate Ophthalmol Visual Science* 1984;25:771-773.

[2] J. Flammer, S.M. Drance. Correlation between color vision scores and quantitative perimetry in suspected glaucoma. *Arch Ophthalmol* 1984;102: 38-39.

[3] G.M. Chioran, K.L. Sellers, S.C. Benes, M.Libow , S.J. Dain , P.E. King-Smith. Color mixture threshold measured on a color television - a new method for analysis, classification and diagnosis of neuroophthalmic disease. *Doc Ophthalmol* 1985;61:119-135.

[4] K. Gunduz, G.B. Arden, S. Perry, G.W. Weinstein, R.A. Hitchings. Color vision defects in ocular hypertension and glaucoma. Quantification with a computer-driven color television system. *Arch Ophthalmol* 1988;106:929-935.

[5] A.J. Vingrys, P. Ewen King-Smith, S.C. Benes. Color perimetry can be more sensitive than achromatic perimetry. Clin Vision Sci 1989: 4: 197-209.

[6] C. Macaluso, A. Lamedica, G. Baratta, M. Cordella. Color discriminant along the cardinal chromatic axes with VECPs as an index of function of the parvocellular pathway. Correspondence of intersubject and axis variations to psychophysics. Electroenceph clin Neurophysiol 1996: 100: 12-17.

Medical Informatics Europe '97
C. Pappas et al. (Eds.)
IOS Press, 1997

RHINE-AM
An Inter-Regional Health Information
Network for Europe

P.H. Ketikidis[1,2], B.V. Ambrosiadou[1,3], A. van der Werff[2],
N. Maglaveras[3,] C.Pappas[3]

[1] *Department of Computer Science, CITY Liberal Studies,*
Thessaloniki, Greece
[2] *The SOCRATES Network, Health & IT Consultants, Netherlands*
[3] *Laboratory of Medical Informatics, Aristotelian University of*
Thessaloniki, Greece

Abstract: RHINE is an inter-regional network in Europe having as an aim, the promotion of know-how transfer in the area of Information Technology methods and tools in the regions involved. The RHINE network's significance will be demonstrated in the health sector. Within the main scope of the project, the aims and objectives of RHINE and the participating partners encompass the extension of the nucleus network and the furtherance of Information Technology research. Application areas include distributed data base and knowledge base technologies for open regional information systems supported by other technologies for business processes.

1. Introduction

The health policy framework and its basic strategies - first published by WHO in 1985 - has been adopted by all Regions of the European Union[1]. Major areas of health data and indicators that have been recognised are: lifestyles and health, risk factors affecting health and the environment, reorientation of the health care system itself, and, finally, the political, management, technological manpower, research and other support necessary to bring about the desired changes in the patient management and provision of quality health services in Europe[2].

Within this framework, a number of projects have been initiated in the European Union in order to provide the necessary infrastructure for medical information system development and to promote the application of information technology in the European Health System[3-7]. Examples of such projects are: the IRIS, for the promotion of Information Technology in a number of sectors including the environment and health in less favoured regions; EURO-ISDN for Health Care network to support local administrators and care providers; SHINE and STAR for the development of open systems frameworks for telematic services networks at community level; DIABCARD for the provision of smartcards with telematics functionality; I4C for the development of a platform for distributed databases demonstrated in cardiology and other.

RHINE has found a niche in the midst of all the European projects in that it aims at the formation of a European network for the dissemination of the results and the integration of theoretical structures and methods for the development of a composite set of tools for applying Information Technology in important sectors such as that of health[8,9]. The co-ordinating responsibility for particular sectors, including health, has been delegated to the Regional Authorities in most European countries. A representative group of Regions has therefore been formed in order to collaborate on a trans-European basis in the field of Information Technology applied to the health system in a joint action, called 'RHINE'. This paper outlines the scope, objectives and expected impact of RHINE in the European health system and it provides a detailed presentation of the results at each stage of the project development.

2. Scope, Mission and Objectives

The major target groups of RHINE Accompanying Measure (AM) are Europe's 250 Regions, as well as the IT, telematics and services industries, in particular SMEs in these Regions. Although health is taken as the focal point for the AM, the results will be applicable in other sectors such as environment, social and economic affairs, social services, social security, education, public administration, and resource management. In this way a substantial repeat business potential for the participating IT industries and spin off activity will be created.

The long-term ultimate goal or mission of RHINE is the achievement of appropriate unlimited information exchange and interoperability of data systems within and across European Regions. This project is a first step towards such a goal, and its scope and objectives are therefore restricted to a **General Accompanying Measure** (RHINE AM) consisting of a **European User Group** in which European Regions (i.e. the users) collaborate with IT industries combined with a **Concerted Action** for **stimulating the effective and efficient uptake of distributed data base technologies** for open regional information systems **supported by technologies for business processes**[8,9]. Health has been selected as the major application area of this AM.

3. Information Systems Objectives for the Health Sector within RHINE

Health data and indicators have been recognised by the Regions as crucial input for regional action in health and health related sectors. Major areas of health data and indicators are health status (life expectancy, mortality, morbidity etc.), diseases and prevention, population groups (children, elderly, disabled etc.), life styles (nutrition, tobacco consumption, sexual behaviour, alcohol abuse, etc.), environment (pollution, working environment, accidents etc.), socio-economic (education, income, pharmaceuticals, cost, etc.).

The objectives of information systems for Regions are to support regional authorities, their representative bodies and communities in providing the information needed for their decisions, in the areas as indicated above.

4. Health Information Systems - Basic Requirements-Applications

The major general requirements of information systems are the following:

First, to meet specific needs of different units. The deliverable of the RHINE project is an integrated distributed information system for data and knowledge interchange among users at different levels (medical doctors/patients) and in various geographical locations all over the regions. The systems will comprise software installed on computers in different physical locations. **Modularity** and **interoperability** are therefore major requirements and the application of distributed software technologies is implemented. Regional information systems should therefore offer **Region-wide coverage** and provide **interconnectivity** between the data bases concerned. Similarly, Regions could protect their investments in existing products (legacy systems) if this would function satisfactorily, and avoid replacement. Hence, regional information systems should ideally be built on the basis of **common 'integration' platforms, independent from machines and vendors, enabling the interconnection with already existing solutions using different technologies. Such an information infrastructure should not only include networking aspects, but also the basic 'common' software layers.**

Second, stepwise development. This is because regions are under constant budgetary pressure. Therefore the Regional authorities prefer to develop information systems stepwise, incrementally integrating additional applications in accordance with expressed needs and budgetary possibilities.

Finally, health monitoring and management of quality and cost From the viewpoint of health management regional information systems should enable **monitoring** (and surveillance) **of health and disease, and support 'geographical epidemiological' analyses of the differences in the incidence and prevalence of disease between and within Regions, in all relevant areas**. The health situation, quality of care and cost can only be measured if the desired levels can be defined, against which achievements can be compared. Regional information systems should therefore provide information for such analyses, **identifying reasons for variation**. **Knowledge base and decision support systems should be part of regional information systems as well.**

5. RHINE and the Region of Northern Greece

Northern Greece (2-3 million inhabitants) is considered by many historians and politicians as Europe's gateway to the Balkans, Eastern Europe and Asia. Thus, due to excellent economic and political perspectives, telematics have started developing already at both regional and local levels. In particular, in Thessaloniki, the Aristotle University has one of the most advanced networks in the country (FDDI with perspectives to become ATM broadband in the next year). Also in Thrace the University is developing its network, and the two Institutions are part of the Greek National Host for ACTS named HESTIA. Because of the recent development, certain health indices pertinent to quality and management of health care and epidemiology can now be measured for the whole area of Northern Greece through the use of telematics. More specifically, the four areas proposed for implementation in this telematics proposal are the following: hospital efficiency monitoring system for better health care management; accident monitoring for the continuity of health care; health monitoring system for measurement of health inequalities across the region; health monitoring system for health condition of moving people (e.g. tourists);

The priority areas of the RHINE project will therefore be the development, and validation of: health education of the public; improvement of linkage between the health services at primary and secondary level; connectivity with the outside world, and interregional and cross-border health issues of the population.

Common base, open architecture will be applied to provide for Europe-wide interworking, and Internet World Wide Web-applications will provide for European retrieval services. With regard to administrative and professional use 'security servers' will be built in for confidentiality and data protection and for separating access. The basis for the public network will be multi-channel ISDN, whereas in addition also users of X-25 networks (PSDN) and other networks should be offered the opportunity of sharing the services. Furthermore, common base, open architectures will be applied to provide for Europe-wide interworking, and Internet World Wide Web- applications will be provided for European retrieval services.

The approach that will be adopted by the project covers the following areas: data bases, documents bases, image bases; new generation of information systems oriented towards health outputs and outcomes; easy to use technologies, and open, configurable screens; modular applications in conformance with user requirements and open systems technology offering vendor independence, flexibility, scalability and interoperability; use of basic telecommunication services, including E-mail, file transfer, interactive digital multimedia transmission; choices on physical infrastructure made from ISDN (include EURO-ISDN), ATM.

6. The RHINE Information System Platform

The result and technologies used in the RHINE internetwork should be downward compatible to existing health networks. In the regions of the consortium usually PSDN-networks are used to exchange Text-Data. Actually some of the networks (Bearer services) used in national health of administrative networks are upgraded to ISDN speeds. The partners will contribute the results of RHINE to national activities concerning multimedia communications.

6.1 Technical basic concept of RHINE

Basic concept of the "RHINE" network is a "two level" network[7]. That means, that there are different access levels provided for professional users from the health and administrative area and a public community (interested citizens).

For this reason security facilities inside the network guarantee the privacy of distinct health data have to be installed and used. To make use of bandwidth higher 64 kbps, ISDN and multichannel ISDN is foreseen as the basic public network technology to be used. But besides, also users with X.25, leased lines and other networks in use, must be integrated into the user scenario. EURO-ISDN seems feasible as it provides an integrated PSDN access.

After setting up the regional parts of the RHINE network, the construction of transeuropean network connections has to be done. This is a very important topic : to achieve a high degree of acceptance the Transeuropean Network supporting RHINE must be easy-to-use, and offer a high availability, reliability and security. Possible

Networks used will be, public ISDN (include. X. 25), ATM-Services (later) or special private network services.

6.2 The Technical Aspects of RHINE

Specification and development of Database System and User Application Software - it is planned to base the information system on concepts of "Open Systems".

Network architecture and specification and development of Multinetwork Access Facilities - network access via different public available networks must be provided. Security facilities must be foreseen in the network level by use of mechanisms like encryption and authentication.

Specification and implementation of a Remote Operating Centre for the RHINE services and for "Help-Desk" Support - during the user-trials, user-validation phase, and demonstrations-phase the network must be operated. This should be done most efficiently by means of a "remote operating centre".

Technical Systems Integration and operating services - the work of systems Integration covers the following topics: network and systems configuration plus management system; setting up the network (ordering PNO services,...) national / international; integration with applications;

7. Summary

This paper has outlined the RHINE project which aims at providing a European group of Tele Health Regions. The User Group will act as a permanent platform for collaboration between Regions and IT-Industries which will be further expanded and used for transfer of know-how and IT products as applied in the areas of business process reengineering and distributed database technologies, demonstrated for the European health system . The project RHINE will also serve as a pilot for new initiatives in the European medical informatics area.

References

[1]   CEU, Treaty on European Union, 1992.
[2]   CEU, Growth Competitiveness, Employment - The Challenges and ways forward into the
        21st   Century (White Paper), 1993.
[3]   C. Cordon, J.P. Crhistensen, Health Telematics for Clinical Guidelines & Protocols, IOS
        Press 1994.
[4]   J. De Maeseneer, L. Beolchi, Telematics in Primary Care in Europe, IOS Press 1995.
[5]   Jesus Villasante, Telematic systems for health in Europe - a look towards the future,
        Health Informatics in Europe, June 1993.
[6]   M.F. Laires, M.J. Ladeira, J.P. Christensen, Health Care Telematics for the 21st Century,
        IOS Press 1995.
[7]   Albert van der Werff, Community Care: Towards a trans-European telematics services
        network for health surveillance and early warnings, *Health Informatics in Europe*, March
        1993.
[8]   J.E. De Cockborne, C. Berben, P. Scott, Telecommunications for Europe - the CEC
        sources, IOS Press 1995.
[9]   K. Cheng and T. Ohta, Future Interactions in Telecommunications Systems III, IOS Press
        1995.

Medical Informatics Europe '97
C. Pappas et al. (Eds.)
IOS Press, 1997

Organisation, Transmission, Manipulation of Pathological Human Organs on the WWW*

Meleagros A. KROKOS[1], Gordon J. CLAPWORTHY[1], Michele CRUDELE[2],
Giuliano SALCITO[3], Nikos VASILONIKOLIDAKIS[4]

[1]*Department of Computer & Information Sciences, De Montfort University,
Hammerwood Gate, Kents Hill, Milton Keynes MK7 6HP, United Kingdom*
[2]*Campus Bio-Medico Di Roma, Libero Istituto Universitario,
Via Longoni 83, Rome 00155, Italy*
[3]*CITEC S.p.A., Via Alessandro Farnese 3, Rome 00192, Italy*
[4]*Neuroware Ltd.,12 Alitsis Street, Athens 10433, Greece*

Abstract

The paper describes an integrated methodology for the development of a WWW computer system which addresses issues of the organisation, retrieval and manipulation of 3D volumetric models of pathological human organs. The library of organs is distributed on the WWW since medical expertise and needs are typically expensive resources and also because many pathological conditions are often restricted to local diffusion. Users are provided with a WWW viewer for interactive manipulation of the models of the organs. The system supports low-cost MS-Windows 32 platforms and requires no specialised hardware. Early results demonstrate that the compression techniques employed provide near real-time response for retrieval/manipulation, not only over high-speed expensive network lines, but also over low/medium network connections.

1. Introduction

One of the major contributions of computer graphics to the biomedical sciences has been to provide tools for reconstructing 3D volumetric models of anatomical structures, typically from 2D cross-sections captured by Computed Tomography (CT), Magnetic Resonance Imaging (MRI) or Single-Photon Emission Computed Tomography (SPECT) scanners. Computer applications are required to offer increasingly-advanced visualisation and manipulation techniques for realistic, intuitive and interactive displays of the reconstructed 3D volumetric models in order to decrease patient care cost and facilitate medical training. With the use of computer graphics spreading rapidly in medical environments, the emerging need is to organise systematically both 2D information and 3D models and to make them globally available on-line to the largest possible community of medical professionals and students.

Currently, the majority of medical visualisation computer systems are either localised and/or stand-alone, for example in the environment of a particular hospital. Frequently,

---

* The work described in this paper has been carried out under the project IAEVA (HC1025HC) funded by the Fourth Framework Programme of the European Commission.

they are based on static CD-ROMs containing 2D cross-sectional images of 3D volumetric models and are expensive and difficult to expand (often only possible by purchasing additional CD-ROMs). Many medical visualisation systems have the additional disadvantage of running only on high-cost computer platforms.

On the other hand, WWW servers are easily expandable and merely require low-cost connection hardware and software. However, medical visualisation systems currently found on the WWW often contain rather unorganised 2D radiological images and offer extremely impractical response times for downloading, thus making interaction difficult, or even impossible.

The aim of the project is to construct an intuitively-organised WWW reference library of 3D volumetric models of pathological human organs and to provide efficient mechanisms for their retrieval and interactive manipulation. The paper describes the integrated methodology employed for these purposes. An extensive survey was undertaken regarding the needs of prospective users to identify relevant preferences and trends; this is outlined in Section 2. Using the survey results and the currently-available technologies as a basis, the individual components of the computer system were designed and implemented, as described in Section 3. Section 4 discusses the operating scenario of the system from the user's point of view. Finally, Section 5 identifies possible extensions and future directions.

2. User Requirement Survey

This section will describe the preferences identified by the collection of requirements from the prospective users of our system - medical students and medical professionals (including general practitioners). The questionnaires concentrated particularly on the database (the nature and structure of the data to be included, search procedures, etc), the image synthesis (3D reconstruction techniques) and the expected functionality of the system (interface, interactivity specifications). Because no comparable WWW system is currently available (except for a limited number of high-cost and highly-localised ones), the medical community has little knowledge of the performance, function choices and trade-offs applicable, so in most interviews, only qualitative and/or partial answers were obtained.

Analysis of the questionnaires identified great interest in a computer visualisation system that serves as an educational tool, for training/practice of medical students and for continuous updating of medical professionals. Interviewees expected to be able to compare 3D volumetric models of human organs in normal and pathological states. Orthopaedists expressed strong interest in "virtual tours" of human organs to support the planning of surgical intervention. Generally, students requested a simplified system incorporating some auto-guiding mechanisms, while professionals required flexibility, involving sophisticated search mechanisms. The majority of interviewees expected low-cost equipment, e.g. standard Windows95 PCs equipped with popular Internet browsers. Rapid response times for downloading the 3D models was identified as essential, especially since many people had already experienced slow downloading times when using the Internet. Finally, emphasis was expected to be given to the understanding of diseases through 3D computer-graphics models - annotations were expected to be brief and have supporting functionality.

3. System Components

Based on the general requirements outlined in Sections 1 and 2, a WWW computer-based system for organisation, transmission and manipulation of pathological human organs was developed. This consists of three main components (Fig. 1):

- a database containing 3D volumetric models of pathological human organs, and related textual information; a Solid Model Producer (*SMP*) to generate 3D volumetric models from CT, MRI or anatomical 2D cross-sectional images; a Resource Manager for the input of 3D volumetric models into the database;
- a Database Connectivity Module (*DCM*) to enable a WWW server to communicate with the database engine;
- a Solid Object Viewer (*SOV*) to visualise and manipulate (rotate, zoom in/out, dissect, etc.) the 3D volumetric models in the database.

The design principles of the system were :
- the system architecture is open (i.e. non-proprietary components);
- any existing standards in the fields of computer graphics and database technologies are followed scrupulously;
- the system software should allow room for expansion (object-oriented technology is mostly employed) and not be built around any particular Relational Database Management System (RDBMS).

The database is relational and distributed on the WWW, that is it resides on multiple WWW servers which are not, necessarily, physically located at the same Internet site.

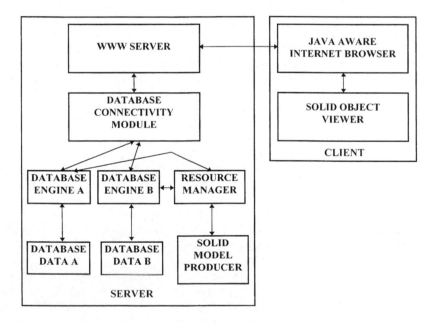

Figure 1. *Component configuration of the system for the organisation, transmission and manipulation of 3D volumetric models of pathological human organs on the WWW.*

Previous work on international standards was carefully examined (ICD-IX or ICD-X for pathological classification, SNOMED for topological classification, MESH for medical concepts, UMLS) to decide upon the retrieval procedure within the system. It was considered that the requirements of our system do not justify as wide an approach as that implemented by UMLS, and that SNOMED currently meets most of our needs as it includes a classification of topography, as well as disease and diagnosis. The inclusion of veterinary terms may be considered as a future addition to the system (it may be of interest, in the future, also to have 3D reconstructions of animal organs in our database).

The Solid Model Producer (SMP) generates 3D volumetric models of human organs from 2D cross-sectional images; it is implemented as C++ classes on top of the freeware libraries of the Visualisation Toolkit (VTK) [1], and employs OpenGL [2]. Early test data demonstrate encouraging results, and the main effort has been concentrated on speeding up rendering operations. Once the raw data collected, the 3D models produced by the SMP, and associated structure data are entered into the database using the Resource Manager.

The main functions of the Database Connectivity Module (DCM) are as follows : to receive data entry requests from the user; to translate these into SQL format: to pass them to the RDBMS; and, finally, to move the results back and present them to the user.

The Solid Object Viewer (SOV) is an independent component which can read a 3D volumetric model (from a file) of a human organ and render it. The SOV can co-operate with Mosaic/Netscape to enable prospective users, not only to view, but also interactively to manipulate, 3D volumetric models of human organs. The SOV provides a two-fold functionality that VRML viewers, in general, cannot offer : firstly, it provides special support for 3D models of human organs; secondly, it supports the interactivity which is necessary for our system. The SOV is also based on the VTK, and the main effort has again fallen on accelerating rendering operations and shrinking file sizes using some recent mathematical techniques based on wavelets [3] and polygon reduction [4].

4. Operating Scenario

The operating scenario for our system is described in this section. Once users connect to one of the WWW servers of our database, they are provided with two alternatives : for inexperienced users, the system provides automatic presentation of the WWW server contents, while more experienced users can use a free-text searching tool. Users may search directly into the database by employing search forms on various attributes of the organ and pathology; typing a word, or a set of words, connected with AND/OR operators, results in a database search to find all the codes containing these words. The resulting code list is then matched to the image database to retrieve all of the descriptors which appear in the database; users are able to choose which descriptors they wish to visualise. A navigation tool for moving in the topological tree of SNOMED is also provided.

Now, the user can elect to view a particular 3D volumetric model. The WWW server interrogates the database and retrieves the URL of the filename of the 3D volumetric model; this action initialises the operation of the SOV.

The SOV reads the file, processes the data, prepares it, and renders the image to the computer screen. Early results demonstrate that response times are between 30 seconds and 1 minute. The SOV performs incremental rendering, that is, the user is rapidly provided with a relatively crude image, and thus given a feeling that something is happening, and the image is continuously refined as the server transmits more detail and the user remains connected. This approach also enables the user to determine, at an early stage, whether the correct model has been retrieved and whether the viewing parameters are as desired.

The user can send requests for interactive manipulation (rotation, zooming in/out, extraction of orthogonal planes corresponding to axial, sagittal and coronal cross-sections, etc.) at any stage, and the viewing process is then repeated.

5. Further Development

The service is at a very early stage of development, and there are many possibilities for improvement in terms both of the available data and of the technological infrastructure.

Existing sites will continue to add more data (both 2D slices and 3D models), and the partners are interested in finding new sites to support the database.

In terms of software development, it is intended to support the reconstruction of 3D volumetric models from multi-modal imaging sources (bone structures are described better by CT, while soft tissues properties are better represented by MRI), the introduction of stereo viewing and the regular enhancement of the viewing system by the inclusion of state-of-the-art graphical procedures.

There is also much work to be done in the file design and modelling procedures for storing 3D models of human organs to produce further data compression and thus improve data transmission speeds.

Finally, the partners are interested in broadening the applicability of the system : firstly, as an advanced teaching tool by encompassing medical techniques, in addition to the physical and functional structures of the various organs, for example colonoscopy, arthroscopy etc.; secondly, as an intelligent tutoring system to give prospective users of the system educational support, structured tuition, etc.

6. Conclusions

The paper has described an integrated methodology for development of a computer-based system for the organisation, retrieval and manipulation of pathological human organs, based on the WWW. The primary purpose of the system is educational, but it can also be used as a virtual reference library to provide cost-effective solutions for medical care, with a focus on updating of particular pathological cases. The associated database is dynamic and can be easily updated with, for example, data from newly-discovered pathologies.

Prospective users are provided with a WWW viewer (a plug-in for popular WWW browsers) for manipulation (rotation, zooming, dissection) of 3D volumetric models of human pathologies. The system supports low-cost MS-Windows 32 platforms and requires no specialised hardware, thereby allowing accessibility to the widest possible audience. Early results suggest that response times for retrieval and manipulation are near real-time, not only over high speed expensive network lines, but also over low/medium network connections. This capability is provided by the incremental transmission of compressed data from a WWW server to the user's WWW viewer, involving a newly-developed flexible/incremental and low-volume file format for 3D models.

As far as we are in a position to know, no comparable computer systems for PC-based 3D synthetic-image illustration currently exist. To illustrate the benefits of such a system, in Histology the physiological histological structure of the organs has normally been taught to students in medical schools by the use of photonic microscopes, requiring the continuous presence of a specialised doctor who is able to use the microscope and provide all necessary explanations. Translation of the histological pictures from the microscope into 3D structures on the computer screen will mark a new era in medical education.

References

[1] W. Schroeder *et al.*, The Visualisation Toolkit: An Object-Oriented Approach to 3D Graphics, Prentice Hall, 1996.

[2] T. Reynolds and K. Danielson, Programming with OpenGL: An Introduction, SIGGRAPH '96 Course Notes, 1996.

[3] E. Stollnitz *et al.*, Wavelets for Computer Graphics: Theory and Applications, Morgan Kaufmann, 1996.

[4] H. Hoppe, Progressive Meshes, SIGGRAPH '96 Proceedings, 1996, pp. 99 - 108.

Medical Informatics Europe '97
C. Pappas et al. (Eds.)
IOS Press, 1997

Supercomputing in Cancer Research

Kurt BÖHM

DKFZ, Im Neuenheimer Feld 280, 69120 Heidelberg, Germany

Abstract: *Human Genome Analysis and Image Processing are part of the 'Grand Challenges' in High Performance Computing. The traditional mainframe has become insufficient for these applications in Biocomputing. Scalable parallel processor systems have entered the marketplace with superior price/performance. The evaluation process of such a system by an application-oriented benchmark test suite is described. Meanwhile a large system is integrated in the client/server structure of the Deutsches Krebsforschungszentrum where the traditional mainframe is completely replaced by scalable systems.*

1. Grand Challenges

In the USA 'High Performance Computing and Communication' became a Research and Development program monitored by the US Office of Science and Technology Policy. The total expenditure for the program were $ 650 million in 1992, $ 800 million in 1993 and $ 1100 million in 1994. The aim of this tremendous effort was to lay the basis for the solution of fundamental scientific problems. Problems which only can be solved by the use of computing power, clearly surpassing the performance of today's multi vector processors by orders of magnitude. These problems therefore are called 'Grand Challenges'.

They comprise, e.g., the prognosis of global changes in climate, long term weather forecast, fluid dynamics and turbulences and they require extraordinary capacities for simulation. The demand for performance is measured in Gflops (= billions of floating point operations per second). In the field of applications in biocomputing there are to be mentioned at the same level of complexity:

- Molecular Modeling/Drug Design
- Bio Informatics
- Quantum Chemistry
- Image Processing
- Polymer Physics

These applications are building blocks of the Human Genome Analysis Program in which the Deutsches Krebsforschungszentrum (DKFZ) is highly involved. The result is an imperative demand for High Performance Computing capabilities that exceeds the computing power available at present by far.

2. High Performance Computing Applications in the DKFZ

The Deutsches Krebsforschungszentrum in Heidelberg is one of the 16 big national research institutions in Germany that are organized in the 'Helmholtz Gesellschaft der Forschungseinrichtungen' (HGF). Our main topic of work is basic research on cancer. Today, the priorities of interdisciplinary research in the DKFZ are:

- Etiology of Cancer and Cell Differentiation
- Risk Factors for Cancer and Cancer Prevention
- Diagnostics and Experimental Therapy
- Virology and Immunology of Tumors.

In this framework the IT department is established as one of the central divisions that report directly to the Chairman of the Board. With 25 persons and an annual budget of six million DM all disciplines are supported with computing power, file and network services, consulting and education in applied informatics.

Following the special focus of the cancer research program on molecular biology and genetics, the applications of biocomputing have become most important. Since ten years self-developed programs are in use to analyse the structure of human genes and proteins. The results are stored in different databases of DNA and protein sequences and exchanged regularly in an international cooperation. Thus DKFZ is part of the world-wide 'Human Genome Analysis Program' which is declared by US government as one of the 'Grand Challenges'.

In this program the DKFZ serves as the German node in the European network for Molecular Biology (EMBnet) as a nation-wide offer for about 3000 scientists. EMBnet consits of about a dozen of national biocomputing centres, collaborating in data and software exchange and communication within Europe. With all these activities in biocomputing, most of the computing power is spent on applications for Genome Sequence Analysis and their data bases as well as for commercial chemical application software packages, e. g., to create computer models of DNA molecules or to simulate the effects of cancer drugs.

With this type of applications the traditional mainframe (IBM) and even additional vector processor systems (Convex) were permanently overloaded. Reasonable help was to be expected with the new generation of scalable parallel processor systems that entered the marketplace in 1994.

Another important and more spectacular type of applications in the Deutsches Krebsforschungszentrum is image processing in diagnostics and therapy. Imaging techniques make it possible to detect tumors and metastases that are larger than one or two centimeters. Due to physical and biophysical limitations, however, it cannot be expected to enhance the resolution in the near future. Today the evalution of the tumor size, its structure, and its functional performance is improved by advanced radiological methods. For example Magnetic Resonance Tomography (MRT) is used to scan a specified portion of the body slice - by - slice; the slice images can then be evaluated by the physician.

Parallel to and supplementing MRT, the tumor tissue is also examined with Positron Emission Tomography (PET). PET renders slice images of the distribution of radiolabeled organic substances within the body. Both methods enable the physician to measure, e.g., the effect of cancer drugs in the tumor.

However, if the physician wants to interpret these image series, he has to mentally reconstruct a three-dimensional image from the sequence of individual sections. Only a well trained radiologist is capable of gaining a more or less clear picture of the scene. Therefore three-dimensional reconstruction and visualization simulated by the computer is helpful for the planning of surgical operations and radiotherapy [4].

For example, in stereotactic irradiation of a brain tumor, the patient's head is fixed and the tumor is irradiated from various directions with highly collimated photon beams. To concentrate the dose within the tumor and spare the healthy tissue in the neigbourhood, the precise detection of tumor localisation is important. This is the field of image processing and 3D reconstruction. Supported by more powerful parallel RISC processor systems, there is a chance to come to nearly real time processing with these applications, that require High Performance Computing capabilities.

3. Structure of Computing Facilities

With the introduction of the client/server model, the traditional focus on one single mainframe disappeared, and was replaced by a hierachy of three levels of computing supply [2].

On the first level, spezialized (vector) computers are used as servers for computational intensive applications; applications as mentioned before, that surpass the performance and storage capacity of any single workstation by one order at minimum. Other computers are dedicated as file or communication servers to support network file systems (NFS), centralized backup and data archiving.

On the second level of hierarchy there are about 200 RISC workstations running UNIX for application development, hardware control of medical devices (i.e. computer tomographs) and image processing. They are mostly clustered in departmental networks and connected to the first level servers by an FDDI-based LAN.

The third level consists of the whole bunch of about 1000 desktop computers at the individual working places with a wide range of use, e.g., control of devices, word processing and graphics. They are part of a PC Network (Novell) and have access to the upper computer levels via Ethernet.

This hierachy of computing supply had to be upgraded on the first level by a system that should allow high performance computing. For the reasons of price/performance it was obvious to concentrate on the new parallel processor systems. In the following, the evaluation process of the system will be illustrated by some application programs, forming the benchmark test suite.

4. Evaluation Process for a Parallel Processor System

In *Molecular Modeling*, research activities include as main projects [6]:

- Combined use of modeling and NMR data for the elucidation of the 3D structure and conformation properties of molecules.
- Understanding chemical and biological effects at the molecular level.
- Computer-aided drug design.

Modeling of the molecular structure of drugs, receptors and their complexes using computer simulation has become a popular method in the field of drug design. This approach aims at the elucidation of structure - function relationships at an atomic level. It serves as a guidance for the design of new molecules with specific pharmacological activity, e.g., different speeds of resorption into the blood for varieties of Insulin.

Relevant commerical software packages for these applications are the molecular dynamics programs DISCOVER and AMBER as well as the semiempirical quantum chemical program MOPAC and some molecular mechanics programs. In molecular simulations the computation time depends first on the number of timesteps simulated and second on the square of the number of atoms in a molecule. Due to the classical approximation, the number of timesteps must be one order less than the typical oszillation time of the atom (about 10^{-15} seconds). Since relevant periods for the simulation last in the order of seconds, one gets an impression of the computation power principly needed, but is not available with today's methods.

For the benchmark test DISCOVER package was selected with two very different examples: one molecule consisting of more than 5000 atoms (but only 500 timesteps) and another one with only 150 atoms (but 10 000 timesteps). Parallelizing in MD programs means that the calculations on a certain part of the molecule are dedicated to one of the processors available. So the efficiency of parallelism depends more on the size and geometry of the problem than on the architecture of the computer system. Best results of elapsed time were found on the 8-processor versions of SGI's shared memory 'Power Challenge' and IBM's distributed memory 'SP2' system. On 16 processors the efficiency of parallelism became rather poor, already.

In *Quantum Chemistry*, research activities are directed to the electronic properties of molecules, their interactions and reactions, equivalent to the principles of theoretical physics, especially Quantum Mechanics [5]. The mathematical models of Quantum Chemistry describe the electron wave function of molecules (Schrödinger equation) and become extremely complex. For ab-initio - methods the computation time increases by the power of five with the number of electrons.

Depending on the size of molecules, in the Deutsches Krebsforschungszentrum different methods are in use:

- For small molecules (with 15 to 20 first row atoms) ab-initio - methods of high quality (post-SCF methods) will be used as implemented, e.g., in GAUSSIAN and GAMESS software packages.

- For medium size molecules (containing 20 to 50 first row atoms) different versions of density functional theory will be applied.

- For large molecules (50 to 100 first row atoms) semiempirical quantum mechanical procedures will be utilized as implemented, e.g., in the MOPAC package.

- For very large molecules the electron wave function cannot be calculated at all, today.

The benchmark test suite also comprised three application sets of GAUSSIAN as well as GAMESS. The rather poor performance of the parallelized version of GAUSSIAN on the SGI and the existance of only a single-processor version of GAUSSIAN on the IBM SP2 was disappointing. So alternatively throughput rates were measured for this application that detected an advantage for the SP2 configuration because of its powerful single processors.

For GAMESS the efficiency of parallelism turned out to be even better than those of DISCOVER software; it showed more than 80% on all tested 8-processor configurations and even 70% on IBM's 16-processor system.

Extremely high computational power and storage capacity is also required for other relevant applications in DKFZ:

- The numerical simulation of the dynamics of polymers, e.g., DNA-protein, growing with the length of molecule chains to thousands of CPU hours.

- The analysis of the complete sequence of the three billion nucleotides in DNA of the human genome and its storage in different data bases for on-line access in world-wide computer networks.

- The 3D realtime reconstruction of slice images produced by different types of tomographs [3].

For these key applications, described above in more detail, special software packages were developed. Different application sets composed by their programmers supplemented the benchmark test suite.

Though these codes are hardly parallelized yet, they are representative for the present demand for High Performance Computing. Their results also confirmed the leading performance of the 'Power 2' processor in IBM's SP2 system (see also [1]).

5. Scalable Systems

As a starting configuration an IBM SP2 with 14 processors, 2 GB memory and 20 GB disk storage was installed in 1994. The users are content with this decision which in the described field of applications gives the best value in price/performance for a compute server. This layed the ground for an expansion by another 10 processors, 3 GB memory and 52 GB disk storage in 1995.

Looking back on the evalution process, we were lucky to exclude several candidates rather early, who catch the eye today by bad news, e.g. KSR, TM, DEC. The systems finally selected and tested in detail: SPP (HP-Convex), Power Challenge (SGI), SP2 (IBM) have properties that make them superior to any mainframe, especially in High Performance Computing.

These criteria are:

- High Performance
- Simple Maintenance
- Low Cost of Ownership

- Broad Spectrum of Application Software
- Open Connectivity
- True Scalability

where the last point 'scalability' is one of the most important.

During the era of mainframes, the term 'modularity' was used to describe the ability to upgrade a system in principle. In practise it meant an investment of DM 500 000 to add one processor or of DM 100 000 to add a pair of disks.

What a decisive change of that situation comes with the new scalable systems. By use of standard components - taken out of the shelve from mass production - it now only requires an investment of DM 50 000 for an additional high performance processor or DM 1 000 for an additional disk drive. This demonstrates the extreme reduction of the cost of hardware by a factor of 10 in minimum. And even more astonishing, each of the new components offers a multiple of the performance or capacity compared to the mainframe equipment! Here another factor of 10 can be calculated so that in total the price/performance relation of scalable systems has changed since legacy systems by a factor of hundred. This is the real 'secret' behind the success of scalable systems.

For the Deutsches Krebsforschungszentrum, the reinvestment of the former expenditures for the traditional mainframe equipment into new scalable systems creates an enormous gain both in computational power and efficiency of storage. This strategy led the poor starting configuration of 1994 to a computing facility ready to contribute a respectable share to the 'Grand Challenges'.

With the expansion in 1996 the SP2 today consists of 78 processors (20.7 GFLOPS peak performance) with 12.5 GB memory and 320 GB disk storage.

In this configuration the parallel processor system IBM SP2 of the DKFZ belongs to the group of the most powerful supercomputers in Europa and is comparable to the SP2 systems in the National Institute of Health (NIH) in USA or the cancer research center of Japan.

6. References

[1] Bachler, G. et al.: Benchmarking the parallel FIRE code
     on IBM SP1-2 Scalable Parallel Platforms.
     In: High Performance Computing and Networking.
     Eds.: B. Hertzberger, G. Serazzi, pp. 640-645
     [Springer, Berlin, Heidelberg, 1995].

[2] Böhm, K.: High Performance Computing for one of the Grand Challenges.
     In: High Performance Computing and Networking.
     Eds.: B. Hertzberger, G. Serazzi, pp. 496-501
     [Springer, Berlin, Heidelberg, 1995].

[3] Meinzer, H.-P. et al.: Raytracing of medical 3D tomographies.
     In: New Frontiers of Biomedical Engineering, 5.
     Eds.: J.H. Nagel et al., pp. 41-42.
     [IEEE, Orlando, 1991].

[4] Schlegel, W. et al.: Computer systems and mechanical tools for
     stereotactically guided conformation therapy with linear accelerators.
     Int. Journal of Radiation Oncology, Biology and Physics 24 [1992], 781-787.

[5] Suhai, S.: Structural and electronic properties of infinite cis and trans
     polyenes: Perturbation theory of electron correlation effects.
     International Journal of Quantum Chemistry 42 [1992], 193-216.

[6] von der Lieth, C.-W.: Spectroscopic Information and Molecular Modeling.
     Chemometrics and Intelligent Laboratory System 8, [1990], 53-58.

Medical Informatics Europe '97
C. Pappas et al. (Eds.)
IOS Press, 1997

BEAM@Net: Telematic Services for Clinical Engineers and Medical Physicists

Cees Zeelenberg[1]., Zoi Kolitsi[2]., Vassilios Kapsalis[2]., Chris Van Nimwegen[1].,
Nicolas Pallikarakis[2]

[1]*TNO, Prevention and Health, Leiden, The Netherlands*
[2]*INBIT, Institute of Biomedical Technology, Patras, Greece*

1. Introduction

BEAM II is a follow up to BEAM/AIM Project which has addressed issues related to the Biomedical Technology sector and has demonstrated its contribution to the domain by introducing front-end telematic technology to the service of professionals that share involvement in the distribution, use and follow - up of medical devices. The main objectives of BEAM II are: a) to extend the existing application by creating, validating, installing and commissioning BEAM services over Europe's Information Highway, b) to upgrade, populate and widely evaluate the BEAM tools, in preparation for commercial development. A significant impact in the field is anticipated. From providing the platform for the new approach to the management of biomedical technology, based on standardization and compliance with the EU directives and standards, but also on communication, sharing and exchange of knowledge, ideas and information, towards achievement of common goals within the European Union. The BEAM@Net is a an integrated information network with user and device related information. The purpose of BEAM@Net is to support professionals in the field of Clinical Engineering and Medical Physics by providing them with a facility for exchange of information and access to a collection of data and news on a variety of issues of interest. As such, once it has undergone a substantial level of population. it will comprise a valuable tool for interaction, as well as collection and dissemination of information to professionals. For this reason, the relevant associations have expressed a strong interest in assuming the responsibility of maintaining and running the services after the life time of the project.

2. Description of the system

For the user, BEAM@*Net* is conceived as a WWW site comprising a road map and four information sectors, depicted schematically in Fig.1. The sectors are differentiated by both type of information and access policy to the information. These actions are also under the responsibility of different structures, with regard to the quality and the integrity of the information they contain. The purpose of BEAM@*Net* is to support professionals in the fields of Clinical Engineering and Medical Physics by providing them with a facility for exchange of information and access to a collection of data and news on a variety of issues of interest and additionally to obtain specific information of medical devices on the

European market. Two professional associations, IFMBE and EFOMP, have already confirmed their involvement in taking the responsibility of using the communication services for their members.

For the user, BEAM@*Net* will be conceived as a WWW site with 4 sections of information, depicted schematically below. These sections are differentiated by the type of information dealt with, and the access policy to this information. These actions are also under the responsibility of different structures, with regard to the quality and the integrity of the information they contain.

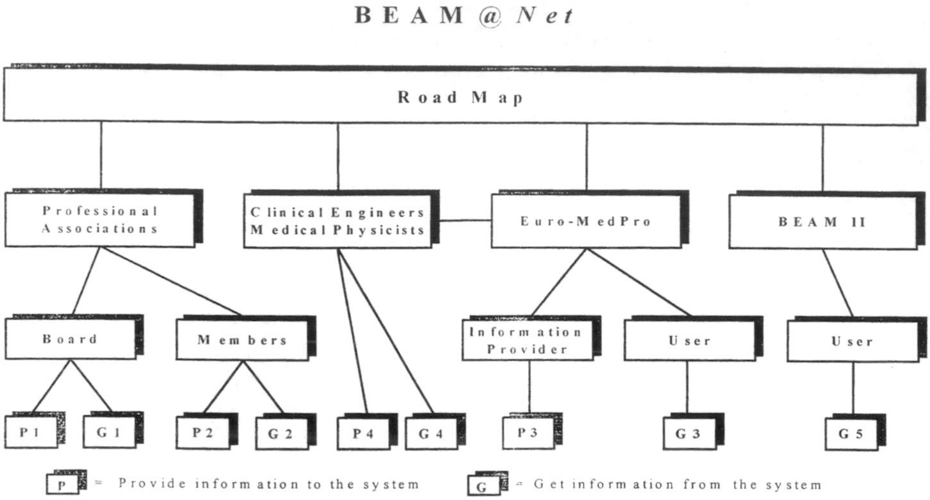

B E A M @ *N e t*

Figure 1: Structure layout for BEAM@Net services

The basic BEAM network services will be offered to users on all hardware and software platforms, capable of supporting a suitable World Wide Web browser. Such browsers are now available on a wide range of hardware/operating system platforms. At a later stage, additional facilities maybe offered to those with advanced browsers, but this will depend on feed back from users during early stages of evaluation.

2.1 Road Map

The first section will be of public access and will include a road map to the BEAM services, project information, with demos of the BEAM tools and services, information on the professional societies hosted under BEAM@*Net*, announcements for conferences, events, etc.

2.2 IFMBE/CED & EFOMP

A second section will be made available to the professional associations for the exchange of information with their members and the committees. Two such associations will be hosted during the course of the project; however, the facility is of a generic nature, such that any other society could also use it later on, apart from the IFMBE/CED and the EFOMP. These services will cater as close as possible to the specific needs of the associations for communication with their members, dissemination of information, as well as collection - and possibly pre-processing - of information before making it available to their members.

The services will also include tools for facilitating the production, presentation and distribution of the associations newsletters and journals, in an electronic form. The associations will have the ultimate responsibility for the quality and the validity of the information residing in this part and they will employ the necessary mechanisms for the maintenance of this information. Access to this part of the BEAM services will be granted to the members of the professional societies, respectively.

According to the functions performed at the FINE Database, three different types of users can be identified, each accessing the Database with a different intent. Table 1 summarizes the FINE functions available to each type of user.

Table 1: FINE functions per user type

USERS	FUNCTIONS
1. Member	1.1 Gets and provides information
	1.2 Has access to Official Information
	1.3 Participates in Discussion Groups
	1.4 Submit articles
2. EFOMP	2.1 Creates Official Reports
	2.2 Creates Directories & Listings
	2.3 Creates SIGs & Discussion Groups
	2.4 Creates E-Magazine & Newsletters issues
	2.5 Registration of users
	2.6 Send messages
3. FDB Administrator	3.1 System Administration
	3.2 FDB Logger
	3.3 FDB Statistics

Members of the associations are able to get and provide information by inserting and retrieving *User Reports* and *Announcements,* retrieving *Official Reports*, participating in *Discussion Groups,* submitting articles for the *E-Magazine* and receiving the issues as soon as they are available.

The associations (e.g. EFOMP) compile and handle information (insertion, modification, deletion) in the form of *Official Reports,* create *Directories & Listings,* create the *E-Magazine* and transmit messages to their members. EFOMP is responsible for the creation (and the update) of *SIGs* and the assignment of each user to one or more *SIGs* (and consequently to the corresponding *Discussion Groups*) during the registration phase. The creation of the *E-Magazine* is under the responsibility of an editorial board, which selects the articles to be published (from the articles submitted by the members), reviews them and creates new issues that are available to be downloaded by the subscribers.

The FDB Administrator is responsible for the overall system management in order to keep the system operational, monitors the Database traffic and logs information about all users' activity.

On the basis of the above task analysis we can identify three major categories of information contained in the Database, i.e. user information (Member's corner), official information (EFOMP post) and information related to the operation of the System (FDB Administrator).

3. Euro-MedPro

The third sector concers medical devices related data and information. Euro-MedPro is a database mainly covering medical equipment, which is intended to support clinical engineers, medical physicists and others involved in medical instrumentation with information on (i) the local market concerning medical devices belonging to 65 device groups: makes and models, suppliers, characteristics and features; (ii) quality aspects of medical devices in the form of single test reports and comparative test reports; (iii) incidents and accidents with medical devices in the form of published hazard reports and (iv) standards concerning medical devices.

All data are related to the Universal Medical Device Nomenclature System (UMDNS) published by ECRI in the USA. This nomenclature will be a provisional standard in Europe during the period that CEN/TC 257 will develop a standard for a European nomenclature. To be able to consult the database through the Internet, a user interface will be designed using the HTML forms mode. The Figures 2 and 3 show examples of two forms presenting data from the database.

For each device stored in the database (make and model), a survey can be obtained of data and information related to that device. Depending on the availability of details, information items like 'Alerts', 'Tests' etc. will be underlined. The underlined information items will be linked to surveys with more detailed information.

Fig. 2 shows an example of a 'market survey', a table presenting a number of characteristics and/or features of (in this case) defibrillators offered to the market. The relevant makes and models are displayed vertically and the characteristics and features belonging to the device group under consideration horizontally. The symbol '4' in the table points to standard features, while the symbol '+' means that a feature is available as an option. Clicking on 'Info' in the left hand column leads to a Fig.2 like survey of device related data and information. It is possible to store in the database device related data from the markets of various countries and to restrict data presented to devices available on a country's local market. Through a language option it will be possible to consult Euro-MedPro using various languages.

During the course of the project, the BEAM II consortium will assume the responsibility for the quality and the validity of the information residing in this part and will establish the necessary self-sustainable mechanisms for the maintenance of this information, after the end of the project. Access to this part of the BEAM services will be granted to the subscribing members only.

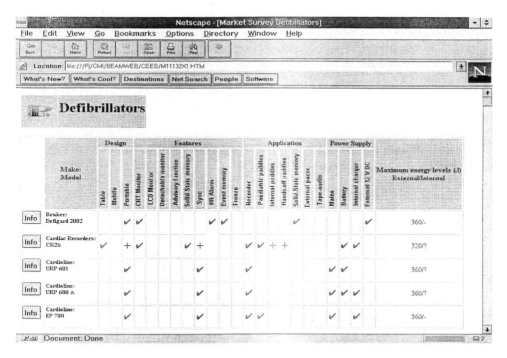

Figure 3: Example of a market survey table with characteristics and features of defibrillators

4. BEAM II

This section will be devoted to the BEAM II project. It will contain details of the partners, the projects, workpackages, services. It will serve both as a shop window for BEAM services and as an information resource. This section will be publicly accessible although it may lead to a limited-access section for the partners to share information.

References

[1] J. Boter and Chr. Van Nimwegen; Report on the Development of a Medical Devices Database and on the Inclusion of Other Databases; Deliverable #4 [WP01:DBs], AIM Project Number A2001 (BEAM), 30-06.92.
[2] J. Boter, Chr. Van Nimwegen and W. Cavens; Intermediate Report on the Status of the Medical Devices Database; Deliverable #19 [WP01:DBs], AIM Project Number A2001 (BEAM), 30.09.93.
[3] N. Pallikarakis, Z. Kolitsi, C. Zeelenberg and Chr. Van Nimwegen; BEAM demonstrator 1995 on CD-ROM; ISBN 90-5412-030-4, 1995.
[4] Eric Tilton; Composing Good HTML (Version 2.0.8); http://www.cs.cmu.edu/~tilt/cgh/, 1996
[5] Tim Berners-Lee; Style Guide for online hypertext; http://www.w3.org/pub/WWW/Provider/Style/All.html, 1995
[6] Gareth Reese; Style guide; http://www.cl.cam.ac.uk/users/gdr11/style-guide.html, 1996
[7] Rick Levine; Guide to Web Style; http://www.sun.com/styleguide/tables/Printing_Version.html, 1995

UN/EDIFACT based Medical Documentation and Messages

Dimitar TCHARAKTCHIEV[1], Borislav GEORGIEV[2], Petar TZONOV[3], Anton DIMITROV[4], George DIMOV[5], Vladimir KIROV[4], Alexander SHINKOV[1]
[1]University Hospital of Endocrinology and Gerontology, 6 Damian Gruev str., 1303 Sofia, Bulgaria; [2]BULPRO-BCCI, Ministry of Trade and Foreign Economic Cooperation, 12 A Batenberg str., 1000 Sofia; [3]National Center of Medical Information, 15 Dim. Nesterov str., Sofia; [4]Macrosoft Ltd 24 Kamen Andreev str., 1606 Sofia, [5]ACSIOR Ltd, 8-B Hristo Georgiev str., 1504 Sofia

Abstract. New documentation and messages conforming to the rules of EDIFACT are created and an attempt is made to follow internationally standardised and wordwide available commercial experience. A set of medical documents, aligned with United Nations Layout Key for trade documents is designed. The approach is to develop a set of paper documents and to standardise the data which are filled in these documents. There is a possibility to fill the data directly in medical documents and to print them from the Clinical Information System in our University Hospital.

1. Introduction

The implementation of the Clinical information system "Medica" in our University Hospital nine years ago was confronted with the inability of standard printers to print on the medical documentation used in the clinics (1). For this reason we started the development of a set of medical documents for clinical practice, that could be filled either manually, by typewriter or computer printers. We implemented the methods for simplification of the process of production and use of documents (2). The quality of clinical documentation was improved.

The other problem posed initially was to prepare the grounds for the exchange of the messages between our institution and the externals pharmacies, specialised centres and non-medical institutions.

2. Material and Methods

All documents (paper based information forms) are designed on the basis of the standard-form of ISO 6422 for trade documents. We use the set in accordance to ISO 3535 and the format in conformity with ISO 216 (3,4,5). This set of documents is related to the computer modules of our Clinical Information System, that can capture the data directly from the databases and fill in the forms.
The messages based on the information of paper forms can be generated

autmatically.The general rules and structure for the construction and implementation of electronic messages are based on UN/EDIFACT and European pre-standards of CEN/TC251 are respected (6,7,8.9).

3. Results and discussion

3.1. Description of the forms

All forms have 2 identical boxes of data allocated in the left and right upper parts of the paper sheet. All identical pieces of data are allocated in the same place in the different documents.

The information related to the hospital and the physician is filled in the left upper box In the right upper box of the forms, related with one patient are located the number and the date of the form, the names, sex, age and personal identification number of the patient.

On the first page of the form Case History (A4) after the first 2 boxes are placed 2 identical boxes with social-demographic data for the patient. The next two areas contain the important medical data and information related to the current hospitalisation. In the next field are filled all clinical diagnoses. In the following two areas are recorded the results of hospitalisation, after that the data concerning the ability of work and the recommendations for continuation of the medical care in another hospital or as an outpatient are inserted. In the last two areas are filled the names and signature of the clinic's chief and the physician in charge. The original form in Bulgarian is presented on figure 1.

The following samples are presented in English - Medical assignment, Medical certificate and partially the Case History and Discharge Letter (fig. 2).

A List of required medication, a Request for laboratory tests and a Request for image diagnostics are included in the set of documents too.

3.2. Implemented principles

The first implemented principle is the strong relation between clinical information system and the paper forms. At first stage all data is registered in the information system and after that printed on the forms with standard dot-matrix printers. We have used the concept of penless technology - the law in Bulgaria imposes imperatevely the availability of paper medical record. There are legal obstacles to apply the paperless technology.

The second concept is the implementation of standard forms. The new design of the forms has not changed the information content of the documents. Due to the legal reasons the data set included in the old forms must be included in the new forms as well. The new forms are universal - the new structure gives the opportunity to fill it manually, by a typewriter or all types of printers.

ИСТОРИЯ НА ЗАБОЛЯВАНЕТО

Здравно заведение ЕКПОУ	N° Дата	
Отделение Стая Легло Лекуващ лекар	Пациент Пол Възраст ЕГН	
Народност Гражданство Образование Сем. полож. Близки - име, адрес, тел.	Адрес Месторабота Тел. Професия	
Насочен от: Постъпил: час gama Причина за хоспитализация ☐ Лечение ☐ Изследване ☐ Социални индикации ☐ Експертиза ☐ Друго ☐ Прием по спешност Прием: ☐ Първично ☐ Последващо	**АЛЕРГИЧЕН КЪМ** Инфекции и вирусоносителство: Паразити: Санитарна обработка:	КРЪВНА ГРУПА Rh фактор
ДИАГНОЗА Изпращащото заведение Приемен кабинет Клинична: а) Предварителна б) Окончателна в) Усложнения г) Придружаващи заболявания		МКБ ⊔⊔⊔⊔⊔

Болният е:	Час	Дата	ИЗХОД ОТ ХОСПИТАЛИЗАЦИЯТА	
☐ Изписан ☐ Приведен ☐ ПОЧИНАЛ ☐ АУТОПСИРАН			☐ оздравял ☐ без промяна ☐ с подобрение ☐ с влошаване **ПРОЛЕЖАНИ ДНИ**	

ТРУДОСПОСОБНОСТ
☐ Възстановена
☐ Временно изгубена - отпуск
     ☐ до постъпването   дни
     ☐ при изписването   дни б. лист N°
☐ Изгубена трудоспособност
     ☐ частично   ☐ пълно
☐ Насочен към ТЕЛК
			НАСОЧЕН ЗА ЛЕЧЕНИЕ
			☐ Амбулаторно
			
			☐ Болнично
			
			☐ Санаториално
			
			☐ Друго	

Лекуващ лекар *Подпис*			*Зав. отделение* *Подпис*	

© /Проектm^{57}/ПЧ/БГ

Figure 1

CASE HISTORY

HEALTH CENTRE CODE (MEDICAL INSTITUTION)		N° DATE
WARD (CLINIC)	BED ROOM	PATIENT'S FIRSTNAME, SURNAME & FAMILYNAME
PHISICIAN IN CHARGE OF CASE		SEX AGE ID N°
MARITAL STATUS RELATIVES' ADDRESS		DISCHARGE LETTER

Health centre (Medical Institution) Code		ID N° (Case History N°) Date
Ward (Clinic)	Bed Room	Patient's Firstname, Surname & Familyname
Physician in Charge of Csae		Sex Age ID N°
Adressed to Code		Adress MEDICAL ASSIGNMENT

Medical Institution Code	N° Date
	Patient's Firstname, Surname & Familyname
	Sex Age ID N°
Adressed to Code	Adress
	Employed at Tel.
	Occupation

Request for	Diagnosis
☐ hospitalisation ☐ consultation ☐ medical examination (analisys, tests) ☐ health resort therapy	MEDICAL CERTIFICATE

Medical Institution Code	N° Date
	Patient's Firstname, Surname & Familyname
	Sex Age ID N°
Certificate Issue to Serve Before Code	Address
	Educational Institution Attended
Diagnosis in good health/ill Health status	Patient in need of Duration of sick-leave
Infections Diseases Sustained	
Contact with Infected Patients - Diagnosis YES NO Date	
Phisician Position	Date Signed Stamp

Figure 2

The third concept is that the new documentation is open for further development - electronic data interchange between the health centres connected in community, national and internationals networks.

The structure of forms and data give the possibility for future UN/EDIFACT implementation. For example the first developed healthcare message (Personal Identification) achieved global approval. The first implementation of the developed in Europe prescription message (MEDPRE) in US is going live in Wisconsin (10). In Denmark the quality of EDI-prescriptions has invariably been better than the quality of other forms of prescriptions (11).

We are aiming at UN/EDIFACT future implementation of the messages MEDPID (Patient Identification Details), MEDPRE (Medical Prescription), MEDREQ (Medical Service Request), MEDRPT (Medical Service Report), MEDRUC (Medical Resource Usage/cost), MEDADR (Adverse Drug Reaction message), MEDDIS (Discharge Summary message).

4. Conclusion

New documentation and messages conforming to the rules of EDIFACT are created and an attempt is made to follow the internationally standardised and wordwide available commercial experience. A set of medical documents, aligned with United Nations Layout Key for trade documents is designed. The approach is to develop a set of paper documents and to standardise the data which are filled in these documents.

References

[1] D. Tcharaktchiev, A. Dimitrov, G. Dimov, P. Tzonov, B. Bajkushev, Vl. Kirov, B. Georgiev, MEDICA - 9 years of Development and Use of a Clinical Information System in the University Hospital of Endocrinology and Gerontology - Sofia. In: J. Brender et al. (Eds.), Medical Informatics Europe '96, IOS Press, Amsterdam, 1996, pp. 458-462.
[2] P. Tsonov, Turnover of documents in medical practice. Social medicine, 2:30-33, 1994.
[3] Trade Data Elements Directory, UNITED 1990, United Nations, New York, 1990.
[4] La formule cadre des Nations Unies pour les documents commerciaux, United Nations publication F.81.11.E.19.
[5] B. Stoven, Actualite de la "Formule-cadre pour les documents commerciaux". Simprofrance, No 11:2-4,1992.
[6] Messages for Exchange of Laboratory Information, preENV, Project Team leader: Dr. Georges De Moor. CEN/TC 251/Medical Informatics/N94-068.
[7] Method for the Development of Healthcare Messages, CEN Report, Project Team leader: Mr. Dirk Segers. CEN/TC 251/Medical Informatics/N95-249.
[8] Message Specification Report Health Care Spell Message, NHS Executive, Birmingham, Reference IMG 5114, 1995.
[9] Message Implementation Guidelines, NHS Executive, Birmingham, Reference IMG 5115, 1995.
[10] B. Love, Status Report from Western European EDIFACT Board Message Decelopment Group 9. CEN/ TC 251/Medical Informatics/N95-127.
[11] S. Sorensen and S. Korsgaard, Test of EDI Prescriptions. In: J. Brender et al. (Eds.), Medical Informatics Europe '96, IOS Press, Amsterdam, 1996, pp.137-140.

Medical Informatics Europe '97
C. Pappas et al. (Eds.)
IOS Press, 1997

Intranet and HTML at a major university hospital
- experiences from Munich

M. Dugas
University of Munich, IBE, Marchioninistr. 15, 81377 Munich, Germany

Abstract. Intranet-technology is the application of Internet-Tools in local networks. With this technique electronic information systems for large hospitals can be realized very easily. This technology has been in routine use in 'Klinikum Großhadern' for more than one year on over 50 wards and more than 200 computers.

The following clinical application areas are described: drug information, nursing information, electronic literature retrieval systems, multimedia teaching und laboratory information systems.

1. Introduction

Availability of up-to-date information is a real challenge in a big hospital. Using paper-based communication, this goal cannot be achieved with a reasonable effort. The drug list of our local pharmacy for example contains more then 1000 drugs and is revised several times a year. The nurses need information about more than 200 diagnostic and therapeutic standard procedures; the department of clinical chemistry offers more than a thousand laboratory procedures. With an electronic information system on the wards the necessary information can be provided up-to-date. HTML-based systems are easy-to-use and efficient.

2. Technical background: Access to databases using Intranet-technology

Because the data (e.g. drug data) is complex and extensive, it is reasonable to use a database. Flexibility and ease-of-use is an important issue; for this reason an HTML-based system has been chosen. The information is stored in a relational database; the user sends his queries with a WWW-Browser (e.g. Netscape Navigator®, Internet Explorer®) to a WWW-Server (e.g. NCSA-/Apache-/Netscape-/Oracle-Webserver). The Server queries the database and sends the result back to the user.

By collecting the Log-File of the WWW-Server it is possible to evaluate which information is asked most frequently and from which computer. This is important to improve the quality of the service.

3. Drug information

The *local drug list* contains all drugs which are in regular use at our medical facul
It covers around 1000 different drugs, which are structured in groups of indicatic
using the ABDA-system. The list has generic and proprietary names, information
how to administer the drug, the price and a comment text.
This service is queried approximately 500 times a month, see [4].
The *Rote Liste®* [2] is the directory of all drugs which are manufactured
companies of the 'Bundesverbandes der Pharmazeutischen Industrie' (association
German pharmaceutical companies). It covers around 9000 drugs and conta
proprietary and generic name, indication, side effects, interactions, contraindicatio
dosage, administration and references.
The Rote Liste® is queried around 1500 times a month and the ratio of nurses
doctors is about 5:1.
Our pharmacy has around 70 self-produced articles. The information on how to t
these products is published in our intranet.

4. Nursing information

The nursing service at the Klinikum Großhadern employs about 1200 people a
trains around 60 - 70 new nurses each year. The nursing service has developped
extensive collection of information about medical procedures and hygien
(approximately 400 pages). This nursing information is divided into different sectic
such as endoscopy and radiology and contains an overview of the medi
procedures such as coloscopy and phlebography. Each sheet has three parts: 1)
administrative data (e.g. telephone number, schedule, required records etc.); 2)
necessary preparation of the patient (e.g. dosage of laxatives); 3) how to take care
the patient after the procedure (e.g. check for vital signs). The nursing informatio
provided with the 'Pflegeinformationsnetz' (network for nursing information). Th
are about 3200 requests to this system per month.

5. Electronic literature retrieval systems

The library of our university provides on a central server a collection of medi
databases (Medline®, Embase®, Current Contents®). These databases can
queried with a WWW-interface (Webspirs®). Using intranet-technology this exter
information source can be integrated very easily.
In addition there is a separate system for Medline with Knowledgefinder®.
Recently more medical books are published as CD-Rom, usually containing sing
user, platform-dependent programs. In a large hospital with many differ
computers, such solutions are useless and client-server technology is required.
this reason we cooperated with a medical publisher who provided two well-kno
books in raw data format; we successfully converted these books to HTML and t
are now on-line on our Intranet.

6. Multimedia teaching

By converting the existing teaching material for medical students to HTML (*online-script*), recent versions can be provided. E.g. a textbook of clinical chemistry has been converted to HTML. By this means our students can access this information from any computer within the medical faculty. The major advantage of this approach, in the context of teaching, is that for each topic there can be links to more detailed contents; the student can find the information fast and explore as deeply as needed.

By cooperation with Dartmouth Medical School and the Technical University of Munich (neurology) a set of *interactive learning programmes* has been developped (e.g. Parkinson's disease) using intranet-technology. Text, graphics, audio and video have been integrated. A carefully controlled study from Dartmouth Medical School showed that CBI (computer based instruction) can improve learning efficiency [5].

7. Laboratory information systems

The service of clinical chemistry of our faculty offers more than a thousand different analyses. For each parameter there is a reference value and a comment (how to interpret results, common errors etc.). With an electronic list for procedures in clinical chemistry it is possible to provide the most recent information on the wards.

8. Future directions and conclusions

Similar to the service for clinical chemistry, we want to provide relevant medical information for other departments on our intranet-server. Access to patient records using intranet-technology is under development in our hospital. The extensive use of our intranet-server indicates that there's a need for such information systems on the wards. Physicians and nurses must, however, be trained to use these services.

9. Summary

Five areas of HTML-applications using intranet-technology were presented, which are in routine use in our hospital: drug information; nursing information; electronic literature retrieval systems; multimedia teaching and laboratory information systems. For a more detailed description see [3].

The basic concept is an integration of commercial databases and local information. All applications are hardware-independent with the same user-interface and all use client-server-technology. By a central update it is ensured that everybody gets the most recent information.

As a result of these efforts synergy has developed, communications have improved and we are cutting costs. The training of the medical staff is supported which helps to improve the care of the patients.

10. References

[1] Jones, R.; Nye, A.: HTML und das WWW: Selbst publizieren im WWW. O'Re International Thomson Verlag 1995

[2] Bundesverband der Pharmazeutischen Industrie (eds.): Rote Liste 19 Aulendorf/Württ., Editio Cantor 1996

[3] Dugas, M.: HTML-Anwendungen im Intranet - Erfahrungen im Klinik Großhadern.
In: Koehler, C.O. (eds.): Medizinische Dokumentation und Informati Handbuch für Klinik und Praxis. Landsberg, ecomed-Verlag 1997

[4] Dugas, M.; Maag, K.: HTML-Anwendungen im Intranet am Beis Arzneimittelinformationssystem. In: Klein, H.-G; Seidel D. (eds.): Resea Festival '96. München, MMV Verlag 1996, 190

[5] Lyon, H.C.; Healy, J.C.; Bell J.R.; O'Donnell J.F.; Shultz E.K.; Moore-West Wigton R.S.; Hirai F.; Beck J.R.: Plananalyzer, an interactive Computer-Assis Program to Teach Clinical Problem Solving in Diagnosing Anemia and Coron Artery Disease. Acad-Med. 67/12, 1992, 821-828

Medical Informatics Europe '97
C. Pappas et al. (Eds.)
IOS Press, 1997

ORGANISING HEALTH SYSTEMS FOR BETTER CARE AND PERFORMANCE BY OPEN INFORMATION TECHNOLOGY

Albert van der Werff

The SOCRATES Network, Health & IT Consultants
Woubrugge, The Netherlands
Tel.: 00 31 172 518910, Fax: 00 31 172 519204, E–mail: avdwsocr@pi.net

Abstract.   In this document the application of open information technology to assist in reforming healthcare systems of countries is being discussed. Present technologies demonstrated by HANSA in Western and Eastern Europe enable the integration of electronic patient records in existing systems, provide for flexibility and support the interoperability of different applications. However, computers and IT must not drive the required process of change. This is the responsibility of top management.

Introduction

Health is by its very nature an intensive user of information. The application of advanced technologies to the collection, storage, retrieval and communication of this information will be one of the critical success factors for the health services in countries. Those responsible for the provision of healthcare understand that it is possible to improve the quality of patient care and the cost–benefit equation by the effective **introduction of information technology (IT), which will ultimately transform the traditional structure of healthcare provision.**

Reforming Healthcare

National health systems have come under strong and growing pressures to institute major structural reforms. While conditions vary in different countries, the source of these reform pressures is remarkably common across most nations. They are confronted by externally generated demands from: demography, technology and economy. National policy makers are in turn insisting that existing patterns of health services be modifiied to achieve higher levels of responsiveness, efficiency and effectiveness. In response to these demands, many countries have set out to develop a new health system framework, re–balancing the public–private mix. It is worth mentioning that countries are in a process of reform irrespective of their initial starting point: states with a tax–based national health service are moving towards market orientation and competition, whereas countries with a health insurance–based system are implementing more regulation and measures for cost containment. 1)

In this respect we will consider an information framework as a change agent. The process of developing an information framework should in itself be the unifying force that would draw the actors in healthcare into cooperative creation of an infrastructure designed to meet their needs on a continuing basis. Each actor has essential information to contribute, and each needs information from the others. Collectively their information would have even greater value. All actors should also understand that they own a very valuable resource, valuable not only to themselves and to healthcare, but also to other sectors (Karen A. Duncan). 2). Priorities of making transformation a reality are the integration of electronic patient records in existing systems and the realisation of open, modular healthcare information systems that offer flexibility.

Healthcare Information

Healthcare is becoming increasingly complex, requiring many different professionals, i.e. physicians, nurses and others to collaborate in the care of a single patient. They require access to a common set of information and support by knowledge–based tools. Patient care supporting (or clinical) hospital information systems should therefore be multi–disciplinary, enabling collaborative work with regard to patient care, and be equipped by a multi–purpose knowledge base. This will improve the quality, effectiveness and efficiency of patient care. IT can help to achieve these benefits.

Improving the Use of Healthcare Information and IT

Most hospitals now have computer systems, particularly for administration and finance, and considerable investments have been made. However, these investments have generally failed t benefit patient care. The data are often of poor quality because the clinical staff, who collect them, get little benefit from their use. Data must be collected in a form that is useful for physicians, nurses and other professionals, and checked before use. The introduction of the electronic patient record will help solving these problems. However, these new patient care supporting systems differ fundamentally from the traditional management support systems as they have to be comprehensive, covering all areas of patient care and hospital activity, be accurate and precise, be on line and in real time, and be shared only by authorised users. Moreover, data capture must be made as easy as possible. And, finally, information and knowledge increasingly need to be integrated with primary care and other services. Today ma systems are not linked, are out of date, are not flexible and difficult to use. Future healthcare information systems must therefore be developed within a wider, and long term strategy, and primarily be designed to improve the delivery of patient care. Procurement, design and development of systems need to be led by users. 3)

Integration Strategies

The introduction of the electronic patient record will shift present emphasis on the application of information technology for administrative purposes towards a more balanced situation in which data in the first place are used to support patient care, but also to monitor clinical and business performance. As hospitals, and in general health services as well as IT vendors, want to protect past investments, integration of electronic patient records in existing systems is of particular importance. Current practices can be grouped in three global strategies:

– Integration of electronic patient records into already 'existing' generally administration–oriented information systems;
– Building integrated 'patient record–based' information systems 'from the outset';
– Integration of patient record systems through the application of 'open' systems technology, based on European standards.

In the present situation the first approach is generally adopted. The standard offering is a transaction system (order entry and registration), a clinical repository equipped with interfacing tools to assist in populating the repository from disparate systems, and a graphical user interface to access the information. However, these systems remain administrative in basic design. A complete redefinition of the data would be required to automate satisfactorily the patient care process. Moreover, the critical applications as care planning and knowledge tools are usually missing. These problems can be avoided by integrated 'patient record–based' information systems that are designed that way 'from the outset'. Such systems are currently offered, but need considerable re–investments to enjoy all its benefits. The third strategy is to migrate present systems to a new environment through the application of 'open' system technology, based on European standards. This solution, which is also on the market, is avoiding re–investment and is specifically designed for integration of electronic patient records. Integration is therefore easier, and cheaper.

Open Healthcare Information Systems: Results available from RTD Development in the European Union

Started in 1987 a series of research and technology development projects have been undertaken in Europe on the basis of international collaboration of hospital and healthcare organisations, governmental and non–governmental IT agencies, health IT consultancies, IT industries and the CEU. The total activity is representing an investment value of USD 40 million of which up to 50% was co–funded by the Commission. Today (end of 1996) we can conclude that **'real' open healthcare information systems are a reality in Europe.** 4)

Present projects under the umbrella of HANSA (an acronym for Healthcare Advanced Networked System Architecture) are demonstrating and transferring the new technology both in the EU Member States (HANSA WEST) and in Central and Eastern Europe (HANSA EAST). Currently 60 organisations participate and demonstrations are provided in over 20 sites in 12 countries.

Open healthcare information systems will have to be built on a 'common unified base' or: 'reference architecture', conformant with the new European standard: CEN TC251/WG1/PT013/N95-285. The key feature of this architecture is its layered structure:

– Level of applications, serving the individual users (patient management, nursing or ward systems, medical care, medical support services, ancillary services systems);
– Level of the middleware of common services, enabling the functional procedural integration or interworking of the individual applications from different software vendors at the top layer;

– Level of the technological platform, responsibe for the transparent connection of
different hardware.

The applications and the middleware of common services provide the input to the patient recor
and general management systems as well as to public health statistics or indicator systems.

The middleware can be used, both for:

– integration of application software and/or migration of existing systems towards the
new, open environment, and
– development, respectively production of software for entirely new, open information system

The HANSA Consortium has decided to publish the middleware APIs, i.e. the interfaces that
connect the application software through the middleware of common services. This strategy is
enabling users to choose products from different vendors, to make the best use of existing
products, and to replace or to add application software in accordance with their needs. On this
basis **flexibility is provided, as well as interoperability of the different components that
make up a healthcare or hospital information system.**

The benefits of open systems technology are equally important

– for health IT users to gradually put to use open information systems through a free choice
from the best of breed software, built on a common base according to specific needs and at
affordable costs;
– for health IT suppliers to develop, produce, market, install and maintain different
competitive solutions based on European standards;
– for health IT authorities to issue vendor independent IT policies and strategies of
implementation, including standards in order to guide developments.

The Responsibilities of Management

Patients, health professionals as well as management will ultimately receive great benefits fro
open patient record–based information systems both within hospitals as between hospitals an
primary care and other services. However, as may have become clear from above, managers
and administrators must realise that such systems **will affect the entire organisation and in**
areas, i.e.: its basic philosophies, organisational principles, patient care processes and
supporting workflows, interdisciplinary collaboration, handling of knowledge, methods of
measuring clinical and business performance as well as hospital management. **Computers an**
IT must not drive the required process of change. This is the responsibility of top
management: administrators, health services and hospital chief executive officers, and senio
managers.

Top management must acquire a broad understanding of health information, openly
acknowledge the importance of information and give a clear lead to other staff through active
involvement. The responsibilities of management refer to the improvement of the quality of

healthcare information, as well as of its use by IT, and ensuring success in procurement and implementation of systems. In all this, **involvement and commitment** of the users themselves, i.e. of **the professional staff, as well as their education and training are crucially important**.

First and foremost, healthcare systems must have a **plan for their information technology that is firmly rooted in their information strategy, and which is regularly reviewed and up‐dated**. Generally speaking the plan should focus **both on patient care support and operational, administrative systems**.

Just buying IT and introducing systems will result in not more than reproduction of existing information and continuation of existing care processes. Only some, small benefits may be expected in such a case. According to good practice, first a general commitment must be built by a review of existing care processes, followed by an identification of information flows and completed by adjustment of the need for information. Strategy development should be a part of the process of introducing new systems. On this basis an overall, long term strategy must be developed for the selection of IT solutions that indeed fit. Such systems will **produce necessary information**, applied by **new care processes**. It is common experience that **only in this way significant benefits can be achieved**.

References

1) Tomas Varhclyi: Healthcare Reform: The New Possibilities Offered by Informatics, MIE96, 1996
2) Karen A. Duncan: Health Information and Health Reform: Jossey‐Bass Inc, San Francisco, 1994
3) NHS, National Report of the Audit Commission, HMSO, London, 1995
4) CEU Projects: RICHE Nr 2221, ISA Nr 2267, EDITH Italy Nr 7508, EDITH Ireland Nr 7507, HOSPITAL2000 Nr 7509, AIDA Nr 20867, COBRA Nr 20908, HANSA WEST Nr HC1019, HANSA EAST Nr 960096, RHINE Nr 22669

Medical Informatics Europe '97
C. Pappas et al. (Eds.)
IOS Press, 1997

ITHACA
Telematics for Integrated Client Centred Care

Mrs Vasiliki Karounou
*N.T.U.A., Division of Computer Science, Dept of Electrical & Computer Engineering, 157 73 Zographou,
Athens, GREECE*

Dr Leslie Boydell (on behalf of the ITHACA Consortium)
*ITHACA Project Manager/Consultant in Public Health Medicine, South and East Belfast Trust,
Knockbracken Healthcare Park, Saintfield Road, BELFAST*

Abstract: ITHACA is a project supported by the healthcare telematics programme of the European Commission's Fourth Framework Programme. The user organisations involved in ITHACA shared a philosophy of community based care that focuses on the client and development of the multi-disciplinary care team, involving a range of professionals delivering care to clients in their own homes or community facilities. The focus of ITHACA system is to support client case management which includes client assessment, care planning, delivery and evaluation of care outcomes. System analysis and design process identified that practices and procedures in health and social care are very similar throughout the diverse sites represented in ITHACA and they are represented in a generic model that describes the great majority of local health and social care requirements. The ITHACA demonstrator will consist of a client/patient centred community care information system, which is distributed across a number of community care centres within a given region and covers the homes of selected clients.

1. Introduction

ITHACA is a project supported by the healthcare telematics programme of the European Commission's Fourth Framework Programme. The project commenced in January 1996 and will end in December 1998. Health authorities in Europe are facing similar challenges in providing community health and social care [1], including:

- Rising costs of care within institutional settings and the need to develop primary care.
- An expectation by the citizen to be able to make choices about their own care.
- The need for agencies to work together to provide co-ordinated care for vulnerable people in the community.
- The need to provide care which is effective, outcome-oriented and demonstrates value for money.
- A shift in demography with an increasing proportion of elderly people in the population.

It is the need to address these challenges that has lead to the creation of the ITHACA project to seek common solutions.

The user organisations involved in ITHACA have a shared philosophy of community based care that focuses on the client of the services and development of the multi-disciplinary care team, involving a range of professionals delivering care to clients in their own homes or community facilities. Care provided should be goal-oriented with the involvement of the client in setting their own objectives in negotiation with professionals. The goal of care for very frail or vulnerable clients is to help them maintain their autonomy within home care settings and the use of telematic solutions may provide the means to do this. The focus of ITHACA is on support for case management which includes client assessment, care planning and delivery of care. The demonstrator will consist of a client/patient centred community care information system, which is distributed across a number of community care centres within a given region and covers the homes of selected clients. The core functionalities of the system will be: assessment, care planning, care delivery, optimisation services for management/administration and home telecare services

2. Objectives of the Project

The overall aim of the ITHACA project is to achieve improved quality of care and quality of life, access to services, empowerment and choice for patients and clients through support for:

- client focused care
- multidisciplinary and inter-agency working
- improved access to information

and for health care provider organisations:

- secure better value for money
- support new models of care/re-engineered processed
- provide more care in the community
- impact on European strategy
- develop an market for products

To achieve this high level aim. a number of specific objectives have been defined, These are:

- *To implement and validate demonstrators based on generic functional specifications for mental health, maternal and child health and elderly incorporating the generic concepts and components of EPIC.*

User requirements have been collected from all of the ten sites involved in the ITHACA project using a common methodology. This information has been consolidated into a common user requirements functional model with the common requirements for all client groups and sites identified. This has been used to develop generic functional specifications for the demonstrators for the four lead sites (Andalucia, Belfast, Porto and Turku).

- *To tailor the system developed to new pilot sites with different primary care systems using the experience of the existing sites to provide further validation of the system.*

All ten sites have been involved in the description of user requirements so that their needs could be included within the functional model and any differences identified. The new sites. termed replication sites. will be offered the opportunity to chose the application from any of the four lead sites that best meets their needs following verification and early validation.

- *Agree common values and standards for care in the community and achieve consensus on assessment, care planning and outcomes.*

A multidisciplinary users' group has been formed from all ten ITHACA sites, including doctors working in the specialities of mental health, elderly care and maternal and child health as well as general practitioners, nurses, social workers, health service managers and other allied professions such as occupational therapists and physiotherapists. The users' group has worked assessment and the development of generic multidisciplinary assessment, care planning, confidentiality and security, critical success factors and the re-engineering of services, relevant to ITHACA.

- *Survey and integrate existing tools which will improve the effectiveness and efficiency of services e.g. data access tools for professionals working from the clients homes.*

A survey of existing technologies relevant to ITHACA has been completed. Based on the user requirements, candidate technologies for integration with ITHACA are being selected, for example, the use of hand held computers and bar coding for health care workers visiting clients a home.

- *Integrate home telecare management and evaluate its value in maintaining dependent people at home.*

For the elderly, home telecare services will be integrated within ITHACA. This means that the home telecare operators operating a 24 hour alarm service will have access to information held within the clients community care record and that the report of any event dealt with by the alarm operator will be available to the professionals normally responsible for the care of individual clients.

- *Investigate the potential of existing technologies to analyse information on client centred database and optimise services using executive information systems and geographical information system.*

An important aspect of ITHACA is the opportunity provided by a person centred information system to aggregate and analyse the information within the system to improve the services provided. Working with Ordnance Survey, Northern Ireland, a demonstrator of the possible uses of a geographical Information System for the management and planning of community services using data from a person centred information system will be created and the potential scenarios for this demonstrator have been described.

- *Create common products.*

To ensure that a working demonstrator is provided at each of the lead sites, one developer is working with each of the lead sites. Each developer is working from the generic functional specification and have collaborated in the design and modelling of the ITHACA prototypes to identify those software objects which have a common definition and behave in a consistent way within a core data model.

- *Provide adequate mechanisms for confidentiality, security and privacy.*

The importance of confidentiality and security has been recognised by the project and the users have undertaken a security risk analysis for ITHACA. Further work of agreeing access rights will be undertaken locally.

3. Progress of the Project

The first year of the project has been mainly devoted to the collection of user requirements. the development of the functional specifications and identification of suitable technologies and software tools for service optimisation and home care. A great deal of effort was given to the development of the functional specifications and the system high level which defines a common community care framework that is applicable to all ITHACA client groups (Elderly, Mother & Child and Mental Health) at all 10 user sites around Europe and Canada.

The diagram below shows the steps, the activities and the approach that resulted to system specification and design.

SYSTEM SPECIFICATION AND DESIGN

Site specific user requirements for the above mentioned client groups at the ten user sites around Europe and Canada were collected using a common methodology. They were processed. evaluated and *consolidated into a generic report of user requirements* across all client groups and sites. A *system prototype* was developed and translated to the language spoken in every user site. It was *evaluated* and adopted to local requirements. *Re-engineering requirements* for managing and operating community client centred care services were identified by managerial and health and social professionals. An iterative process between the activities described in the above diagram resulted to the *high level functional specification and design models* of the ITHACA system. The *high level functional specification and design* models are tailored to meet the *site specific requirements* of the four demonstration sites.

One of the aims of the ITHACA project is to identify best practice in community health and social care throughout the EEC. using the countries and sites involved as representative samples of different European practices. Through the modelling process it was identified that practices and procedures in health and social care were very similar throughout the diverse sites represented in ITHACA and they could be represented in a generic model that describes the great majority of local health and social care requirements.

The development of the application software for the demonstrators, based on the ITHACA generic models, will take place during the first half of 1997 and the verification and early validation of the demonstrators will take place during the second half. During 1998, the demonstrators will be implemented in all sites and full demonstration and validation of the ITHACA system will take place.

4. Concluding remarks

The Community care functions and tasks described in user requirements appeared to suggest unique requirements at local sites, however by a long iterative process of modelling and abstraction, it has been identified that there are essentially generic. Furthermore, the exercise of modelling the user requirements was highly instructive in providing a forum for particular ideas to be tested in a wider context, regarding better ways of practice and re-structuring particular processes of the community care system.

The success in defining an applicable generic model has implications within and beyond the ITHACA project. There is a reference model that can be used for the evaluation of any local healthcare procedure, facilitating the identification of 'best practice' and supporting the endeavour of re-engineering healthcare processes where appropriate. Prototype and system development benefits from having a well-defined structure for all the key software components that is needed in end-user applications. Finally, commercial system developers have an added incentive for developing applications that have a pan-European scope.

5. ITHACA Consortium

- South and East Belfast Health and Social Services Trust, Northern Ireland (Co-ordinators)
- Systems Team Group, U.K.
- Irish Medical System, Republic of Ireland
- Ordnance Survey, Northern Ireland
- Federation des Associations de Coordination Sanitaire et Sociale de L'Oise, France
- ETC - Societe Anonyme, France
- Azienda USSL, Italy
- TSD-Projects, Italy
- Servicio Andaluz de Salud, Spain
- Empresa Publica Hospital Costa del Sol, Spain
- Ingenia, Spain
- Health Office City of Turku, Finland
- Tampereen Tiedonhallinta Oy, Finland
- VTT Information Technology, Finland
- City Council of Gothenburg, Sweden
- Administracao Regional de Saude do Norte, Portugal
- Instituto de Engenharia de Sistemas e Computadores, Portugal
- Maternidade de Julio Dinis, Portugal
- Hospital Magalhaes Lemos, Portugal
- National Technical University of Athens, Greece
- Hellenic Red Cross, Greece
- Municipality of Amaroussion, Greece
- Grupo de Bioingenieria y Telemedicina Universidad Politecnica de Madrid, Spain
- Prodimed, Spain
- Saskatchewan, Canada

6. References

[1] L. Boydell. European Commission health telematic projects: The Belfast Experience. *British Journal of Health Care Management*, 1995, vol. 1, No 6, 297-301.

Medical Informatics Europe '97
C. Pappas et al. (Eds.)
IOS Press, 1997

TELENURSE - Nursing Classifications, Quality Indicators and the Electronic Nursing Record

Hendrik D. Jorgensen and Tommy M. Nielsen,

*Kommunedata, The Centre for Health Information Services, Lautrupvang 3,
DK-2750 Ballerup, Denmark*

Abstract. In the area of nursing, national and international clinical databases are practically non-existing. The lack of common nomenclatures and classifications is the main reason for this situation. This article elaborates on the TELENURSE project's two objectives which focus on improving that situation. The first objective concerns the "The International Classification for Nursing Practice" (ICNP) and methods for implementation of ICNP electronically in nursing modules of electronic patient records. The second objective concerns the development of a clinical nursing database in which clinical data collected from electronic nursing systems can be stored. On the basis of this data storage, nursing indicators can be developed, which in the long term allows for comparison of nursing interventions across Europe.

1. Introduction

In the nursing community, there is considerable interest in recording nursing activities in a structured manner and in being able to use the structured data for assessment and comparison of the quality of nursing care provided at local, regional, national - and even international - levels. Due to the lack of internationally accepted nomenclatures and classifications, which provide a framework for suitably structuring nursing information, it has until now been very difficult to effectively satisfy this interest. Additionally, the limited use of electronic nursing records by nurses in their daily work makes the provision of structured and standardised nursing data almost impossible.

It is within the framework of the TELENURSE project to address these issues, relying on the latest developments in classifications and electronic health care records.

The TELENURSE project is an accompanying measure under the EU Telematics Applications Programme for Health. The project is co-ordinated by the Danish Institute for Health and Nursing Research (DIHNR), and the project participants come from practically all EU countries.

The focus of this article is on the TELENURSE project and the relation between nursing classifications, quality indicators and the electronic nursing record. In the following, the TELENURSE project will be briefly described. Furthermore, the developmental activities within the project, including a description of the NUREC-DK demonstrator and the clinical database, will be elaborated on.

2. The TELENURSE Project

The primary purpose of the TELENURSE project is to promote consensus in Europe on the International Classification for Nursing Practice (ICNP) [1]. The ICNP was initiated in 1990 by the International Council of Nurses (ICN) as a long-term project to advance nursing care throughout the world. More specifically, the objective was to establish a common language for nursing practice to be used for describing the nursing care in a variety of settings in such a way that it may be compared across populations, settings, geographical areas and time. Through the TELENURSE project, the EU has funded the promotion of ICNP in Europe and a field test of an alpha version of the classification.

A secondary purpose of the TELENURSE project deals with the implementation of the ICNP in small scale demonstrators of nursing modules of electronic nursing records in different countries in Europe. Furthermore, TELENURSE deals with the illustration of how data entered in the electronic nursing record can be extracted for use in clinical databases - in the first instance at local and national levels, but in the long term also at the level of a European clinical nursing database. This allows for comparisons between nursing activities in different countries in Europe.

It should be noted that the demonstrator developed in the TELENURSE project should not be seen as a complete electronic nursing record. The demonstrator should be seen as selected parts of an electronic nursing record. These parts are necessary in order to be able to implement and validate the ICNP for documentation of nursing activities and for illustration of the potential of ICNP as a means of comparing nursing activities between different organisations and health care institutions.

3. The Developmental Activities

To successfully implement a new classification and define the contents of a European clinical database, which can form the basis for a commonly approved set of indicators for monitoring nursing activities, is a difficult task. For the outcome of this task to be a success, the problems should be approached in a step-wise and iterative manner, which allows for continuous improvement based on user inputs. Therefore, the project has carefully ensured that the development activities support this process and provide an avenue for new concepts to be discussed, defined and tested.

The concepts and their interaction are illustrated in figure 1 below, and the following sections will describe an example of one of the electronic nursing records in TELENURSE, the NUREC-DK demonstrator, the clinical database and their interdependence with the nursing indicators.

Nursing Systems   Clinical Database   Nursing Indicators

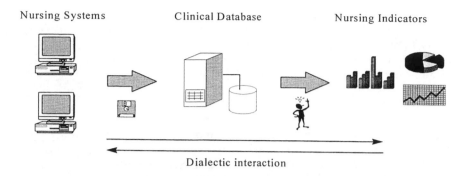

Dialectic interaction

Figure 1 - Context of the Clinical Database

As it is illustrated above, there is close connection and interdependence between the nursing systems, the clinical database and the nursing indicators. Only data which is actually recorded in the electronic nursing record can be transmitted to the clinical database, and the nursing indicators can, of course, only be based on data which is actually available in the clinical database. Consequently, the three components have to evolve in a dialectic interaction. For instance, a demand for a certain nursing indicator could have an impact on the data entries made into the nursing systems, whereas the introduction of new data items in the nursing systems may lead to the formulation of new indicators. This dialectic interaction is a continuous process to which the TELENURSE project provides an important and efficient avenue for new concepts to be discussed, defined and tested.

3.1. The NUREC-DK Demonstrator

Specifying the design of an electronic nursing record involves both a specification of the sort of information which should be contained in the system, of how the information should be presented and of how the user should interact with the computer. Considerable effort has gone into resolving these issues in the TELENURSE project.

The design of NUREC-DK is based on the concepts and informational contents in an existing Swiss demonstrator developed by the Swiss partner in the TELENURSE project, "Hopitaux University de Geneva (HUG)". The Swiss demonstrator, "Group d'Etude pour un Processus de Soins Informatisé (GEPSI)" [2], was developed in 1991-1992 and has been verified in several wards in the University Hospital in Geneva.

The general design of the user interaction with the system is built on a theoretical framework for computer-based medical records founded in cognitive modelling [3,4]. The overall idea is that in addition to the potential advantages of the computer-based system, the computer-based medical record has to retain the advantages of the paper-based medical record. With the purpose of obtaining a basis for the design of a user interface for reading the medical record from a computer screen, the framework is primarily based on a study on how the paper-based medical record is, in fact, used by the physicians and nurses today.

NUREC-DK will be implemented through the use of DocuLive®EPR which is the software tool which was developed by Siemens Nixdorf in Norway as a result of the NORA project [5]. The general design of the user interaction in DocuLive®EPR is based on a paper metaphor: The record is presented as imitations of paper pages. The pages are organised in bundles which are dynamically connected to scrollable index lists. The navigation in and presentation of the pages are fundamental concepts of the interface. The user interface is designed and will be implemented on a workstation with a 19-inch colour screen with the page size as close to A4 as possible. In this way, it is anticipated that the project will achieve, as its primary goal, a design of the user interface for an electronic nursing record which is smooth and efficient for routine use by the nurse and which, on the basis of ICNP, supports the structured documentation of nursing activities.

3.2. The Clinical Database

Today, the number of relevant national and international clinical databases which contain data on outcomes of nursing interventions is very modest. This is, as mentioned above, primarily due to the lack of common nomenclatures and classifications. However, a few initiatives related to clinical databases in nursing have been made. The two most important of these initiatives are the approach applied by Katholieke Universiteit Leuven, Centre for Health Services Research, on the management of Belgian nursing activities [6], and the findings in a project on clinical quality in nursing undertaken by DIHNR and the Danish validation site in TELENURSE, Odense University Hospital [7]. These initiatives have been taken into account and have served as inspiration in the logical design of the clinical database in TELENURSE.

In the TELENURSE approach, data for the clinical database will be provided as an extraction from the NUREC-DK demonstrator developed in the project. Furthermore, in preparation for meeting the long-term objective of making nursing data comparable on a European scale, the data set for a European clinical nursing database will be specified in TELENURSE.

It is important to recognise that the system is designed so that the data for the clinical database can be automatically extracted from the electronic nursing record. Thus, the clinical database will impose no extra burden on the clinical staff at the hospital - the data in the clinical database is simply generated from data which the nurse enters in NUREC-DK as a natural and integral part of the daily work routines. This means that data will only have to be entered once - in NUREC-DK - and there will be no need for a separate system to capture the quality data. This is not only time-saving, it will also ensure correctness and timeliness of data in the clinical database.

The difference between clinical databases and the electronic nursing record is that the purpose of data recording in the clinical databases is primarily focused on a retrospective evaluation of the treatment, whereas data recording in the electronic nursing record focuses on the patient needs in the course of a treatment. However, it is important to realise that the data is the same, and it differs only in terms of structure and level of aggregation.

Another important component in the context of clinical databases is the nursing indicators. Until now, the amount of valuable internationally comparable information on nursing activities has, as mentioned, been very limited, primarily due to lack of structured and comparable nursing data in an electronic form. Furthermore, the definition of a commonly approved set of indicators on nursing activities has not yet been formulated. The clinical database will provide structured and comparable nursing data. In the course of the project, this data will be analysed, and through the use of available analysis and manipulation tools it will be turned into a wide range of meaningful nursing indicators. It is expected that the experiences from the analysis and use of the data in the clinical database will lead to the formation of a formalised and commonly accepted set of indicators for monitoring nursing activities across Europe.

4. Conclusion

The long-term objective of the TELENURSE project is to obtain the ability to analyse and compare nursing quality data. As described above, this objective will be reached through the development of ICNP towards a validated and generally accepted classification for description of nursing activities as well as through the use of this classification in electronic nursing records and in a common European quality database which receives data from the electronic patient records. Thus, this quality database constitutes the data basis for the required nursing indicators. The development activities which take place at the moment are important steps in the right direction. As regards implementation of ICNP in the Danish demonstrator, the important factors for successful implementation of an electronic nursing record can be comprised under three points:

* The development is based on verified concepts and experiences from the existing Swiss demonstrator (GEPSI) and on the theoretical framework for the development of electronic patient records.
* The development will - to as great an extent as possible - comply with the European standard for electronic patient record architecture (EHCRA - European Healthcare Record Architecture) and it will, together with the theoretical background, form the best possible basis for the integration with the complete common electronic patient record.
* Finally, the work is organised in a step-wise approach and in close co-operation with a user group, all of which ensures the most effective use of the resources available in the TELENURSE project and which will render it possible that the result of the development will prove to be satisfactory to the users.

As regards the clinical quality database, it is important to note that the design, which is specified in the project, is to be seen as an alpha version. Through experimenting with, combination and analysis of this data and creation of nursing indicators, it is anticipated that one step further is taken in the right direction towards establishment of an internationally recognised set of indicators for monitoring nursing activities.

References

[1] RA. Mortensen (ed), The International Classification for Nursing Practice ICNP. ISBN: 87 88635 54 6
[2] Assimacopoulos and A. Borgazzi., An Electronic Patient Record Combining Free Text And Coded Nomenclature: Application To The Nursing Process. In: MEDINFO 92, K.C. Lund et al. (eds), Elsevier (North-Holland), 1992:746-751.
[3] E. Nygren, Modelling and Analysis of Human Work Situations as a Basis for Design of Human-Computer Interfaces (Licentiat Thesis), Uppsala University, Uppsala, 1992.
[4] E. Nygren et al., Reading the medical record, *Computer Methods and Programs in Biomedicine*, 39 (1992) 1-12.
[5] Knut Skifjeld, Gunvald Harket, Petter Hurlen, Jo Piene, Sigbjørn Skjervold: A Document Architecture for Health Care Records Integrating structural and semantic aspects.
[6] W. Sermeus et al., The Nursing Minimum Data Set In Belgium: A Basic Tool For Tomorrow's Health Care Management, Katholieke Universiteit Leuven, Leuven, 1995.
[7] Landsdækkende Database for Klinisk Kvalitet I Sygeplejen - Med Fokus på Resultat/Outcome Kriterier, Odense Universitetshospital, September 1994

Medical Informatics Europe '97
C. Pappas et al. (Eds.)
IOS Press, 1997

C.A.S.M. and C.A.S.T. – Phase Two

Nicola T Ellis

Researcher. Information Management Research Group, Lancashire Business School,
Preston. Lancashire. Great Britain. PR1 2HE

Abstract. This paper outlines the second phase of a research project currently being conducted at the University of Central Lancashire. The aim of this second phase is to construct a computer based toolset for clinical audit, based on the structured method (C.A.S.M.) developed during the first phase of the project. A discussion of the validation of the C.A.S.M. and an outline of the toolset is portrayed.

1 Introduction

This paper describes the second phase of an ongoing project. The first phase of which was presented as a paper at MIE'96.

2 Background

Clinical audit is an investigation into the quality of care received by patients. The Department of Health defines audit as "the systematic, critical analysis of the quality of medical care, including the procedures used for diagnosis and treatment, the use of resources, and the resulting outcome and quality of life for the patient" [1]. However, a review of the current literature pertaining to medical audit reveals that there is a discrepancy between the above stated aim of assessing the quality of patient care and that which appears to occur in practice [2, 3, 4].

Clinical audit differs from medical research in that it is generally well defined and can have clear aims and objectives which are understood at the start of the audit project. The analysis requirements are normally relatively straight forward, typically involving cross tabulations.

The objectives of the first phase of this project were, therefore:

- To consider current practice in audit through literature reviews and evaluation of audits carried out in the four counties, Anglia and Oxford region.
- To develop a structured method (Clinical Audit Structured Method - C.A.S.M.) for clinical audit.

The outcomes of the work undertaken in connection with these two objectives has been published by the author [4, 5, 6]. However, this paper is concerned with the validation phase of C.A.S.M. and the simulation and initial stages of the development of the Clinical Audit Structured Toolset (C.A.S.T.).

2.1 Validation & Verification Of The C.A.S.M.

The C.A.S.M. has been tested using a methodology based upon prototyping. This has been a three stage approach (Figure One):

- Historical Review
- Facilitated Testing
- Independent Testing

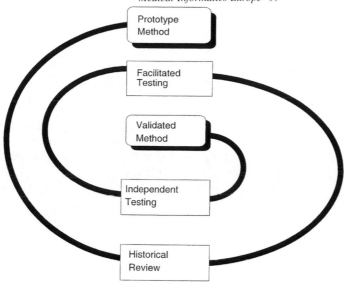

Figure 1: *Testing Methodology* [1]

Historical Review

The first step in testing the C.A.S.M. was to apply it retrospectively to completed audits in order to identify both whether or not the C.A.S.M. could have been used and also where the differences would have been, had the audit been undertaken following the C.A.S.M. Three audit projects have been identified for this purpose:

- Health Visitor Audit undertaken by Oxford Clinical Audit Services. This audit has had the C.A.S.M. applied retrospectively and the results of this written up [7].
- Fractured Neck of Femur. This is part of a national audit and the author is currently waiting for the data collection phase of the Oxford section of the audit to be completed.
- Post-operative Pain. This is a re-audit undertaken by Oxford Clinical Audit Services and the author is currently waiting for the data collection phase of the audit to be completed.

Facilitated Testing

The second stage in testing the C.A.S.M. was to facilitate its use in live audit projects. The author is currently working with the Department of General & Special Surgery at Blackburn Royal Infirmary undertaking multiple audits concerned with the re-organisation of surgical services and day case surgery provision at the Infirmary.

Independent Testing

The third stage in testing the C.A.S.M. was to develop the method as a resource pack [8] and to issue it to health care professionals in both primary and secondary care. Consequently, the C.A.S.M. is currently being tested at various sites through out the U.K. including: Middlesborough General Hospital, Manchester Royal Eye Hospital, the Royal College of Midwives, the East London Medical Audit Advisory Group, the College of Occupation Therapists and a Clinician in Tyneside.

Further health care professionals have also expressed interest in testing the method and resource packs have been issued to them. It is hoped that this interest will provide the basis for a comparative study of the use of the method within a clinical speciality across several regions to be undertaken.

[1] This graphical representation of the Testing Methodology has been developed by A.C. Gillies. The Methodology will be more fully discussed in a forthcoming publication co-authored by the author and A. C. Gillies.

2.2   *Outcomes & Impacts On Users*

Currently, audits are often being undertaken with little thought being taken as to the consequences of such an audit. As a result of which, many audit reports lie unused and wasted. It was hoped that the use of the C.A.S.M. would ensure that all possible consequences and their ramifications would be considered before the audit is undertaken. The use of the C.A.S.M. should make audit easier but, more importantly, improve practice and as a consequence of this improve the quality of patient care. Initial feedback from independent test sites indicates that these hopes are being borne out in practice.

A secondary impact on users is that the C.A.S.M. allows the clinical audit process to be undertaken by the health care professionals themselves, as opposed to management or specific audit personnel, thus providing ownership of the audit project to those for whom audit was originally intended.

3   **The Second Phase**

3.1   *The Problem*

The C.A.S.M. provides a structured approach to the entire process of clinical audit for individual audits. However, it does not provide for a systematic approach to audit planning.

As C.A.S.M. is currently paper-based it is cumbersome and time consuming and it can be off-putting for health care professionals to be faced with, what is after all, only another set of forms.

3.2   *The Solution*

Case Analogy

As the nature of the problem lends itself to a structured approach, Computer Aided Software Engineering (CASE) is being used as an analogy for computer based audits. The revised C.A.S.M. has formed the basis of a simulated C.A.S.T. (Clinical Audit Structured Toolset); the underlying structure of which is portrayed in Figure Two. The C.A.S.T. supports the C.A.S.M. as a CASE tool supports a software engineering method [9].

It is intended that this simulated C.A.S.T. will be evaluated, re-evaluated and refined to produce a full, working version of the method and toolset which will incorporate a strategic planning element (analogous to information systems planning).

3.3   *Proposed Validation & Verification Methodology*

The methodology used to validate the C.A.S.M. has been proven as an effective mechanism and therefore the process of:

- Development
- Historical review
- Facilitated trials
- Independent trials

is being followed again.

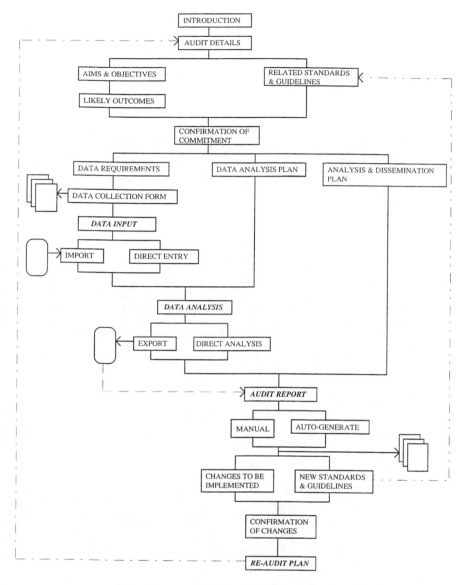

Figure 2:   *C.A.S.T. - Clinical Audit Structured Toolset*

The computer based tool is being implemented in Delphi. The visual nature and flexibility of this programming environment lends itself to a prototyping approach and is compatible with users expectations of information systems development methods.

4   Anticipated Benefits

There are three major benefits anticipated as a result of the development of C.A.S.M. and C.A.S.T.:

1. The development of C.A.S.M. and C.A.S.T. solves a perceived knowledge gap for users.

2. Their development will facilitate the stated aim of the NHS, specifically:
   - to improve patient care
   - the development of standards and guidelines
   - to reduce duplication of effort
   - reduction in wastage of resources

3. The use of C.A.S.M. and C.A.S.T. facilitates comparative audits which are not possible using existing audit methods.

5   References

[1] Department of Health, 1989 *"Working for patients"* **The NHS White Paper,** Cmnd 55., London, HMSO

[2] Ellis N.T., Gillies A.C. 1995a *"The Reality Of Clinical Audit: The Oxford Experience"* **SHIMR '95 Conference Proceedings,** University of Sheffield

[3] Ellis ·N.T., Gillies A.C. 1995b *'The Need for a Structured Method For Medical Audit'* **Current Developments in Medical Computing,** University of Teesside, Middlesborough

[4] Ellis N.T. 1995 *"Audit Of Audit: A Survey Of Audit Practice In The Four Counties, Anglia And Oxford Region"* **Auditorium** v4:2 pp8-10

[5] Ellis N.T. 1996a *'C.A.S.M. & C.A.S.T. : Clinical Audit Structured Method & Clinical Audit Structured Toolset'* **MIE'96 Congress Proceedings,** Denmark

[6] Ellis N.T. 1996b *'Progress Towards A Structured Method & Computerised Toolset For Clinical Audit'* **Innovations in Healthcare Computing,** University of Teesside, Middlesborough

[7] Ellis N.T., Gillies A..C. 1996 *'Evaluating And Improving The Process Of Change In The UK National Health Service'* Submitted for publication **Business Change & Re-Engineering** John Wiley & Sons

[8] Ellis N.T. 1996c **C.A.S.M.: Paper Based Method, Trial Version 1.0** (Resource Pack) Information Management Research Group, University of Central Lancashire 1 October 1996 ISBN 0-906694-72-8

[9] Fisher A. 1992 **Case: Using Tools For Systems Development** John Wiley 2nd Edition

Medical Informatics Europe '97
C. Pappas et al. (Eds.)
IOS Press, 1997

Emergency Health Care Information System For Bucharest-Romania

ROMSYS, Bucharest:

Laura Lazaroiu, Dan Horhoianu, Petre Alexandrescu, Bogdan Birghilescu, Calin Avram, George Dan and Marian Pascu.

Emergency Ambulance Service of Bucharest:

A. Ripanu, M. Oprisan, E. Nemtisor and M. Chiriacescu

Abstract: The Emergency Health Care Information System (EHCIS) in Bucharest provides information about the whole activity of Dispatch Emergency Ambulance Service and Emergency Receiving Room of the 7 Hospitals, providing emergency health care in Bucharest over a MAN (Metropolitan Area Network). In each of these places a local network is located, containing a database server ORACLE. The link among LANs is made via switched lines. The Hospitals collect information only about emergency cases. The microstation represents station for emergency teams of Emergency Ambulance Service of Bucharest (EASB), distributed in all 6 districts of Bucharest. The system is structured accordingly with the working-groups existing in Dispatch, microstations and hospitals:
- registration operators (phone-operators) for administer the emergency requests/calls;
- a location for the medical coordinator which must to choose, in few seconds, the emergency team, accordingly with the case emergency degree;
- radio-operators which communicate with the teams in the field;
- a location for the manager of Dispatch, in order to provide a full-set of real-time medical and resources information;
- a registration operator at each microstation;
- a registration operator at each hospital.
The data are registered in the ORACLE database on the central server. The client/server architecture assures the real time communication among all these locations. The system works 7days/week, 24 hours/day.

The Emergency Health Care Information System (EHCIS) is a "critical-mission system" from the medical point of view, that means surviving chances are decided here. In Romania, the emergency health care medical service has as purpose **diagnosis, statistical evaluation and stabilisation of medical-surgical emergencies**. The components of this system are the following: Dispatch (961) as a part of Emergency Ambulance Service of Bucharest (EASB), EASB Microstations (for districts 1, 2, 3, 4, 5, 6), and Emergency Receiving Rooms in the hospitals which offer emergency medical assistance.

An Information System was implemented for the emergency health care medical system in order to increase the efficiency and service quality in assuring emergency health care.

A real time set of programs has been implemented in the Dispatch, conceived and achieved for automation of EASB activity and consisting in the following activities:

1) **Overtaking the data of pacients identification and standardised ᴜᴠertaking of the symptoms declared by pacients**, which are the base of establish automatically the degree of emergency for each pacient; and the medical staff needed for solving the case. There are 11 of such working locations. Here can also be obtained information regarding the registered case situation.

2) **Register the operating medical staff and the teams** which are working in a shift (1 working location).

3) **Automation of decision act of the medical coordinator**, meaning the association of a free team for each registered case (1 working multiscreen location). This is the poli-criterial decisional process focused on: the emergency degree, the time and place of request solicitation, the place in each is located a free team, the qualification of the medical staff requested accordingly with the presumptive diagnosis. The medical coordinator has access to special functions in the system which allow him the visualisation of same particularly categories of solicitations and teams, and the eventually modifications of automatically associations according with some criteria.

4) **Communication in the field through the radio operator** of information regarding the case and announcing teams that become free.

5) **Communication and printing to the microstation of the medical records** which have to be solved by the teams that are located in the microstation; using modem and leased switched lines.

6) **Automatically print-out of solicitation's list and activities list** performed in the Dispatch, in each shift; and the full-filled form of solicitation record.

7) **Add of final information in the system with real data registered in each case record** by the team which has solved the case (operation performed in the 6 microstations). These way can be obtained statistical situations regarding the diagnosis, centralising, establishing the vital function in dynamic, etc.

8) **Elaborate and print-out the final statistics of the shift** (solved cases, the staff activity, the promptitude of coordination and other events).

9) **Obtaining statistics** regarding the promptitude in solving cases, the diseases the calls are making for, morbidity and mortality, the concordance diagnosis-reason of request, usage of drugs, etc.

A key point of the system is the manner in witch the presumptive diagnosis is automatically established:

1. At the emergency call-phone, on the screen of each phone-operator are displayed 15 general reasons of solicitation.

2. The phone-operator selects a reason, in accordance with the information the pacient communicates.

3. The set of presumptive symptoms associated with reason of call is displayed on the operator screen.

4. The operator selects the symptoms declared by pacient.
5. In this moment, the system establishes automatically a presumptive diagnosis in accordance with the declared symptoms, the age and the sex of pacient. Also, it is automatically associated the emergency degree, accordingly with the seriousness of the diagnosis and pacients' age and it is established the required type of team (emergency team, transportation team, etc.)

The "management and control level" of the system is located at the medical coordinator. Here, there are automatically established the optimal pairs between the cases that have to be solved and the available teams. This is a decisional complex process, in which are taking into consideration the characteristics of each case and team.

The characteristics of registered cases are the following:

- the emergency degree of case (0 - 3);
- the hour and minute of registration;
- the district where the case is located in;
- the set of assignments associated to the case.

The assignment is a number associated to each qualification of staff working in EASB (emergency team with medical-specialist, emergency team with pediatrical doctor, emergency team with emergency medical specialist, emergency team with nurses/assistant, transportation teams).

The characteristics of available team are the following:
- qualification of the medical staff involved in the team or the brand of car in the transportation cases/situation;
- the district in which the team is available.

For taking the decision of coupling case-to-team the system provides an algorithm for search, which analyses the records sorted by the emergency degree (0, 1, 2, 3), and for the same degree the records are sorted by registration order of cases.

The pairs realised in this way are displayed on the main screen. The medical coordinator can confirm the computer proposal or can modify it through commands. If the medical coordinator hasn't confirmed the computer proposal, the pair is automatically confirmed in a minute.

The automatically coupling can be stopped at the request or can be stopped automatically, in the case in which it doesn't exists any other possibility of coupling according with the programmed algorithm (i.e.: there are no unsolved cases or there are no available teams).

The system at Dispatch of EASB - as a part of the whole EHCIS - was conceived as an automatic system which can work perfectly without the existing of an human operator at the medical coordinator location. If there is a person which carry out this role, his tasks are diminuted and the coupling process is much improved from the perspective of association method and response time.

In each of the 7 Emergency Hospitals within the health care emergency system, there are 3 computers connected in a LAN. The link with the central server based on Dispatch is made via switched lines through a modem. The communication protocol is TCP/IP.

The programs working on these computers are carrying out the following functions:

1. **Register the data regarding the pacients which are presenting at the Emergency Receiving Room;**
2. **Transfer the registered data from Hospital to the server of EHCS** and make the reverse operation, in order to allow the Hospital to obtain certain information from the server through;
3. **Elaborate and print-out of statistics useful for Hospital or EASB;**
4. **Represent a starting point** in a global information system of Hospitals;

The Technical Characteristics of IT System in Emergency Health Care

1. Client/server architecture (ORACLE);
2. Distributed software application (50 users);
3. "Real-time" communication among applications;
4. Critical-mission system;
5. Open system, easy to be integrated in an Internet/Intranet architecture (ORACLE+TCP/IP);
6. Expert system for automatically coupling;
7. Automatically managing (LOG) for the functionality of the whole system;
8. Full functional software system;
9. 7days/week 24 hours/day running system.

Work Configuration

Both the SCO-UNIX server and the ORACLE database are located at the EASB. All processing are performed here. At the Dispatch are localised 16 workstations and 3 printers, other 4 workstations and 2 printers being located at Statistics and Management of EASB. At each microstation there is a WINDOWS/NT server connected via modem to the central server. Also, there is a workstation linked with server and a printer.

In each Emergency Hospital, there is one WINDOWS/NT server and an ORACLE local database which is connected to the central server via modem and switched lines. There are also two workstations and 2 printers linked with the local server.

Earnings Obtained through the "Live Operation" of Emergency Health Care Information System

- Improving the concordance between solicitation reason and diagnosis per case **from 65% to 82,5%**;
- Protection of the "real emergency", which means that the promptitude in coordination (the interval between the time of registration of record and the time of team's distribution) **has been increased 60 times**;
- Optimisation of the balance between competency and distance;
- A fast and correct decision support for the complex situation in the district;
- A superior management of involved resources in health care emergency assistance (ambulance, active medical staff, etc.) through a daily evaluation of the reports;
- Availability of real-time tools in the Hospitals, for measurement of emergency health care's efficiency.

Medical Informatics Europe '97
C. Pappas et al. (Eds.)
IOS Press, 1997

Evolution of a Regional Health-care Information System - the design phase

László Balkányi*, Gábor Magyar**,
Géza Lakner*, Éva Orosz***

*HIETE University of Health Sciences,
Dept. of Medical Informatics, Budapest, e-mail: h13208bal@ella.hu
**KFKI, Budapest, ***ELTE University, Dept. of Sociology, Budapest*

Abstract In 1996 a program of the Soros Foundation was launched to study a *regional* health care model Main stake holders of health care financing and providing in three counties in South-Western Hungary. found the idea appealing and the *Soros Model Region Program* was started. *This paper outlines the activity of the second sub-project of the model region program: the development of a regional health care information system.* The build-up of a data and knowledge base serving the differing needs of mentioned goals is based on international standards. Availability and user involvement is based on different media for presenting the information as printed publications, CD-ROM data bases and World Wide Web availability. A congruency and coherency principle is maintained by a unified data model used for different purposes and a planned unified communication protocol among all participants in the model region program. Studies regarding health care status, economics and financing on regional level show that a better fitting health care services profile and a more flexible resource management might be achieved based on the mentioned regionality principle.

1. Introduction: background and goals of the regional information system

In 1996 the Soros Foundation launched a program to study the possibilities of establishing a regional health care model where financing and providing of health-care services are optimized upon the principles of regional decentralization in contrast with todays´ institution oriented, centrally administered budgeting in Hungary Main stake holders of health care financing and providing of three counties (Tolna, Somogy, Baranya) in South-Western Hungary found the idea appealing and the Soros Model Region Program was launched. Research activities exploring population health status, related environmental factors, health care providing infrastructure, modeling of region oriented health care political decision making started, all requiring extensive and intensive informatics infrastructure. Studies regarding economics and financing on regional level show that a better fitting health care services profile and a more flexible resource management might be achieved by the mentioned regionality principle To serve the above mentioned outlined wide range of health care system research and development activities, an information system was envisaged, that can serve the following specific needs:

- storing large amounts of health-, and health care-related data in a structured way,
- enabling retrospective data surveys,
- enabling design of new parameters / health care indicators for prospective data collection
- creating data views according to international standards and quasi-standards for international comparability and analysis: OECD (Eco-Sante), WHO Health for All by 2000 data set mirrors
- providing user friendly way different sort of information services as
  - differently structured information for experts in sociology, epidemiology, for health care managers, for practicing doctors and for the public
  - a "Yellow Pages"-like general information service on health care services, providers, organizations and institutions in the model region

2. Methods and means

2.1. building an architecture

The regional information system (RIS) is developed according to the ISO 3-layer architecture: bitways, middleware and application. Forthcoming CEN/TC251 standards (mainly HIF - Health-care Information Framework) are also taken in account. The RIS is conceptually designed object-oriented for future extensibility. In it's implementation it has been "downgraded" to an affordable relational database structure.

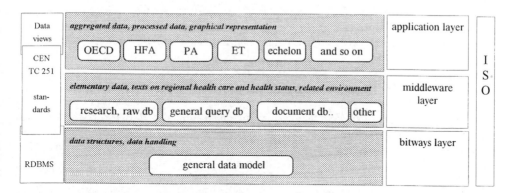

Fig.1. regional information system architecture
(see explanation for abbreviations in the text below)

2.2. designing information system views for the end user

The following "information views" are generated from the common, integrated data base:

- *OECD* > Eco-Sante provided data set of health indicators applied for the region enabling international comparability
- *HFA* > Health for All by 2000 data set - WHO health indicators applied for the region

- *Echelon>*   Echelon view - a systematic approach to visualize and discuss health care
              organizations / institutions and health care services / tasks
- *"Whois">*   Information service on health care services, providers, organizations and
              institutions in the model region
- *PA>*   Pannon almanac - a comprehensive data set about the region (environment,
              social status, health state of Hungarian inhabitants, risk factors, prevention
              programs, morbidity, nursing, health services, health care resources,
              health care financing, health care informatics)
- *ET>*   Health Plan / Health Status Assessment - structured data about education,
              employment, social handicap, home budget, physical environment, lifestyle-
              health behavior, demography and mortality, occupational health care, health
              status self-assessment, mentalhygiene, disability and rehabilitation, social care,
              alternative care/homeopathy, local health politics and resource management,
              civil groups and organizations

2.3. methodology of communicating with end users

To communicate with end users the following aspects has to be considered: wide availability
of data, usability in different environment, techniques to maintain up to date status. Three
methods were chosen to present the results of data collection and processing: (i) printed
material of partial results for wide availability, (ii) CD-ROM versions for flexible handling of
large amount of data and (iii) World Wide Web availability for interactivity and updating.

3. Results and discussion

Designing a multipurpose, but consistent database used by different actors with differing
methodology is not a trivial task. In the following we shall discuss a few principles that we
found worth to consider.

3.1. object oriented architecture features

The conceptual model of the regional health care information system has to cover the broad
spectra of health care information. Features of object oriented thinking as application of
inheritance and object embedding to express hierarchy are useful to organize the large
amount of different data characterizing health care.

*3.2. conceptual modeling on the application level is based on a (health care) functional
point of view*

The above mentioned "object-oriented" thinking is used to model the structure of health care
related information. The model below (fig.2.) shows the result of this thinking. The echelon
model is one of the views of the "application layer" aimed at connecting population related
data with health care related data. As shown on this (2.) figure a single layer model is not
sufficient to represent all health related concepts.

3.3. data modeling on bitways layer uses a generalized mode

A common general data model (fig.3.) is developed ensuring congruity among particular
data bases of the regional health care information system.

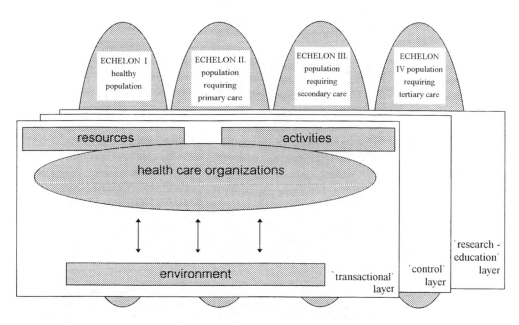

Fig.2 . echelon model of health care related concepts

data model entity	explanation
data abbreviated name	mnemonic abbreviation for data entities, maximal length 8 character
data name	name of data entity
data definition	detailed data description
data classification according to a "data view" and hierarchic position within the given view	The model region program uses the same data for different purposes. For each purpose systematic data views are constructed, as listed in paragraph "*designing information system views for the end user*" A given data might be classified within more data views (resulting in a list), where as default value the position in OECD classification is used.
data conversion to other views	If possible, a conversion algorhitm is given to other classifications instead of the above mentioned list of classification positions.
data type	raw or calculated data
unit of data	if the data is quantifiable, the measurement unit is given here
data sources	name and availability of the data source
validity characterization	time or time span of validity, specificity and sensitivity of data measurement method, predictive value if relevant
frame of reference	as e.g. date, time period, geographic area, specific population

Fig3. the unified data model

4. Summary

The paper describes the design phase of establishing a regional data base to support research and development leading to better health policy making. Cogent handling of the broad spectra and large amount of data requires a clear and consistent conceptual framework. A three level ISO inspired architecture, object-oriented concept handling and a unified data model are serving the above mentioned goals.

Medical Informatics Europe '97
C. Pappas et al. (Eds.)
IOS Press, 1997

Does TISS pave a way towards the nurses care documentation ?

Bürkle T[1], Michel A[1], Horch W[2], Dudeck J[1], Schleifenbaum L[3]

[1]*Department of Medical Informatics, University of Gießen, Heinrich-Buff-Ring 44, 35392 Gießen, Germany*
[2]*Head Nurse, University Hospital Gießen*
[3]*Medical Intensive Care Unit, University Hospital Gießen*

Abstract. New functions have been integrated in the Gießen Hospital Information System WING to support the classification of all intensive care patients into the Therapeutic Intervention Scoring System TISS. The use of those functions has been pushed by legal requirements which made it essential to assess the staffing of intensive care wards in comparison with the accumulated TISS scores. This paper describes the experiences made within two years of TISS scoring. We think that TISS gave a major impact to the construction and implementation of nursing documentation into our HIS.

1. The problem: How to introduce electronic nurse charting

Some German hospitals have tried to introduce electronic nurse charting. Various systems have been used, but the results have not been totally emphatic [1,2,3,4]. Good success could be achieved under ideal conditions, on well staffed intensive care units, using bedside computers. Under such circumstances, complete replacement of the paper based record (At least it was only printed from the computer and not maintained manually) has been reported [5]. Many other observers however report only partial usage of the information system, missing advantages and sometimes even discontinuation [6,7,8,9].

At Gießen University Hospital a HIS called WING is actively serving about thousand clinical users on more than 700 clinical workstations which are provided in almost every ward, outpatient clinic and doctor's office throughout the widespread hospital campus [10]. WING is an in-house-developed system, running on a Tandem Himalaya mainframe. The central clinical data is stored in a Tandem NonStop-SQL RDBMS. Approximately 400 IBM-compatible PC's have access to WING via terminal-emulation, some 300 Macintosh PowerPC run a graphical user interface which is also connected to the same central WING functionality's in client-server fashion [11].

This system however did until recently not offer specific support for nurse charting and documentation. Nurses did use WING functions to retrieve laboratory data for ward rounds and to classify patient care on normal wards (just 2 numbers per patient and day specifying a level between 1 and 3 of general nursing care respectively special nursing care). A nursing specific departmental application had been experimented in one ward, offering support for nursing interview, nurses work schedule and nurses work report as well as for bed and staff assignment [12,13]. This application however for various reasons did not find acceptance within nursing staff and has been discontinued [14].

2. The TISS score

The Therapeutic Intervention Scoring System TISS is an intensive care score dating from 1974 which allows to classify patients into severity categories by means of medical and nursing interventions performed [15,16]. It has been actualised in 1983 for new intervention types and is used for acuity scoring of diseased patients or calculation of patient-nurse relations in intensive care units. 75 types of typical intensive care interventions are associated with between 1 and 4 TISS-points. An acute resuscitation within the last 24 hours counts for example 4 TISS points. The same count of TISS points is awarded to an emergency bronchoscopy, whilst a minor intervention like central venous pressure metering is rated with 2 points.

3. TISS at the Gießen University Hospital before 1996

The Gießen University Hospital, a tertiary care hospital with approximately 1500 beds, has 6 intensive care units (anaesthetists ICU, cardiovascular ICU, neurosurgical ICU, medical ICU, neurological ICU and paediatric ICU) and 3 intensive monitoring units (medical, neurological, and orthopaedic IMU) with a total of 109 registered beds.

The medical intensive care ward had been using paper forms for several years to monitor patient acuity according to the TISS scheme. Statistics had been made for staffing purposes mainly. This ward, equipped with bedside computers already for laboratory results and drug prescription, requested in 1994 if the TISS entry and the statistical calculations could be integrated into the WING hospital information system. Together with staff of the medical ICU a WING-module for data entry was developed and integrated into WING. Monthly statistics could be performed with another WING module, showing the workload in terms of patients grouped in different severity groups.

During introduction into routine we could then demonstrate a markedly increased quality of documentation data [17]. In addition to this the data storage in an electronic database revealed advantages for individual statistic interpretation of data. We examined for example if initial high tiss scores were predictive for bad patient outcome. Such statistics had not been made before, since the individual TISS scoring forms had been destroyed after compilation of the monthly summary statistic. Within nearly 2 years of continous routine use some 6500 entries for approximately 1200 different patients have been recorded on the medical ICU. Documentation quality has been further improved by checking with knowledge based functions for incorrect TISS entries. According to the TISS scheme for example only one entry of either controlled ventilation under relaxation (4 points), or controlled ventilation (4 points), or continous positive pressure ventilation (3 points) or assisted ventilation (3 points) is allowed. This and similar exclusions are checked and incorrect entries are refused (See figure 1).

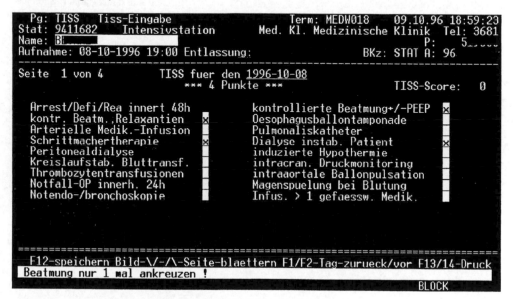

Figure 1   One of four entry screen pages of the first TISS module:
Two interventions which are mutually exclusive (kont. Beatm. /Relaxantien and kontrollierte Beatmung +/-PEEP) have been marked. The program interacts directly with the user issuing a warning in the message line (bright background at the bottom of the screen).

4. The Legal Push

German legal bodies have within the last couple of years restructured the legal foundation of hospital financing. The intention is to establish cost effective treatment strategies in order to avoid increasing health insurance premiums [18]. Hospitals have to prove that they work cost effective and in future part of the reimbursement will be case based (similarly to the DRG's) instead of just covering the accumulated expenses on base of a patient-day-treatment price [19]. Within the surge of such legal changes hospitals are required to give exact account about their delivery of care. In 1996 Gießen University Hospital was undergoing tests of the medical services of the health insurance (MDK) to evaluate if the intensive care units were correctly classified. In this situation the head nursing department could offer to deliver complete TISS statistics for all ICU's and IMU's. In the German state of Hessen, TISS has been officially translated by the state ministry of social care to serve as a guideline for hospital ICU's. The offer was therefore accepted by the MDK. Within just a couple of months TISS was also integrated into the Macintosh WING applications and extended statistical functions have been implemented collecting data about all intensive care / intensive monitoring units.

5. Problems and their solution

Practical introduction on all ICU's and IMU's however posed some problems. Numerous minor problems regarding for example the timeframe for which the TISS-score would be valid and the time of recording TISS-scores had to be solved. The bare legal terms of TISS interventions needed written explanation which had again to be certified by the MDK. Most of the other ICU's did not have bedside workstations, so the data entry had to be done on a single workstation only. Having not documented TISS scores at all before, some ICU staff found it difficult to keep track of all patients to be entered into TISS scoring. The original TISS module on terminals of the medical ICU had offered a semiautomatic reminding service to check for missing TISS entries. This could not be immediately offered on the other ICU's. Missing TISS entries influenced heavily the statistics, showing varying daily workload. Two issues helped to overcome the problem: During a certain time period in May 1996 the MDK asked for paper printouts of all TISS scores for each individual patient. Samples of those paper printouts have been randomly compared with the full paper based medical record to ascertain the correct scoring. During this time period regular „tissing" was manifested as a routine care documentation method in all intensive care units.

Typical results can be seen in figure 2. On average more than 3000 TISS scores have been recorded each month since May 1996 within the 9 ICU's respectively IMU's of the university hospital. Patients have been grouped into the acuity categories 0 (No Tiss-points available), I (1-9 Tiss-points), II (10-19 Tiss-points, III (20-40 Tiss-points) and IV (> 40 Tisspoints). Altogether nearly 500.000 individual nursing respectively medical interventions have been recorded for more than 5000 different ICU-patients. On average 14 different interventions have been stored for each patient per day which have then been accumulated to a TISS score.

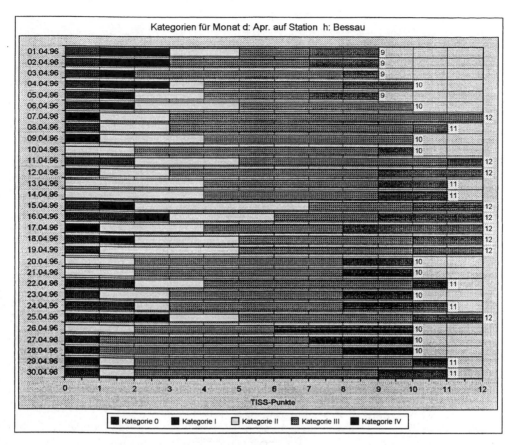

Figure 2   An Example for daily TISS scores on an intensive care unit
Patients are grouped into 5 severity categories ranked according to the TISS points awarded. IV is the
highest category.

6. Discussion

Integration of electronic nurse charting into daily routine is not an easy task. Numerous experiences of other hospitals have shown that often only partial aspects of nursing information systems have been used or that the use has been discontinued altogether due to missing advantages and increased workload [6,7,8,9]. In many places electronic charting was only achieved after bedside workstations had been established [5,20,21,22]. Similar experiences have been made in Gießen [14].

This paper described the process of introducing a marginal care documentation system on 9 intensive care units and intensive monitoring units of an university hospital. On average 14 medical and nursing interventions per patient and day have been documented for more than 5000 patients in the Therapeutic Intervention Scoring System TISS. That implies that the electronic nursing care documentation has been firmly established on all ICU's and IMU's. We think that, even though TISS documentation in Gießen was heavily pushed by legal requirements, it nevertheless shows positive effects on computer based documentation. Nursing staff becomes increasingly aware of the necessity to document their own activities in an electronic patient record. First steps have been made and scores such as TISS offer additional means to follow up patients during their clinical stay. Even consequences for clinical treatment can arise. The head nursing department is intended to continue this development in order to achieve a complete electronic nursing documentation at Gießen University Hospital.

References

[1]   Opitz E., Informationsverarbeitung im Pflegebereich - Checkliste und Marktlage. In: Haas et al. (eds)
      Praxis der Informationsverarbeitung im Krankenhaus. Ecomed Verlagsgesellschaft Landsberg (1996)
      123-130.
[2]   Opitz E. et al., Nursing Information Systems in Germany and Europe. In: Prokosch, H.U. and Dudeck
      J. (eds) Hospital Information Systems: Current Status and Future Trends, Elsevier, Amsterdam
      (1995) 153-174.
[3]   John J. et al. Entwicklungsstand und -perspektiven rechnergestützter Informations- und
      Kommunikationssysteme in der stationären Krankenpflege. In: Prognos (ed.): Auf dem Weg aus der
      Pflegekrise ? Edition Sigma, Berlin (1992) 89-125
[4]   Bürkle, T. et al. Pflegeinformationssysteme Eine Literaturübersicht, Informatik, Biometrie und
      Epidemiologie in Medizin und Biologie 25 (1994) 199-215.
[5]   Schillings H., Experiences with an HIS Subsystem in Intensive Care. In: Prokosch, H.U. and Dudeck
      J. (eds) Hospital Information Systems: Current Status and Future Trends, Elsevier, Amsterdam
      (1995) 79-98.
[6]   Hofmann et al. Evaluation von Stationssystemen. GMDS '96 Proceedings Abstract Band (1996) 326.
[7]   W. Schoner, Zum Abbruch eines Projektes zur Einführung eines EDV-gestützten
      Krankenhauskommunikationssystemes. In: Pöppl S.J., et al. (eds.): Medizinische Informatik Ein
      integrierender Teil arztunterstützender Technologien, MMV Medizin-Verlag München (1994) 62-67.
[8]   Malik B. personal communication München (1994)
[9]   Schrader U. personal communication Gießen (1995)
[10] Prokosch H.-U. et al., WING - Entering a New Phase of Electronic Data Processing at the Gießen
      University Hospital, Meth. Inform. Med. 30 (1991) 289-298.
[11] Michel A. Migration Steps from a Mainframe Based HIS Approach to an Open HIS Environment In:
      Prokosch, H.U. and Dudeck J. (eds) Hospital Information Systems: Current Status and Future Trends,
      Elsevier, Amsterdam (1995) 267-286.
[12] Bürkle, T. et al. Florence, ein integriertes Abteilungssystem für die Pflege In: Kunath H. et al. (eds):
      Medizin und Information, MMV Medizin-Verlag München (1994) 95-98.
[13] Bürkle, T. et al. The Impact of Introducing Computers on Nursing Work Patterns: Study Design and
      First Results. In: Greenes R.A. et al. (eds) Medinfo 95 Proceedings HC & CC Healthcare Computing
      and Communications Canada Inc (1995) 1321-1325.
[14] Kuch R. Evaluation der Einführung eines EDV-Arbeitsplatzes auf das Arbeitsumfeld von
      Krankenpflegepersonal, Medical Dissertation Gießen (1996).
[15] Keene A.R. et al., Therapeutic Intervention Scoring System Update 1983 Crit Care Med 11, 1 (1983)
      1-3.
[16] Nauck-Kreiten E., Personalberechnung mit dem Therapeutic Intervention Scoring System (TISS).
      Deutsche Krankenpflege-Zeitschrift 6 (1993) 411-415.
[17] Bürkle, T. et al. (1995) GMDS '95 Abstract Band (1995) 42.
[18] Fahrbach J. Krankenhaus der Zukunft - Fachtagung des Ministeriums für Arbeit, Gesundheit und
      Soziales des Landes NRW. Medizintechnik 115 (1995) 53-56.
[19] Neubauer G. and Rehermann P. Fallkosten im internationalen Vergleich - Eine Hilfe zur
      Preisfindung in der Bundesrepublik. Das Krankenhaus 12 (1994) 563-567.
[20] Kuperman G. J. et al. (eds) Help: A Dynamic Hospital Information System. Springer Verlag New
      York (1991).
[21] Johnson D. et al. Nurse Charting on the HELP System. Medical Informatics Europe '87 Proceedings
      (1987).
[22] Grewal R., et al. Bedside Computerization of the ICU, Design Issues: Benefits of Computerization
      versus Ease of Paper & Pen. 15th SCAMC Proceedings IEEE Computer Society Washington DC
      (1991) 793-797.

Medical Informatics Europe '97
C. Pappas et al. (Eds.)
IOS Press, 1997

Seamless Care in the Health Region of Crete: the Star☆ Case Study

Michalis Blazadonakis[1], Vassilis S. Moustakis[1,2] and Giorgos Charissis[3]

[1]*Institute of Computer Science, Foundation for Research and Technology - Hellas, Science and Technology Park of Crete, Vassilika Vouton, P.O Box 1385, 71110 Heraklion Greece*
[2]*Department of Production and Management Engineering, Technical University of Crete, 73132 Chania Greece*
[3]*Director, Pediatric Surgery Clinic, University Hospital of Crete*

Abstract: Seamless collaboration and medical information exchange among health care experts is an open question on existing health care systems. The patient record is usually scattered all over the health care network making access to crucial medical information troublesome. The Star☆ (Seamless Telematics Across Regions) project provides a set of solutions towards this direction which will soon be applied at Crete. Initially two health care structures will be involved in the process but later on and after tests have been completed successfully in real world applications, results will be defused over the whole health care region of Crete.

1. Introduction

In our days care for patients is increasingly more demanding and should meet the needs of reliability and effectiveness. In most health care networks immediate supply of medical information and experience is troublesome causing waste of valuable time to health care experts, and economic deficit to the resource providing authorities. The same situation also applies at Crete which consists of a lot of remote and rural areas where immediate access to main health care providers located at urban sites is some times difficult and time consuming. On the island, there exist four prefecture Hospitals, one University Hospital located at Heraklion and several Health Care Centers which are scattered across the various sites. A patient may enter the health care network contacting various points of reference, sharing medical information and expertise among the various health care experts involved in such a process, is more than necessary. Lack of such information may cause waste of time to health care experts not to mention the fact that a lot of results may be reproduced across the various sites of the health care network.

At Crete, we approach seamless care through the use of Star☆ (Seamless Telematics Across Regions) project. The Star☆ is a 4th Frame Work European project that has selected key regions across the Europe to demonstrate the benefits of information sharing among one or more hospitals and their surrounding health care providers [1].

2. What does Seamless Care mean?

Unfortunately there is a gap when it comes to communicate among the various health care experts and institutions while information still flows on paper fax and telephone. With the increased use of specialist care and pressure of immediate access to valuable medical

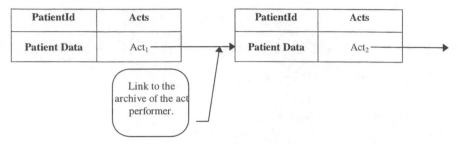

Figure 1: Management of Acts

information there is a clear requirement to replace the paper-based communication with something more efficient. We need a technology where experts will be able to inter-work with each other seamlessly, that is, they should be able to access information independent on where the information is located on as well as be able to publish information anywhere within the health care network.

The term Seamless is used to describe the inter-working of linked information systems. Based on the principles of act management and distributed patient dossiers, the Star☆ servers provide the mechanisms for act negotiation and patient record event linkage across different enterprises. Seamless access to data merits special interest in the following situations:

1. Each time a patient enters the health care network, an act has been initialized with a specified life cycle which ends when the patient eventually exits the health care network. The life cycle of an act then may be viewed as a succession of events within the health care network (see Figure 1).

2. Health care experts involved in the process should be able to follow the links and access information. This is achieved within the Star☆ project through the Act Management Server.

3. The health care experts should also be able to view the various parts of the patient dossier which may be scattered across the health care network through a set of links to the appropriate locations. This is achieved within the Star☆ project through the Patient Reference Dossier (Figure 2).

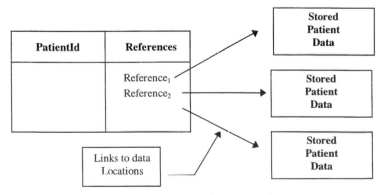

Figure 2: Management of Patient References

3. The Star☆ project Structure and mission statement

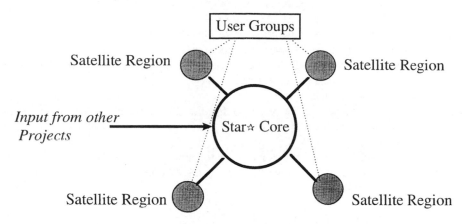

Figure 3: The Star☆ Project Structure

The mission of Star☆ is *to develop and validate open common telematic systems and services that enable a continuum of care for patients.* This overall goal breaks down into four main objectives:

1. To understand and deliver through demonstrations, the benefits of seamless care to patients and providers.
2. Integrate and develop close to market telematic service products.
3. Produce generic open system solutions for heterogeneous legacy systems
4. Produce publish and promote protocols and guidelines for interoperability.

The Star☆ demonstrator sites are called Satellites. This reflects the project structure and also shows that all the developments (within the core of the project) are driven by the user and business requirements of the satellite demonstrator sites. The overall project structure is shown in Figure 3. For more information on the users requirements at Crete, refer either to the Star☆ home page on the WWW [3], or to the home page of the Institute of Computer Science, FORTH [2]

4. An Architecture for implementing seamless care based on Star☆

As presented in section 3 the Star☆ core group provides a set of services for remote access and interoperability to the Star☆ satellites which are then called to integrate their implementations using those services. The services provided by Star☆ core group are the following (see also Figure 4):

1. *The Authorization Server (AS):*
   - Provides Controlled access to the Star☆ telematic Services
   - Provides security and privacy to the data
   - Provides control in the access of services.
2. *The Patient Reference Dossier (PRD):*
   - The Patient Dossier is seen as a set of acts performed for a given patient.
   - Provides links to the various acts performed for a given patient (See Figure 1and Figure 2).
3. *Act Manager Server (AMS):*
   - Concerns the management and keeping track of the activities within the health care network.

- Provides links to data of the various activities concerning a patient, in most of the cases the data is distributed across the health care network.

4. *Enterprise Manager Servers (EMS), Local or Regional*:
- Describes the health resources provided at local or regional level.
- Management of resources at local or regional level.
- Describes the health care activities that may be performed in the health care organization of the health care service provider.

5. *Patient Reference Manager (PRM):*
- References to the acts performed for a specific patient are maintained by the patient reference manager.

6. *Booking Server (BS):*
- Provides interactive process demands for appointments.

For more information on Star✩ project, refer to Star✩ home page [3].Figure 4 shows the general Star✩ architecture.

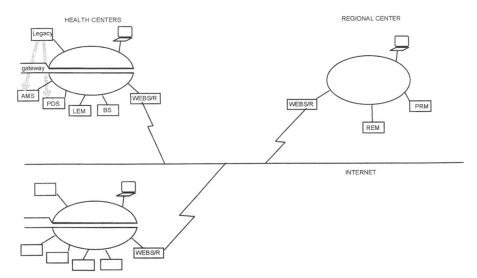

Figure 4: The Star✩ Architecture

5. Case study Pediatric Care at Crete

The Star✩ architecture will be applied and tested on the island of Crete to provide telematic services for the Pediatric Surgery Clinic of the University Hospital of Crete at Heraklion and the Health Care Center of Kastelli Kissamou at Chania.

The Pediatric Surgery Clinic is already using an electronic patient dossier software, which runs in Macintosh environment on the Omnis Data Base and is now migrating in ORACLE. The health care center of Kastelli at Chania will be in short time using an electronic patient dossier software implemented also in ORACLE. The main goal of Star✩ at Crete is to make those health care structures to inter-operate with each other. The Internet will be used to connect those two sites together while information exchange will be achieved via SQL, HTML and CGI scripts. SQL stands for Structured Query Language, HTML refers to Hypertext Mark-up Language and CGI to Common Gateway Interfaces.

This main goal breaks down into the following sub-goals:

1. An expert located at Kastelli Kissamou (Requester) should be able to refer a child to the Pediatric Surgery Clinic.
2. An expert located at the Pediatric Surgery Clinic(Performer) should be able to receive the referral and have access to the contents of the patient record located at Kastelli.
3. After the referral has been conducted and the child has entered the surgery clinic the requester should be able to view the contents of the patient record located at Heraklion.
4. An expert located anywhere at those two sites should be able to view and search for a patient located anywhere within this network.
5. An expert should be able to view specific contents of the patient record independent from its location

Work for the first year of the project have been conducted towards 1st and 2nd sub-goals. The Star☆ servers involved for the accomplishment of the above task are the Patient Reference Dossier (PRD), the Patient Reference Manager (PRM) and the Act Manager Server (AMS).

6. Conclusions

Evolution on technology has a direct impact on the way health care has been delivered. There is an urgent need for the synchronisation of health care, a very crucial social factor, to be able to meet the needs and requirements of a modern society. At Crete there is a clear requirement to replace the paper-based communication, between health care experts, with something more efficient. The Star☆ project seems to be a good solution towards this direction. Our main interests in future work is to implement and test in real world applications all the tasks referred in section 5 and when proven to be successful to expand this implementation to include more Hospital, Departments and Health Care Centers located across the island.

References

[1] B. Frandji and P. Cooper, Seamless Telematics Across Regions-Star☆, evolution and practical approach of open, modular, patient based health care solution, *In proceedings of MIE* '96, Copenhagen.
[2] Reference material mey be found on the World Wide Web at: http://www.ics.forth.gr
[3] Reference material mey be found on the World Wide Web at:
      http://www.compulink.co.uk/~haystacks/star/

Medical Informatics Europe '97
C. Pappas et al. (Eds.)
IOS Press, 1997

Spreading the clinical information system: which users are satisfied?

M.C. Mazzoleni[1], P. Baiardi[1], I. Giorgi[2], G. Franchi[1], R. Marconi[1], M. Cortesi[1]
[1]Medical Informatics Service, [2]Psychology Unit,
Salvatore Maugeri Foundation, IRCCS, Medical Center of Pavia, Italy

The present study deals with the assessment of the perceived usefulness and perceived ease of use of the clinical core of the HIS we are building, and progressively spreading into the medical centre, through the use of two questionnaires. The differences in subjective perception among clinical units and professional roles have been analyzed. Results show that the system, in use on a mandatory basis, has been accepted. Most of the users are satisfied, and probable removable causes of dissatisfaction have been identified.

Introduction

The assessment of information technology in health-care is a more and more important problem, particularly as regards hospital/clinical information systems (HIS). Direct use by physicians has traditionally been a goal difficult to be achieved, and failures are common experiences. On the other hand the potential utility of such systems is now out of discussion.

The satisfaction of the users is a necessary condition to the survival of an information system, and hence to the full realization of the medium- and long-term benefits.

Spreading the HIS we are developing inside the medical centre, and evaluating if, where and how to continue, we are interested into how much the HIS fits the needs of the users, how it is perceived by the users, and which are the weak points of the global system composed by the information system, the users, the context in which they use it.

The system

The HIS we are building[1], that is in use on mandatory basis, integrates administrative and clinical data for a small (177 beds, 5 clinical units) medical centre. It operates in the Windows environment with its standard graphic user interface, and consists of a set of modules providing, at present, for
- collection of demographic data
- entry and retrieval of encounter clinical data
- management of laboratory, radiology and nuclear medicine data, from the generation of requisitions (typically handled by nurses on physicians' indication) to the reporting and review of results
- creation of composite time-oriented view of data
- printing of discharge documents, and reports
- selection of patients matching user-defined conditions

At present the system covers the nephrology unit (N), the dialysis service (D), the general medicine unit (MG), and the oncology unit (O).

Methods

In order to assess the acceptance of the HIS by the users (physicians and nurses), we have developed two questionnaires in Italian, starting from those (fig.1,2) developed by Davis[2], aimed to the inspection of the constructs of perceived usefulness (PU) and ease of use (PEU) of information technology. From Davis study[2], reliability was tested through Cronbach alfa (.98 and .94 per PU and PEU respectively), and the factorial validity of PU and PEU was confirmed by factor analysis. The questionnaires are domain and technology independent, and have been used across industries, health-care included for commercially available software[3]. Each item was measured on a seven-point Likert scale, ranging from "Strongly disagree" (value -3), to "Strongly agree" (value +3), through the indifference (value 0).The usefulness score (SCU) and the ease of use score (SCE) are the equally weighted sum of the six individual items for each scale.

Confidential pen and paper questionnaires were distributed to all the personnel of the clinical units where the HIS was available, 6 months after the installation. Each person had to compile a sheet of general data, including age, clinical unit, professional status, previous experience in use of PC and self-reported personal frequency of use of the system.

1	Using [Technology X] allows me to accomplish tasks more quickly
2	Using [Technology X] improves my job performance
3	Using [Technology X] increases my productivity
4	Using [Technology X] enhances my effectiveness in the job
5	Using [Technology X] makes it easier to do my job
6	Overall, I find [Technology X] useful in my job

fig. 1 Items of the Perceived Usefulness Scale

1	Learning to operate [Technology X] would be easy for me
2	I would find it easy to get [Technology X] to do what I want it to do
3	My interaction with [Technology X] would be clear and understandable
4	I would find [Technology X] to be flexible to interact with
5	It would be easy for me to become skillful at using [Technology X]
6	I would find [Technology X] easy to use

fig. 2 Items of the Ease of Use Scale

The sample

81 of the 85 questionnaires returned, and hence the sample represents the 95% of the users and it is constituted by 22 physicians and 59 nurses.
Age is distributed in the range 21, 61 years with mean 34.4 ± 9.8.
45% of the users had previous experience in the use of PC: particularly 82% of the physicians and 30% of the nurses.
86% of the physicians declare they use the system many times a day, and the 14% once a day, while 27%,30%,32% of the nurses use the system respectively many times a day, once a day, many times a week.

Results and discussion

1. Global results

As regards the questionnaires, reliability was tested through Cronbach alfa (.91 and .92 per PU and PEU respectively).
No relationship has been found between SCU, SCE and age: according to other previous studies[4], in our centre the age of the uses is not a problem, but simply a commonplace.
Moreover, no significant differences have been found between experienced and inexperienced users for SCU,SCE, and particularly as regards learning to operate and becoming skillful at using the system (item 1st,5th PEU scale).
In the following, the results are detailed for scale, role of the user (physicians and nurses use different modules of the system) and clinical unit (for nephrology and dialysis units, physicians are gathered in a single group, since they work by turns in both the ward and the dialysis service).

2. Usefulness scale results

2.1 Physicians

Table 1 (like all the following tables) summarizes the percentages, referred to each clinical unit, of the negative, indifferent, and positive answers to the items of the usefulness scale, and the calculated score. Fig 3 shows the distribution of the answers on the Likert scale.

	1st item			2nd item			3rd item			4th item			5th item			6th item			SCU		
	<0	=0	>0	<0	=0	>0	<0	=0	>0	<0	=0	>0	<0	=0	>0	<0	=0	>0	<0	=0	>0
MG	40	30	40	0	20	80	80	20	0	40	20	40	60	20	20	10	20	70	60	0	40
N,D	14	14	72	0	43	57	14	43	43	0	43	57	14	0	86	0	0	100	14	0	86
O	80	0	20	0	0	100	40	20	40	0	20	80	0	40	60	0	0	100	20	0	80
Tot	41	18	41	0	23	77	50	27	23	18	27	55	32	18	50	5	9	86	36	0	64

Tab. 1: Results (%) of PU questionnaire and SCU score for physicians

Considering the physicians as a whole, the percentage of positive answers (86%) to the last item (Overall, I find the system useful in my job) is higher than the one of SCU (64%). We think that they perceive other benefits than those included in the questionnaire, or they had difficulties in including these benefits in the categories proposed by the questionnaire.

This not so good a result for SCU is principally due to the scarcely positive perception in MG unit (only 40% of positive SCU, median 0, range -8,10). As shown in fig 3, the answers are spread over the negative part of the Likert scale more than for the other units. Being MG the biggest unit (10 physicians), the analysis phase of the informatization project has involved only a portion of the personnel: inspecting each user answers, the users who had not participated to the discussion reveal a worse perception in terms of usefulness.

100% of non negative answers for item 2 (...improves my job performance) and 77% for item 4 (...enhances my effectiveness in my job) show that the system is achieving the goal of being a tool to enhance quality in the care delivery process.

Rather less than 50% of the users think that using the system is more time-consuming (item 1st and 3rd usefulness scale), but this doesn't penalize the perception in terms of the usefulness on the whole they have of the system (95% of non negative answers for item 6th). This is particularly true for O unit: it must be noted that the physicians of this unit previously had a small but, accurately tailored to their minimal needs, system, whose use was necessarily less expensive in term of time resources.

On the other hand, 86% of the physicians of N,D unit gave non negative answers to item 1st (...allows me to accomplish tasks more quickly) and 3rd (...increases my productivity) of the usefulness scale: they have always had a heavy need of monitoring and documenting the evolution of chronic patients during long periods, particularly as regards dialysis treatments, lab tests, clinical notes. The interfacement of laboratories and diagnostic services, and the integration of ward and dialysis service in the hospital information system and has relieved them of a certain number of activities.

For MG unit, item 3rd has the highest percentage of negative answers (80%). No particular problems have been identified through PEU questionnaires and a further cause of wasting time could be the often-complained difficult sharing of a workstation by more than one physician.

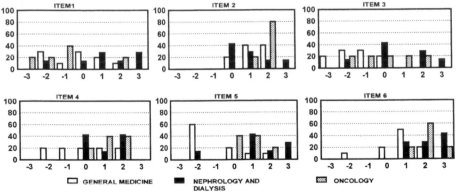

FIG. 3 USEFULNESS SCALE - PHYSICIANS . PERCENTAGES ARE REFERRED TO EACH SINGLE UNIT

2.2 Nurses

Considering nurses as a whole, the percentage of positive SCU (87%) is high and comparable to the one of the positive answers (93%) to the last item of the scale (Overall, I find the system useful in my job).

	1st item			2nd item			3rd item			4th item			5th item			6th item			SCU		
	<0	=0	>0	<0	=0	>0	<0	=0	>0	<0	=0	>0	<0	=0	>0	<0	=0	>0	<0	=0	>0
MG	0	18	82	18	9	73	0	64	36	0	0	100	0	9	91	0	0	100	0	0	100
N	42	16	42	9	8	83	67	25	8	58	9	33	42	8	50	34	0	66	42	0	58
D	0	0	100	14	10	76	24	19	57	14	14	72	9	0	91	0	0	100	14	0	86
O	0	0	100	0	0	100	13	0	87	0	0	100	0	0	100	0	0	100	0	0	100
Tot	8	7	85	10	7	83	25	24	51	17	7	76	12	3	85	7	0	93	13	0	87

Tab. 2: Results (%) of PU questionnaire and SCU score for nurses

All the unit are aligned, with the exception of N whose answers are the most negative for all the items of the scale. As shown (fig.4), the answers are spread on the negative part of the Likert scale more than for all the other units, and SCU is in the range -10,10 with median 1.

Moreover , for most of the items, the answers of MG,D,O unit are grouped around value +2.Since the nurses of N unit use the same modules that are used in O and MG unit, the reasons for this scarcely positive perception of the system must be looked for in the organizational context of the nurses group, and in the workflow following the round the physicians with the nurse in chief perform twice a day. It must be noted also that, as regards the frequency of use, that is consequence of the organization of the unit, in MG 9/11, in O 4/15, while in only N 1/12 of the nurses use the system more than once a day, and a positive relationship exists between SCU and frequency of use[5].

As it occurs for physicians, item 3rd (...increases my productivity) has the worst results (25% of negative answers), while item 1st (...accomplish tasks more quickly) show that nurses save time using the system, being relieved of many routine activities, particularly in D and O, where activities are often standardized.

We would have expected even higher values for the answers of unit D, since a few facilities were implemented particularly to help the staff of the unit to produce administrative report, certifications, etc. Actually these additional tools are used only by two nurses in chief, and their answers are, indeed, over the mean.

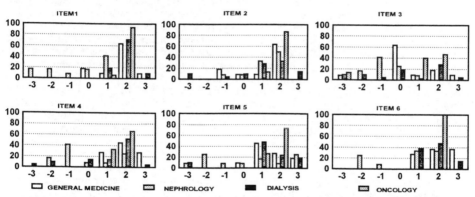

FIG. 4 USEFULNESS SCALE - NURSES . PERCENTAGES ARE REFERRED TO EACH SINGLE UNIT

3. Ease of use scale results

3.1 Physicians

The results for ease of use scale (tab. 3) are substantially all positive.

N,D unit shows a lower percentage of positive SCE (72%) due to item 2nd (...easy to get it to do what I want it to do) and 3rd (...interaction ..clear and understandable), where answers are negative for 43% and 29% respectively.

The physicians of MG unit, whose usefulness perception is the lowest, don't declare to have particular problems in using and interacting with the system , while O unit physicians show an even too positive ease of use perception. Being the last unit to be informatized, probably training and support in the initial period has been supplied with more care, due to the experience matured in the other previous units. Moreover some abruptness of the common procedures had already been smoothed when O unit was integrated in HIS.

No problem with learning and becoming skillful.

	1st item			2nd item			3rd item			4th item			5th item			6th item			SCE		
	<0	=0	>0	<0	=0	>0	<0	=0	>0	<0	=0	>0	<0	=0	>0	<0	=0	>0	<0	=0	>0
MG	20	0	80	30	0	70	30	0	70	20	0	80	20	0	80	20	0	80	20	0	80
N,D	0	0	100	43	0	57	29	14	57	0	0	100	14	0	86	0	29	71	14	14	72
O	0	0	100	0	0	100	0	0	100	0	0	100	0	0	100	0	0	100	0	0	100
Tot	9	0	91	27	0	73	23	5	72	9	0	91	14	0	86	9	9	82	9	9	82

Tab. 3: Results (%) of PEU questionnaire and SCE score for physicians

3.2 Nurses

Good global results as regards ease of use perception also for nurses (tab. 4). The percentages of positive answers are higher than 75% for all the items, except item 2nd (...easy to get it to do what I want it to do). Difficulties in getting the system to do what the nurse wants it to do are common to all of the units, and no relationship with both frequency of use and previous experience has been found. Optimization of the HIS modules used by nurses should be taken into account.

	1st item			2nd item			3rd item			4th item			5th item			6th item			SCE		
	<0	=0	>0	<0	=0	>0	<0	=0	>0	<0	=0	>0	<0	=0	>0	<0	=0	>0	<0	=0	>0
MG	18	0	82	27	9	63	9	0	91	36	0	64	18	0	82	9	0	91	9	18	73
N	8	0	92	25	8	67	0	0	100	25	8	67	17	0	83	17	8	75	17	0	83
D	9	5	86	33	0	67	33	0	67	19	5	76	14	10	76	14	0	86	24	0	76
O	0	0	100	27	0	73	7	0	93	0	0	100	0	0	100	0	0	100	0	0	100
Tot	8	2	90	29	5	66	15	0	85	19	3	78	12	3	85	10	2	88	14	3	87

Tab. 4: Results (%) of PEU questionnaire and SCE score for nurses

Conclusions

The tool we used to inspect the acceptance of the system has the intrinsic characteristic of being oriented to a subjective evaluation of the system and of producing results that are affected by the environmental conditions and the recent past experiences of the users.

Since, at least now, we are interested into how our system fits the needs of our users, this low cost tool has reviled to be useful, letting us know and document the weak points of the global system composed by the information system, the users, the context and the way in which they use it. Focusing on the hospital information system, and particularly to the clinical core of it, we are setting up, the results of perceived usefulness and perceived ease of use questionnaires show that most of the user are satisfied. The fact that the system is integrated in the daily routine activity and is used by physicians and nurses for all the patients and for all the encounters in all the clinical unit that have been informatized can be considered an a posteriori judgment of having achieved at least a medium level of usability.

The often-mentioned problem such as age of the users and unfamiliarity with computers have revealed to be prejudices. Through the analysis of the negative answers, we could identify some probable causes, fortunately removable, of dissatisfaction related to both the system itself, and the context in which it has grown and is used.

Critical aspects in the perception of the system are:

- the knowledge the users have of the system, that can be increased by a broad participation of the users to the analysis phase of the informatization project, and by an intensive use by all the users.
- a good organization of the activities in which the system is involved: no system can solve by itself problems of organization, on the contrary it can underline them.
- the availability of an adequate number of workstations to let the users exploit their time at best
- the consciousness that the feeling of paternity some users have of programs they had used (and sometimes developed too) for a long time can't be erased without effort.
- the identification of functionalities representing an added value for a large number of users.

References

1. Mazzoleni MC. et al Pursuing Usableness and effectiveness in the development of a shared patient centered information system. Proceedings of 18th SCAMC, Washington, DC, 1994; 658-62.
2. Davis F. Perceived Usefulness, Perceived Ease of Use, and User Acceptance of Information Technology. MIS Qarterly,1989; 13:319-340
3. Kattan M.W., Adams D.A. Explaining Information technology Use with Usefulness Scale: A Comparison with User Age. Proceedings of 18th SCAMC, Washington, DC, 1994; 81-85
4. Clayton P. Pulver G., Hill C. Physician Use of Computers. Is Age or Value the Predominant Factor? Proceedings of 17th SCAMC, Washington, DC, 1993; 301-305.
5. Mazzoleni MC et al. Assessing users' satisfaction through perception of usefulness and easy of use in the daily interaction with a hospital information system. Proceedings of 20th SCAMC, 1996; 752-56.

Medical Informatics Europe '97
C. Pappas et al. (Eds.)
IOS Press, 1997

Security of the Electronic Health Record

Francis H. ROGER FRANCE
*Centre for Medical Informatics of the University of Louvain
and St Luc Hospital, 1200 Brussels, Belgium*

Abstract. The Electronic Health Record (EHR) raises new challenges for security. Only authorized persons having a "right to know" can have access to identifiable patient data. Differences between the paper record and the EHR are first described. Several solutions in order to assure confidentiality, integrity and accessibility to patient information are then proposed.

From paper to electronic patient records

For clinicians, as well as for public health professionals, the present contribution of informatics and telematics is a mutation from multiple records in paper to the integrated electronic health record of the patient.

The patient record can be defined as a depository of all information related to a patient, both individual and collective, constantly updated. By integration, we mean the management of medical, nursing and administrative information on a patient through a common data base that can be accessed at distance for various applications.

The traditional paper record is often fragmented by medical speciality or by professional function in many European countries. It is easily unreadable and acts, therefore, mainly as a memory for the individual physician. The access to documents in paper can only be done where it stands, in one physical location.

On the contrary, the electronic patient record (EPR) is made by various health professionals. The registration of identification is obtained by administrative personnel, clinical data are entered by physicians and further notes by nurses and others. Its access is ubiquitous in a computerised network. The record is highly structured, well ordered, and linkage from various data sources can be obtained by using unique identifiers. The EPR can reach many more objectives than the paper record. It is not only aimed at helping delivery of care but allows also to evaluate performance and quality of care as well as to perform clinical and epidemiological research. It is a tool for financing and policy making.

This paper has arisen from the author's involvement in the ISHTAR Project (Implementing Secure Healthcare Telematics Applications in Europe). A Telematics Applications for Health Project (HC 1028) of CEC DGXIIIc.

A strategic choice requiring an adequate structure

The integrated EHR should be seen as a fundamental strategic choice in any health care institution. At the end, only one record can be maintained, because double records are costly to update and raise legal questions (Möhr, 1995) [1].

Furthermore, linkage between hospital care and general practice, as well as between clinical and public health research should be planned and provided.

These objectives could not be reached if an appropriate structure is not set up. In a large university hospital in Brussels (St-Luc) a Board for the management of health informatics has been appointed, under the authority of the general director and the hospital Board.

This Board includes a representative of the direction of the hospital, the head nurse, the coordinator of informatics, and chiefs of staff for the departments of medicine, surgery, radiology, clinical laboratories, medical records, as well as the president of the medical council.

Several advisory committees have been created, among which the "security committee" and a task force on the EHR.

Among the numerous choices that have been made up to know, let's quote :

(1) a distinction between the *"temporary" record* (including new results, provisional diagnoses and current plans) and the *"permanent" record* (archived, after dismissal, including a final report and the financial record of the patient).
The temporary record uses mainly the communication network for direct individual patient care, while the permanent record is managed in a data base that allows the application of results to a large number of patients. In the short and median terms, it will be needed to have access simultaneously to paper, images and electronic data, which implies a double maintenance.

(2) users require *"easy to use" workstations* (Carpenter, 1994) [2]. Workstation computers should be programmed to shut down if left idle. They should be connected to a security system (a chip card for user identification, linkage to a "usher" software referring to a table of allowed accesses, followed by a specific data bank for journaling and protected by a firewall).

(3) *communication standards* should be defined, if possible at the European level (CENTC251) in order to allow data transfer between physicians for health care of individual patients and comparison of information between health practices, anonymously. Following a recommendation by a group of experts to the Ministry of Public Health, to which we participated, it has been proposed to divide the medical record into *sections*. They are used as "headings" by speciality and by period of time, to be declared before any data transmission.

Each section contains a *data set* that has been organised in five types :

* clinical notes and protocols
* laboratory results
* therapeutic orders

* record summaries, allowing to be assembled by patient in a "Master Sheet"
* patient personal notes

In this perspective, the patient is becoming a partner in health care.

Reference systems have to be added, such as a vocabulary server, in relation to uniform coding systems, if possible international.

Decision aids could also be associated to factual data, in order to obtain "evidence based medicine" information systems.

This structure corresponds to the object oriented software. At St Luc, the data base management system is in SQL (Sybase), associated to SQL Windows and C++ for development programs.

(4)   The "architecture" of the electronic patient record has to take into account the multiples levels of specialised information systems that should be integrated harmoniously in the hospital network : administrative systems, laboratories, imaging, clinical departments, medical record archiving system, ...

Security issues

The integrated EHR is a special challenge for security. No clinician in charge of patients will accept it if he cannot be confident in the absence of danger to consult it. Only persons having "the right to know" can be authorized to have access to identifiable EHRecords.

Traditionally, clinicians have been sensitised to patient data *confidentiality*, (e.g. the prevention of access of non authorized persons to identifiable information), which is only a part of *security*. The EHR requires also data *integrity* (e.g. the prevention of modification of information) and *accessibility* (e.g. prevention of lack of availability at the right time). (F.H. Roger France, 1996) [3].

Confidentiality can be ensured by the *identification* of the requester (who ?) associated to its *authentication* (prove it). The technical tool most often chosen is a chip card for these two functions.

Authorization can then be done through tables of access by specific user, where rules should be easy to follow: only a physician and assisted health care professionals in charge of a case can have access to patient data; all other cases have to remain anonymous. For research purposes, a specific contract has to be made. In all cases, patients have to be informed of data collection and uses.

In order to assess if these rules have been well followed, a *monitoring system* has to be designed (journaling) where an appointed security officer has to play his role. Electronic transfer of data through networks requests encryption of health information. Record systems should have internal roadblocks to prevent workers from accessing information outside their job requirements. Organizations with Internet connections should have a "firewall" to deny unauthorized entry.

Physicians and public health concerns

Of great concern is the present use of only passwords that are not sufficient to protect the identification of the requester. Also, several software companies have not provided yet enough security tools to implement basic security guidelines for health care. Local software can often be seen as additional applications that could be bypassed by knowledgeable information specialists.

The most difficult issue is most likely the question of access of the patient to his own record. As this knowledge might make harm to some patients, it is recommended that access should be done through a physician designed by them.

When a national law on the European Directive does not cover some persons (students, external data managers, ...) specific contracts have to be written to overcome some omissions or to clarify some situations.

In order to allow long term integrity and accessibility, archived data should remain accessible in future, which requires a strong management for data maintenance. Information supports vary with time as well as software, such as mass retrieval robots.

References

(1)   Mohr D.N., Carpenter P.C., Claus P.L., Hagen P.T., Karsell P.R., Van Scay R.E.
        Implementing an Electronic Medical Record : Paper's last Hurrah
        AMIA, 157-161, 1995

(2)   Carpenter P.C., *The Electronic Medical Record : perspective from Mayo Clinic*
        Int. J. Biomed. Computing (34), 159-171, 1994

(3)   Roger France F.H., *Control and use of health information : a doctor's perspective*
        Int. J. Biomed. Computing (43), 19-25, 1996

Medical Informatics Europe '97
C. Pappas et al. (Eds.)
IOS Press, 1997

Basic rules for the security of frozen section diagnosis through image transmission between anatomo-pathologists

P. DUSSERRE*, F.-A. ALLAERT**, L. DUSSERRE**

*Centre de Pathologie - 33 rue Bornier - 21000 Dijon France
** Service de Biostatistique et informatique medicale du C.H.U. de Dijon B.P. 1542 21034 Dijon France

Abstract : Telemedicine can provide an alternative solution to the lack of medical resources in areas where the population is no longer dense enough to justify the temporary or permanent presence of certain specialists such as anatomo-pathologists. In the long run certain pre-operational frozen section examinations cannot be carried out without putting the quality of healthcare at stake. The telematic transmission of macro and microscopic images of lesions, under the supervision of a surgeon, to an anatomo-pathologist consultant located off premises allows for the maintenance of equitable care of acceptable quality.

Key words : telemedicine, pathological anatomy, security.

Introduction

Demographic evolution seems to gravitate towards a concentration of the population into urban zones, resulting in a relative desertification of other areas where the density of the inhabitants can no longer guarantee that certain medical specialists will have enough patients to insure their livelihood or that of those who may later replace them.

Telemedicine itself has reached an advanced enough level to fill the gap left by specialists and to maintain an equitable and acceptable access to healthcare by making it possible for patients to be treated from afar.

The biggest difficulties in anatomic pathology could appear in the area of frozen section examinations which require the presence of an anatomo-pathologist who assists the surgeon during the operation. The possibility of transmitting macroscopic and microscopic images of a lesion from a remote place through a telematic line, under the supervision of a surgeon, is a viable alternative to the impossibility of having an anatomic pathologist in person. This technique is therefore referred to as a telediagnosis in anatomic pathology or simply as telepathology. Because these new ways of working (1,2) imply new responsibilities, the systems of security for telepathology, must necessarily be carefully monitored to insure their safety.

After describing the practical aspects of the frozen section examination through image transmission, we will turn to the basic rules needed to guarantee its security.

1. Performing an anatomo-pathological frozen section examination through image transmission

After a review of the pre-operational frozen section examination and its environment, we will consider the role of telediagnosis and its consequences for the patient, the surgeon, the anatomo-pathologist and the healthcare system.

1.1 The pre-operational frozen section examination and its environment

Until recently a patient with a neoplasic lesion was usually operated on in two phases. The first phase consisted of a simple excision biopsy carried out on the affected tissues and then sent to an anatomic pathology laboratory to determine whether it was benign or malignant. When the tumor was revealed to be cancerous after receiving the analysis results a few days later, the second phase consisted of a possible complementary surgical operation.

Over the years however, the pathologist was called more and more often into the operating room by the surgeon to assist in making decisions about the operation by providing a diagnosis during a so-called anatomic pathology frozen section examination.

Because of the progress made in the various techniques used in the preparation of microscopic slices, the field of accessible organs and their possible diagnosis in frozen section examinations has grown considerably and the method has become of unreputable interest and value. Demands have become such that today pathologists can no longer answer all the needs of the clinics and hospitals in a given region. Moreover the pathologist who used to study a preparation had to diagnose alone and within minutes the appropriateness of the operation. It was impossible to ask a colleague's advice on the spot. If unsure, he had to accept the fact that the diagnosis could not be given immediately. Therefore, the surgeon and the patient had to wait for the laboratory results and, if need be, the opinion of several specialists.

1.2 The role of the telediagnosis in the pre-operational frozen section examination

Progress can be made quickly if telediagnostic achievements are used. In order for this to happen the operating room must be provided with the necessary material for adequate microscopic preparations and an image recording system enabling its numerization and transmission through a healthcare network. With its emitting system, the building is connected to the receptors of the telediagnostic network, which allows for the microscopic examination of the removed tissue.

1.3 The methodology of the frozen section examination through the telematic system

There are two possible situations, depending on the presence or absence of a pathologist in the operating room.

1.3.1 The pathologist is present at the time of the operation

In the case of an uncertain diagnosis, the pathologist, because of the telematic network, can directly communicate the images he is unsure about to a consultant at a more or less remote pathology centre. Undisputably there is an increase in the quality and reliability of the diagnosis.

1.3.2 The pathologist is not present for the operation

If the telediagnosis has been planned, the procedure is the following :

The surgeon needing a confirmation of his diagnosis telephones the pathologist he has planned to contact. They simultaneously watch the same macroscopic and topographic image on their respective screens. The pathologist chooses the problem zones on the screen in collaboration with the surgeon and guides the biopsy. The tissues thus obtained are passed on to a technician trained to manipulate cryostat and to use quick dyes. A series of images are sent to the pathologist who discusses with the surgeon, confirms the diagnosis or offers another. In this manner the surgeon can continue the operation with full knowledge of the nature of the lesion. The tissues are then sent to a laboratory to be examined according to the usual protocol.

When a telediagnosis is needed in unforeseen circumstances this means that the surgeon has to face an emergency that he cannot identify. He uses the network to contact an available pathologist and, from a distance, the latter participates through telediagnosis according to the previous modality applications.

2. The security of the anatomic-pathology frozen section examination through the telematic system

For hospitals and clinics that do not have a pathologist present, the frozen section examination through telediagnosis is of utmost value provided that its security can be guaranteed. The three main functions of security - confidentiality, integrity, and availability of information - must be insured at the time that the frozen section diagnosis by telematics is taking place.

2.1 The confidentiality of the frozen section examinations through a telematic system

According to the different standardization organizations, the definition of confidentiality is *the property which assures that only authorized users, in normal conditions can have access to the system*. Consequently, this protects the private lives of those individuals who are subject to give their personal details for automatised treatment.

In a system of tele-expertise, there are numerous possibilities for the violation of confidentiality. This can be in the form of theft (of all or part of the system), manipulation errors, whereby information is sent to people not meant to receive it, unauthorized access, falsifying the user's identity, making unauthorized file copies, intercepting messages, etc. All of these possibilities underline the need for physical and computerized protection of the system.

Physical protection requires that a computer system be placed in a protected zone, ideally in a closed room equipped with anti-intrusion detectors. This zone must have a sealed door and have a lock and a digital style electronic alarm system or a micro-processed card reader. For daily use all of the security elements are rarely found together especially when information systems are located in open structures such as medical services where many people circulate. The basic precaution needed to avoid material theft, simple and effective in most cases, is to attach these systems to their bases.

Computerized security entails the protection of the system through passwords or the much more effective micro-processed card reading mechanism for health professionals. The latter process will soon be widely available in private and public hospitals. It will allow the doctor to identify and authenticate himself as such and to name his diagnostic conclusions. Other complementary devices can be recommended such as the automatic stop which is set off as soon as the system is no longer being used after 1 or 2 minutes. It is then necessary for the user to identify himself in order to restart it. A large number of breaches of confidentiality happen on systems which are left to function without surveillance through thoughtlessness or negligence. As concerns the network, the installation of anti-intrusion devices of the firewall kind also protects against the risks of distant « hacking ».

Whatever the relevance and power of technical solutions used to protect information, they are ineffective if not accompanied by serious efforts to make the staff aware of the importance of respecting confidentiality. They must be warned of the risks and heavy fines which threaten those who contribute, directly or indirectly, voluntarily, or involuntarily, to the disclosure of registered medical information.

It is, unfortunately, the staff users of the information system who is both in charge of its maintenance and protection, and the ones who are usually the source of problems. Careless talk, the loan or loss of an access card and its personal code, or simple laxness about security rules can be considered as serious offences in light of their possible consequences. The members of staff, however, can only be held responsible if they were warned beforehand of their duties in this area, but this is rarely the case. Such information should be considered the object of oral and written explanations at the interviewing stage for the job. To materialize the solemn commitment of the staff towards the ethical code and of medical information rights, a contract could be written up and signed by the future employee.

2.2 The integrity of a system of frozen section examinations through a telematic system

Integrity is the quality which insures that information is only modified by its habitual users in normally provided circumstances.

Checking computer entries requires not only allowing entry rights based on one's identification and authentification, but also a signature for any modification of pre-existing information or of any supplementary data. In a tele-expertise transaction, all clinical information and images sent for advice must in the future be signed electronically through the use of a personal card for health professionals so that the doctor who asked for advice cannot deny his interaction with the doctor referred to in the face of a legal conflict. The latter must also sign his response. To supplement this and avoid all lawsuits for delayed answers or the reception of several confusing responses which could interfere with the process, all messages should include the date and time they were sent. All the features of the tele-expertise transaction - clinical data, images, answers given, dates and times - will then be electronically secured into the computer and recorded on a non-erasable recording device so that they cannot be modified. In the case of a lawsuit this can serve as possible proof. The solution would be to have a trusted third party certifying all transactions. However, on a daily basis, their number and volume are so great that it would be a major task to undertake.

Dealing with all the data which the transmission of images and information requires, also creates opportunities for the breach of integrity. The consequences of these violations depend both on their importance and on the field of study they take place in ; the technical solutions should be adapted depending on how tolerable the violation is. A few missing data bits only slightly alter the transmitted image quality whereas it can fundamentally change the meaning of the numbered results.

When there are no acceptable alterations, cryptographic functions can be an efficient monitor. When the information is sent out, all of it is transformed into a given value by a mathematical algorithm. The same algorithm is applied to the information received. The slightest variation between the information sent and that received creates substantial differences in the numbered results before and after transmission. For this reason it is easy to detect. A more classic method would consist of sending out several pieces of information and checking the equivalence of each piece received. The major problem with this method is that it is time consuming and just as sensitive as the cryptage technique. On the other hand, it allows for the identification of altered information with precision.

Because of the possible alterations to transmitted data, all frozen section examinations put through the telematic system must be validated before being used in order to judge if a possible breach of integrity of information can have an effect on the quality of the service provided. For anatomic-pathologists, a validation of the RESINTEL system took place between Boston and Dijon to show that the diagnosis given from glass slides or transmitted images were the same and that changes due to the transferring process did not affect their intrinsic qualities.

2.3 The availability of a frozen section examination through a telematic system

Availability is the skill of an information system to be used by authorized users in normally provided conditions of access.

An information system's unavailability results either in major breaches of its integrity as concerns its data, application program or materials or a lack of technical and human organisation needed for it to function properly.

The organisation of a system of frozen section examinations through telematics cannot be limited to the installment of a work station linked to a telecommunication network. The medical, paramedical, and technical staff must be prepared to insure the availability of the proposed services. The surgeon asking for advice expects the response of an expert with the necessary qualifications and experience.

Before setting up such a system, serious thought needs to go into putting all the operating conditions into place, making sure that it will be run efficiently and that it is sound in order to insure the system's continuity.

3. Conclusion

Putting a system of anatomic pathology frozen section diagnosis in place through the transmission of images does not only involve laboratory equipment and operation rooms with stations that transmit and receive anatomic pathology images. It also requires a technical environment and administrative organisation which insures its running order in conditions that guarantee confidentiality of exchanged data, their integrity and the continuity of services in the given period. If there is harm done to a patient because of laxness towards these security rules, the hospital and its doctors would be held responsible.

From the start, telediagnosis must be conceived as an alternative solution to a lack of medical resources when taking into account the constraints which result from this and not as a method used when worst comes to worst and which can be more or less improvised.

References

[1] L.Dusserre, F.A. Allaërt, Is telemedicine legal and ethical ? Information and health. Medical information. Legal ethical aspects and public health. "SpringerVerlag", 1996, nb 8, 67-1-6.

[2] L. Dusserre, Legal and ethical aspects of telediagnosis in medicine. Bull. "Ordre des Médecins", nb 6, 1993.

[3] F.A Allaërt, L. Dusserre, Making information systems secure. "Médecins des Hôpitaux ", 1994, nb 41,11-14.

[4] Allaërt F.A., Genestar 0. Physical security of computer systems. Gestions Hospitalières, 1994, nb 339, 646-648.

[5] F. A. Allaërt, D. Weinberg, P. Dusserre, P. J. Yvon, L. Dusserre, Evaluation of a telepathology system between Boston (USA) and Dijon (France) - Glass slides versus telediagnostic TV Monitor. Nineteenth annual symposium on computer applications in medical care. JAMIA. Proceedings SCAMC, 596-600.

[6] F. A. Allaërt, L. Dusserre, Telemedicine and responsibility. Arch. Anat. Cytol. Path. 1995, 4, 200-205.

Medical Informatics Europe '97
C. Pappas et al. (Eds.)
IOS Press, 1997

Implementing Security
On a Prototype Hospital Database

Marie KHAIR (1), George PANGALOS (2), Foteini ANDRIA (2), Lefteris BOZIOS (3)

(1) Computers Department, Faculty of Sciences, Notre Dame University, Zouk Mosbeh, PO Box 72, Zouk Mikael, Lebanon. mkhair@ndu.edu.lb

(2) Computers Division, Faculty of Technology, General Department, Aristotle University of Thessaloniki, 540 06 Thessaloniki, Greece. gip@eng.auth.gr, fanr@egnatia.ee.auth.gr

(3) Information Technology Dept., AHEPA Hospital, 546 36 Thessaloniki, Greece

Abstract. This paper describes the methodology used and the experience gained from the application of a new secure database design approach and database security policy in a real life hospital environment. The applicability of the proposed database security policy in a major Greek general hospital is demonstrated. Moreover, the security and quality assurance of the developed prototype secure database is examined, taking into consideration the results from the study of the user acceptance.

1. Introduction

A hospital is a typical case of a security critical environment [3], [4]. Due to the widespread use of the database technology and its role and nature, database security plays today a significant role in the overall security of health care information systems [5]. The development of a secure database system requires an appropriate multiphase design methodology which will guide the steps of the development and will provide tools supporting the automatic execution of some steps [1]. Such a design methodology has been proposed in [4] and [5].

In this paper we will focus on the problems related to the application of this methodology and the experience gained from its experiment implementation in a major Greek general hospital.

2. Overview of the proposed secure database design methodology

The two most well known database security policies are the mandatory and the discretionary one [1], which both have proved to be insufficient to cover the security needs of the health care environments [5]. The proposed methodology and security policy is based on the integration of mandatory and discretionary security policies [3],[4],[5]. A step by step design methodology with integrated security has been proposed. The responsibility of the role in the application determines the security label (clearance) of the user role. The user roles are assigned a node at the user role hierarchy. According to the data the user roles need to access, security labels (classification) are assigned to data. Polyinstantiation is supported only in the form of cover stories, due to the support of the write down mechanism (with no fear of inference), which is essential for the hospital environment. A detailed description of the proposed methodology can be found in [4], [5].

3. Pilot Implementation of the Proposed Security Policy

The AHEPA general university hospital was used as a testbed for the implementation of our proposed secure database design methodology in a real life hospital environment. There is a long-standing cooperation between the informatics laboratory and the EDP unit of the AHEPA hospital [2], [4], [5]. Following, we will describe briefly the information system of the hospital and the functions which the prototype secure hospital database SEC_AXEPA was designed to serve.

3.1. Implementation of the prototype secure hospital database SEC_AXEPA

The integrated information system of AHEPA hospital covers the patient administration system (inpatient-outpatient), billing, financial, personal management and payroll. It has been running since 1990 and operates on an inter network of distributed databases based on the client-server model. The application SEC_AXEPA has been developed in order to serve the in-patient administration purposes. This implementation will be used as a pilot for the subsequent implementation of the whole secure hospital information system.

The prototype hospital database SEC_AXEPA was implemented on Ingres, a relational DBMS (since there was not a Trusted DBMS available). The data sets loaded on the prototype hospital database are: the nurse record, the doctor record, the personal patient information record , the patient medical record, the laboratory information and the follow-up information. During his/ her hospitalisation, the patient identification is based on a serial number assigned to him/her, when he/she checks in.

Being a relational database management system, Ingres stores data in tables. The labelling of the data sets can change dynamically, if one of the security constraints is satisfied, leading to upgrading and/or fragmentation. The classification level of each tuple of a table was implemented by adding at each table a column, which was only visible to the D.B.A., and contained the tuple classification. That is 1,2,3 and 0 respectively for confidential, secret, top secret and cover story. Another additional column was added to the related medical data tables, containing the flag 'h' (history) or 'l' (last). It is automatically updated, when new data was inserted. This is one of the integrity constraints that were implemented in the prototype database.

When a user accesses the database, a corresponding user interface is automatically presented to him/her, based on the user group (doctor or nurse) where he/she belongs to. We also support two user roles for the nurse group; the special nurse and the normal nurse, which are given respectively a high and a low level of clearance. The use of Ingres rules and procedures, that create convenient cover stories, had made it possible for these user roles to have the same user interfaces in the application. The security labels which were defined during the secure conceptual design phase were implemented using the notions of roles and groups supported by Ingres. After performing a study on the considered users roles (doctor, nurse, and normal nurse), clearance level 3, 2 and 1 were respectively assigned them.

The access types supported from the secure prototype application are: insert, read, update, execute, cancel. Thus, the possibility of deleting information is excluded, not only for reasons of better control of the information flow, but also for reducing the possibility of fatal mistakes. For the better understanding of the implementation, we will describe next the processing of the security constraints.

3.2. Security Constraints Processing

3.2.1. Definition of the security constraints

The security classification constraints are specified by the database designer in co-operation with the application users [6]. Their application and processing may result to fragmentation and/or upgrading of the classification of some data sets in the medical database [5]. It must be noted that we will use the illness HIV (AIDS) as a representative of every sensitive illness and the characterism VIP (Very Important Person) for the people whose medical record is considered sensitive (that is important people, hospital staff personnel, political, and other well known persons, etc.). Moreover we will represent the unclassified level by 1, the secret by 2, and the top secret by 3.

Below we will define the security constraints that have been applied to the secure prototype application SEC_AXEPA. First we present them informally (as they were defined by the users), we categorise them and then we transform them into mathematical language.

♦*Constraint 1*: The sensitivity level of the name determines the sensitivity level of all the patient personal information. Level-Based Constraint, LbC(PAT-PERS-INFO,{*},name).

♦*Constraint 2:* The name of the patient is always considered top secret, so the personal information is always considered top secret. Simple Constraint, SiC(PAT-PERS-INFO,{name},3). Then, SiC(PAT-PERS-INFO,{*},3). stands for both constraints 1 and 2.

♦*Constraint 3*: The data concerning the disease in the patient medical record is considered secret, if the disease is HIV.

Content-Based Constraint, CbC(Diagnoses,{*},Diagnosis,'=','HIV',2).

♦*Constraint 4*: If the lab result is HIV, then the information concerning the lab-test is considered secret. Complex Constraint, CoC(PAT-LAB-EXAMS,{*},LAB-EXAM-RESULT,'=','HIV',2).

♦*Constraint 5*: If the lab result is HIV, then the information concerning the diagnosis is considered secret. Complex Constraint, CoC(Diagnoses,{Diagnosis},LAB-TEST-RESULT,Lab-exam-result,'=','HIV',2).

♦*Constraint 6*: A nurse should always be able to look at the patient's diagnosis (no matter what his/her status is). This is supported, in order he/she to be able to offer convenient care to the patient and at the same time take himself/herself suitable precautions. In the case of a sensitive diagnosis (see constraint 5), a suitable cover story is created.

♦*Constraint 7*: If the patient is a VIP, then no matter the diagnosis for the patient, it is considered secret and a suitable cover story is created, in order to prevent normal nurses to infer sensitive information. Complex Constraint, CbC(Diagnoses,{Diagnosis}, PAT-PERS-INFO,P-status,'=','1',2) AND cover story.

♦*Constraint 8:* The property ICD9-code of diagnosis is considered secret, while the values of ICD9-code, without information as to whom they refer to, are considered unclassified.

Association-Based Constraint , AbC(Diagnoses, {ICD9-code}, 2).

♦*Constraint 9*: The information of the prescription of a doctor to a certain patient is considered unclassified. However, the aggregation of the prescriptions given to a patient is considered secret, since it may indicate the changes in the patient's health condition.

Aggregation Constraint, AgC(Prescribes, {Doses}, '3', 2).

♦*Constraint 10*: The laboratory exam results are considered unclassified.. In that way, a lab staff member can access all the results of the exams, even if they concern a sensitive disease

(HIV). However, if that user accesses the corresponding diagnosis made for the same patient and realise that it is different from the HIV, he/she can infer the existence of cover stories. This problem is solved by assigning to users and data apart from levels of sensitivity, disjoint categories. Inference Constraint, IfC(Diagnoses, {Diagnosis}, LAB-TEST-RESULT, {lab-exam-result}, corresponding category}.

Since we support tuple-level granularity, level-based constraints automatically undertake the entity integrity constraints. We must also note that apart from the security constraints, integrity constraints and availability constraints were also considered during the implementation. However, since we believe that they are rather typical of a hospital database, we have chosen not to refer to them in this paper.

3.2.2. Implementation of the Security Constraints using SQL

For the implementation of the security constraints that were defined earlier for the hospital database, the security features, rules and procedures supported by Ingres were used. We have applied in our experimental implementation all the different kinds of security constraints to the prototype hospital database SEC_AXEPA. We will describe now a typical implementation of each one type of such a security constraint. We note that since we support tuple-level granularity, the level-based constraints and the entity integrity constraints are automatically satisfied.

A *simple security constraint* (SiC) is implemented by creating a rule that is fired each time new data is inserted. This rule executes a procedure that sets the tuple class of the data inserted equal to the desired classification level. The implementation of the *content-based constraint*s is similar. The following example also includes the implementation of the cover story created.

Example implementation of a content-based security constraint and of a Cover Story
SCL: CbC(Diagnoses,{*},Diagnosis,'=','HIV',2) AND cover story
Rule 3: Create rule r_3 after insert of diagnoses execute procedure p_3
(pid = new.p_id, doctor = new.dr_code, diagdate= new.diag_date, diagnosis = new.diag);
Procedure 3: Create procedure p_3 (pid integer4, drcode c(15), diagdate date, diagnosis c(500)) as
begin if diagnosis = 'HIV' then update 'marie'.diagnoses set tc = 2 where p_id = :pid and
diag_date = :diagdate and dr_code = :drcode and diag = :diagnosis;
insert into 'marie'.diagnoses(p_id, dr_code, diag_date, diag, icd9_code, diag_comm, fl, tc)
values (:pid, :drcode, :diagdate, 'Blood disease', '222', 'Take care', 'l', 0); endif; end;

The *complex-constraint* implementation is executed in rather the same way.

Example implementation of a complex security constraint
SCL: CoC(PAT-LAB-EXAMS,{*},LAB-EXAM-RESULT,'=','HIV',2)
Rule 4: Create rule r_4 after insert of lab_test_res execute procedure p_4
(pid = new.p_id, labexams = new.lab_exam_res, resdate = new.res_date);
Procedure 4: Create procedure p_4 (pid integer 4, labexamres c(100)) as begin
if labexamres = 'HIV' then update 'marie'.lab_test_res set tc = 2 where p_id = :pid; endif; end;

An *association-based security constraint* implemented on Ingres is equivalent to an aggregation constraint, since column-level control is supported only in the update access mode in Ingres. An *aggregation constraint* is implemented by setting a limit to the data the user is able to retrieve. Finally, the *inference constraint's* implementation is carried out by assigning different categories to the data, so that a user can not access certain data and infer sensitive information.

4. Study of the User Acceptance

As part of the experimental implementation, we also studied the user acceptance of the system. The first general conclusion is that most hospital users agreed that security is very important at a hospital. They would also prefer to use a more complex and secure information system, provided that they would be trained properly. They defined, however, the notion of database security in several ways. Moreover, they believed that confidentiality and integrity contribute more to the security of a hospital database than availability. As far as the specific database SEC_AXEPA is concerned, most doctors and nurses thought that using it would significantly improve their work. Additionally, they found it easy to use and satisfyingly secure. The support of cover stories and the user role hierarchy were found rather complex, but important and necessary for a hospital database. They all agreed however that it is important to define legally soon the various types of data sets and user roles in a hospital.

To conclude, almost all the users of the SEC_AXEPA hospital database were positive towards the support of the proposed security environment and the prototype secure hospital database itself.

5. Conclusions

The implementation of the prototype hospital database has shown that the proposed secure database design methodology can be successfully applied at a complex real-life hospital environment. It has also been shown that in the prototype hospital database all the three aspects of security were ensured with no significant overheads. More specifically, the secrecy (confidentiality) was preserved by allowing only the doctors to access the patient's personal data and by creating cover stories for important people. Integrity was also preserved by providing for the users with the least possible privileges and by using security levels. Finally, availability was also well preserved; the performance overheads were relatively low, priority was assigned to the user transactions depending on the user's role in the hospital and flags were used to allow the users to have direct access to the most recent medical data .

We believe therefore that the lessons learned from the implementation of the prototype secure hospital database SEC_AXEPA will be useful to other database designers, who will attempt a similar task in the future.

6. References

[1] S. Castano, M. Fugini, G. Martella, P. Samarati, Database security, Addison Wesley publishing company, 1994.
[2] G. Pangalos, M. Khair, L. Bozios, Enhancing medical database security, In: Journal of medical systems, USA, 1994.
[3] G. Pangalos S. Katsikas, and D. Gritzalis, Medical database security guidelines, In: Computers and security journal, 1994.
[4] G. Pangalos, M. Khair, L. Bozios, An integrated secure design of a medical database system,   In: MEDINFO'95, The 8th world congress on medical informatics, Canada, 1995.
[5] G. Pangalos, M. Khair, Design of secure medical database systems, In: IFIP/SEC'96, 12th international information security conference, 1996.
[6] G. Pernul, Database security, Academic Press Inc., 1994.

Medical Informatics Europe '97
C. Pappas et al. (Eds.)
IOS Press, 1997

Medical Liability, Safety and Confidentiality in Maritime Telemedicine - The MERMAID position on issues of importance

P. Ladas[1], P. Giatagatzidis[2], G. Anogianakis[3,4], S. Maglavera[3]

1 Law School, Aristotle University, Thessaloniki, Greece
2 P. Giatagatzidis & E. Metaxaki Law firm, Athens, Greece
3 BIOTRAST s.a., 111 Mitropoleos Str, GR-54622 Thessaloniki, Greece
4 Department of Physiology, Faculty of Medicine, Aristotle University, Thessaloniki

Abstract. Telemedicine dates to the days of "wireless telegraphy". As an "extraordinary" arrangement for medical services delivered at time of need, telemedicine has thus far escaped the developments that have taken place over the last 50 years in the areas of medical liability, safety and confidentiality. Today, however, telemedicine is also used to increase quality and cost effectiveness of healthcare provision. This trend is set by the U.S. where the U.S. federal government funds telemedicine at an annual rate of more than $100 million i.e., at a rate 30 times or more than what the EU does while state and local agency support and private business investment in telemedicine is 3 to 4 times larger than that of the U.S. federal government. In this respect it must be stressed that technology tends to satisfy the relevant demand for telecommunications. Telemedicine is used in diverse areas such as pathology, surgery, physical therapy, and psychiatry. It is expected to revolutionise health care in the coming decade and, therefore, it will certainly take into account requirements for medical liability, safety and confidentiality in the same way as traditional "establishment" medicine does.

1. The Legal Framework for practicing Telemedicine

Healthcare is a major area of applications under the G-7 "information highways" scenario[1]. Furthermore, the recent shift of industrial countries to telecommunications as one of their major economic growth areas means that an unleashing of investment in telemedicine is imminent. It is, therefore, important to maintain a priority for a public service application of telecommunications such as telemedicine. Giving a "top priority" status to telemedical applications is both innovative policy-making and good business. However, neither the legal implications, nor the relevant legal framework are certain, despite the fact that a classification of telemedicine's legal issues is possible into:

- traditional medico-legal issues not unique to the medium;

---

[1] G7 Conference (Building the Information Society for the Citizens of the World), February 1995, Brussels

- issues of the applicable law and/or legal jurisdiction regarding telemedical acts especially as telemedicine tends to amplify conflicts arising from differences of law
- issues unique to telemedicine
- issues concerning equipment

MERMAID is an EU (DGXIII) Healthcare Telematics programme, that intends to provide an untegrated multilingual medical emergency service around the world (1) and use telematics to transfer medical expertise to sea-borne vessels (2, 3). It is a pilot project that responds not only to the real life needs of the maritime workplace but also to the legal requirements that derive (4) from a series of relevant EU Council Directives such as:

1. Council Directive 89/654/EEC of 30 November 1989 concerning the minimum safety and health requirements for the workplace (first individual Directive within the meaning of Article 16(1) of Directive 89/391/EEC)
2. Council Directive 89/655/EEC of 30 November 1989 concerning the minimum safety and health requirements for the use of work equipment by workers at work (second individual Directive within the meaning of Article 16(1) of Directive 89/391/EEC)
3. Council Directive 89/656/EEC of 30 November 1989 concerning the minimum safety and health requirements for the use by workers of personal projective equipment at the workplace (third individual Directive within the meaning of Article 16(1) of Directive 89/391/EEC)
4. Commission communication for the implementation of Council Directive 89/656/EEC of 30 November 1989 concerning the assessment of the safety aspects of personal projective equipment with a view to the choice and use thereof
5. Council Directive 90/269/EEC of May 1990 on the minimum health and safety requirements for the manual handling of loads where there is a risk particularly of back injury to workers (fourth individual Directive within the meaning of Article 16(1) of Directive 89/391/EEC)
6. Council Directive 92/58/EEC of 24 June 1992 on the implementation of the minimum safety and health requirements at temporary or mobile construction sets (ninth individual Directive within the meaning of Article 16(1) of Directive 89/391/EEC)
7. Council Directive 93/103/EEC of 23 November 1993 concerning the minimum safety and health requirements for work on board fishing vessels (13th individual Directive within the meaning of Article 16(1) of Directive 89/391/EEC)
8. Council Directive 92/29/EEC of 31 March 1992 on the minimum safety and health requirements for improved medical treatment on board
9. Council Directive 93/104/EC of 23 November 1993 concerning certain aspects of the organization of working time
10. Council Directive 91/383/EEC of 25 June 1991 supplementing the measures to encourage improvements in the safety and health at work of workers with a fixed-duration employment relationship or a temporary employment relationship

Traditional medico-legal issues therefore not unique to telemedicine are outside the scope of this paper which focuses on issues of legal jurisdiction and issues unique to telemedicine. Thus the following issues are identified as of potential interest to the MERMAID scenario:

- lack of a uniform rules or a universally accepted Code of Ethics for the practice of telemedicine
- lack of international procedures for telemedicine related physician licencing

- absence of a clear cut international framework for resolving questions of medical liability
- lack of internationally accepted rules concerning confidentiality of patient related information
- lack of internationally accepted rules concerning prescription filling

In terms of ethics, it is observed that each new development in health care, whether a medication, a new procedure, a technological advance, or a change in patterns of service delivery, poses ethical and legal issues. Interactive video transmission of medical services is no exception. For maritime telemedicine, the fundamental issue is its net efficacy: Does it do more good than harm? The results are resoundingly affirmative.

Therefore in the case of marine telemedicine the usual dictum of "do no harm," must be replaced by a new ethical consideration: that "ethical hazard arises in the harmfulness of not using telemedical consultation when a telemedical system is available and a patient's condition demands the highest expertise". The failure to employ telemedically available expertise can be harmful and, therefore, might be deemed unethical. Unfortunately, as the MERMAID data demonstrate, failure to use telemedicine is the rule, rather than the exception, aboard ships, irrespective of the cultural or the economic development of their country of origin or the nationality of their crews.

Finally, health care professionals must apply to marine telemedicine networks the elaborate standards, qualify assurance methodology, peer review, and other means they currently use. In effect, telemedical staff at all sites (central and remote) should be expected to adhere to credentialing criteria and review processes.

2.   *Physician Licensing*

Telemedical services present a legal problem should physicians provide their services across borders. All countries have laws which require physicians to be licensed by their own authorities before they are allowed to work within their borders. Within the EU the situation is complicated by the fact that licensing is in effect limiting the physician to practice within the area of jurisdiction of the Medical Board he is registered with! In the future, as EU statutes that promote mobility become more effective, healthcare professionals may be required to register in more than one countries, something that may bring up among other and problems of multiple taxation. Marine telemedicine, furthermore must cope with additional problems, such as:

- ships registered under "flags of convenience" and therefore, not obliged to dilligently enforce "health and safety in the workplace" rules.
- crews that are multinational with a substantial number of the crewmembers of lower rank coming from third world countries.
- crews that are insured by agencies of countries other than their country of registry.

Finally, if telemedicine is to become truly available as an emergency care alternative, arrangements for both transeuropean and global provision of medical and psychiatric services must be made. The need for such arrangements quickly becomes apparent in the event of a hurricane or earthquake, for example, when a telemedical link with neighbouring countries might be able to respond more promptly to victims' medical needs than a country's own more distant health care facilities.

3.   Medical Liability

Regarding Medical Liability, EU law has developed to where health care systems must adequately supervise and credential their staff and independent physicians providing services under their auspices. Videotaping each telemedical examination is a possibility for managing liability risk.

Negligence issues abound in the situation where it is not clear which facility, the host or the remote practitioner (who may ultimately prescribe further diagnosis and treatment based upon the consultation with the host's medical staff), provides medical care.

Another issue relates to "informal" consent. At a first glance it seems clear that the physician who remotely diagnoses and treats patients at a remote location would be required to secure a patient's informed consent to render care. At present, standards for when consent is "informed" vary from country to country.

4.   Confidenciality of Patient Records

Patient privacy is another important issue for telemedicine. Information about sexually-transmitted diseases, mental health, and genetic diseases is among the most private of personal information. Thus, rules assuring the privacy of patient records while providing access to health care providers must be observed. Problems arise when information flows across borders, because of different privacy laws or in the case of health insurance companies that may exclude from coverage risky patients.

Data encryption methods are generally not sufficient but in the case of video transmission things are considered easier on the practical level since it is practically impossible to "wiretap" such a transmission. Of cource when videotapes are made of patients, the tapes should be given the same legal protection as the patient's chart. Finally, it is believed that Directive 95/46/EU will eventually cover matters of patient confidentiality.

5.   Accreditation

In general no real progress has been made on medical accreditation of telemedical practice. MERMAID is thus faced with questions such as:

- if telemedicine networks must focus attention on telemedical proficiency
- if separate standards are necessary for "virtual" practice and
- if there is a duty for hospitals to monitor physicians' telemedical skills.

6.   Prescription

Finally, there is a lot of uncertainty regarding prescriptions transmitted by telemedicine. At present, pharmacists cannot fill prescriptions signed by physicians licensed in another country. This is a serious issue for marine telemedicine and there is no solution in sight other than to expand the medicine chest aboard ships to include non-emergency related medication!

References

1. MERMAID HC-1034 Joint Deliverables D1.3 & D1.4: "Report on issues of Medical Liability, Safety and Confidentiality", Healthcare Telematics, DGXIII, June 1996.
2. David Wright and Leonid Androuchko, Telemedicine and developing countries, Journal of Telemedicine and Telecare, Vol. 2, Number 2 1996
3. George Anogianakis, The New Flying Doctor, Ocean Voice April 96
4. George Anogianakis and Stavroula Maglavera, MERMAID rescues those in peril on the sea, European Hospital Management Journal, Vol. 3 Issue 1 1996

Medical Informatics Europe '97
C. Pappas et al. (Eds.)
IOS Press, 1997

Investment Appraisal of the Protection, Confidentiality and Security Arrangements of Patient Data

Denise Loftus, Tony Carroll
Department of Information Technology
Rotunda Hospital
Dublin 1
Ireland

Abstract

Data Protection and Security issues are reviewed in relevant literature. Policies implemented in relation to the subject matter are discussed in detail. Findings from a review of data protection and security arrangements at a major hospital are presented. Future data protection and security recommendations are outlined.

1. Overview

The Rotunda Hospital established an Information Technology Department in 1994, the primary focus of which was to implement a Patient Information and Clinical Information System or PAS. In addition to the standard suite of typical PAS Modules, the PAS has a number of major clinical modules including Obstetrical Management, Neo-Natal Information and Casemix. The implementation is scheduled for completion in 1997.

The PAS is used by the majority of the hospital's 600 staff. As part of the implementation, each user underwent a basic 10 hour computer course, one module of which was devoted to Data Protection and Security. Over the past 2 years the IT Department has organised seminars on Confidentiality, Data Security, and related medico legal issues. Senior staff together with the general body of users attended these seminars. Prior to each module going live the implementation team issued documentation specifically highlighting end users obligations in ensuring the integrity and security of data.

Security and other related matters were also addressed on a fairly regular basis through internal memoranda, newsletters and within the hospital's corporate IT documentation. In summary the Rotunda has probably done more than other similar sized organisations in promoting data protection and security throughout its population of end users. From this perspective we were anxious to ascertain and review the success or otherwise of our efforts in this area. This review took place in September 1996.

2. Literature Review

There is considerable literature available which addresses the subjects under discussion. This includes the following: Data Protection, Confidentiality and Computer Security are basic requirements for the appropriate introduction and use of information and communications technology in healthcare. The AIM requirements board identified a basic trilogy for the future of health information systems in Europe - Integration, Modulation and Security, together with recommending the six safety first principles. [1] Brennan suggests the confinement of computer security to integrity, confidentiality and availability. [2]

Binchy describes the protection afforded to individuals in relation to personal data kept on computer about them. [3] Bakker sets out the vulnerability aspects associated with computers in hospitals and suggests that without awareness of the risks, measures to reduce them will hardly be accepted or taken seriously. [4] Anderson identifies the risks associated with wide area networks in healthcare and highlights the importance of implementing compartmentation to secure networked healthcare systems. [5] McCafferty points out the importance of the wider issue of internal systems security and integrity, suggesting that they must also be addressed as part of an overall security policy when examining networks and firewalls. [6] Safran et al identifies a procedure whereby patients can have access to those who seen their medical record. [7] Piret et al points out that although strict security policies may be in existence the weak point of the security confidentiality organisation remains the access to applications still governed by a password which can always be divulged. [8] Kohler outlines the importance of patient cards and informational self determination, outlining the patient's legal rights to read, write his own documentation, to correct and to delete data [9].

3. Basic Security Arrangements

The data protection and security arrangements for PAS users at the Rotunda Hospital include the following:

(a) A member of senior management must authorise in the first instance the establishment of a user on the system.

(b) A manual file for each user is created and maintained during the life of the user in the hospital. The security system also keeps track of user movements.

(c) Each new user receives an information pack and user identification at registration and attends the relevant tutorial sessions. The system prompts the user for his/her unique password. Users are not allowed to access the system until basic training has been completed.

(d) As a cross check the personnel and salary records of hospital staff are matched against a current list of users each month to identify starters and leavers who may not have been notified to the IT Department.

(e) The system allows user categories to be established. Currently there are five main user categories which correspond to the key functional grades of staff. Each category has specific rights assigned to it which determines the level of user access to the system. The security system also has a number of other key features including the control and management of passwords, and peripheral device locations, automatic time out and so forth..

(f) The security system allows access to sensitive data to be controlled by additional internal application function checks built into each of the modules so that sensitive data can be restricted. The Patient Master Index allows patient privacy classification to be classified as "restricted", which allows only a restricted category of users to have access to this "restricted" patient data. The restricted patient classification is applied only at the patient's request or at the discretion of the Medical Records Officer. In the Rotunda Hospital it is used for example when a member of staff is admitted to the hospital as a patient. It may also be used for high risk patients.

(g) The security system is managed by the Security Administrator who also manages the audit trail feature in collaboration with Heads of Departments.

(h) Access to the system from outside the hospital is generally restricted to service providers only. Password Protection is used and in order to use the system a line has to be granted to the user. This is controlled by the help desk who log each request, monitor the call and log off users. The reason for system access and the duration of the handshake is also recorded.

(i) The IT Department also has a comprehensive range of other security features normally associated with a typical computer installation including physical security restrictions, housekeeping and general system management functions.

4. Review of Procedures

The hospital has an extensive quality assurance program in operation. This is aimed primarily at identifying weaknesses in data quality and the program is administered by a number of specially trained staff from the various disciplines. The IT Department also operates a help line bleep number to support end users while individual team members have specific responsibilities for performing housekeeping and systems management functions. The hospital has a Complaints Officer who processes complaints from patients and maintains detailed records in accordance with existing legislation. All of these sources provided the majority of information which formed the basis for the review of data protection/security arrangements.

The most common problems revealed from the data quality records included the following mistakes by end users.
- Amending printouts manually but failing to update the system or updating the system and failing to produce revised printouts.
- Failure to sign printouts.
- Several users entering information under one password.
- Signing printouts which contained information which was illogical by best clinical practise.
- Duplication of information in slightly different formats.

One of the most serious and not uncommon breaches was medical staff giving functional access under their passwords to paramedical staff so that tertiary medical information such as Total Parental Nutrition (TPN) could be amended by the pharmacists. This had been happening previously in the manual records apparently unknowns to senior medical staff.

In reviewing the help desk records the main re-occurring items included:
- User lockouts for password violation.
- Users attempts to gain system access via restricted locations.
- Users forgetting their passwords.
- Users performing illegal system functions.

The most common problem was user lockouts associated with password violation. There were a number of reasons for this, the most likely of which was attempting to reactivate the system following user suspension.

The Systems Management Records, including reviews of the audit trail and discussions with relevant staff revealed that the main risk resulted from users either swapping passwords or leaving terminals open for others to use.

In one instance a member of the clerical staff had given their password to temporary clerical colleagues on a loan basis despite warnings that temporary staff had to receive system training before being allowed to use the system.

Another common problem encountered involved the restricted access function which limits access to certain records on the system. Access was restricted to medical and nursing staff to examine some records but when patients arrived for admission, particularly after office hours, the administrative staff were unable to process the admission because they could not gain access to the relevant records.

The problem of illegally copying software continued to be a significant problem particularly amongst Junior Medical Staff who were the main offenders.

In order to determine the level of complaints or queries from the patients, the records of the Complaint's Officer were examined. No complaint had been filed in writing from patients regarding any data protection/confidentiality issue. The Complaints Officer revealed however that the only patients who had specifically objected to their details being entered on computer, were those who were permanent residents of Non European Union countries (EU) most notably the former Union of Soviet Socialist Republics (USSR). Although each patient should be advised under the Data Protection Legislation that information will be held on computer about them, no patient sought clarification despite the fact that this aspect of the legislation is not displayed in any public areas throughout the hospital. In order to ascertain the general level of queries from patients treated in the Irish Healthcare System, the Data Protection Commissioners Office was contacted. Interviews with officials revealed that very few queries had been received to date, possibly because people did not seem to be aware of their rights under the legislation.

5. Discussion

Although the hospital had initiated a fairly extensive awareness program amongst staff, the number of data protection/security violations coupled with data integrity inaccuracies was quite high. The main offenders were in the medical and nursing categories. Patients were either indifferent to their rights or simply did not know them.

These findings raise a number of important issues. The most likely source of medical litigation arises through malpractice, the records of which provide the corner stone for the clinician's defence. The repository which the records provide in treating the patients is indispensable. Because of these factors the ethos enshrined in the Hippocratic oath and the litigation mentality prevalent in western countries like the United States, should be much closer in the information age than they have been in the past. While the computer should bring both together for the betterment of the patient, the reality is that the credibility of treatment is more questionable now than it was twenty years ago because of the deterioration in the standards of basic medical record keeping.

At a time when patients as citizens are more conscious of their rights, the short fall in their understanding or indifference to data protection and security issues is difficult to understand. It may be that the dangers of the information age are not as apparent to the patient as they may be to the patient as citizen in the global village. Or perhaps the social commentators and IT Professionals are creating dangers which in reality are not perceived to be that dangerous by the ordinary citizen.

Institutions such as hospitals have (in addition to their legal obligations) a moral obligation to ensure that their employees act in an ethical manner. They also have a moral obligation to those they treat because issues associated with data protection and security are very much a part of the patient's well being. At the Rotunda Hospital the approach to these matters is being evaluated. In addition to strengthening existing policies and procedures the following agenda items will be explored during 1997.

- To develop a data protection and security awareness program aimed at all patients attending the hospital.
- To independently audit staff usage of both manual and automated clinical records in circumstances where they have no clinical reason to use such records.
- To examine the possibility of extending existing arrangements whereby patients are allowed to take home their obstetrical records.

6. Conclusions

As we race towards the 21st Century the social and environmental pressures of living in an advanced society will take their toll. Already the information age feeds off systems and services which are invisible and beyond the touching reach of those manipulated by them. The weakest members of the information age are patients so it is important therefore that patients along with their guardians are educated to address the apathy which currently exists in the global village in relation to data protection, confidentiality and computer security.

References

[1]   Roger France, FH: The European Challenge in Health Information Systems. In: Data Protection and Confidentiality in Health Informations. Commission of the European Communities, DGXIII/FAIM. IOS PRESS Pgs 1, 65-70

[2]   Brennan, M, The Real Security Threat: The Enemy Within. In: Datamation, July 15th 1995. Pgs 30-33.

[3]   Binchy, W., Byrne, R. Data Protection Act 1988. Annual Review of Irish Law 1988 Roundstall Press Dublin 1988. Pgs 390-399.

[4]   Bakker, A. R. Computers in Hospitals, Vulnerability Aspects. In: IFIP WG 9.2 Meeting at Namur, Belgium, January 11th 1991.

[5]   Anderson, R.J. Patient Confidentiality - At Risk from NHS Wide Networking. In: Current Perspectives in Healthcare Computing. Proceedings of Healthcare 1996. Bernard Richards(ED). BJHC/BCS 1996. Pgs 687-692.

[6]   McCafferty, Clive, Securing the NHS Net in the British Journal of Healthcare Computing and Information Management. Volume 13 No 8, October 1996. Pgs 24-26

[7]   Safran, C. Et al. Protection of Confidentiality in the computer based Patient Record. In: Clinical Computing, Volume 12 No. 3. 1995. Pgs 187-192.

[8]   Piret, Roger France, FH, Pirard, F. Development of a Coherent Policy of Security Confidentiality in a heterogeneous University Hospital Environment in Belgium. In: Medical Informatics Europe 1996, Brender, J., Christensen, JP, Scherrer, JR., McNair, P. (Eds) IOS Press, Netherlands, 1996 Pgs 951-956.

[9]   Kohler, C.O., The patient Cards and Informational Self-determination. In: The future of Health Records Management. Hoffman, U. Et al (Eds) Proceedings of the 12th International Health Records Congress, Munich April 15 - 19th 1996. MMV Medizin Verlag GmbH, Munchen, 1996. Pgs 321-327

Medical Informatics Europe '97
C. Pappas et al. (Eds.)
IOS Press, 1997

A formal, mathematics oriented method for identifying security risks in information systems

Henk U. van Piggelen[1]
Information Technology and Telecommunications Department
University Hospital Maastricht
The Netherlands

Abstract. IT security presently lacks the benefits of physics where certain unifying grand principles can be applied. The aim of the method is to provide a technology independent method of identifying components of a system in general, and of information systems in particular. The need for the proposed method is derived from ad hoc character of theories used in the present formal security textbooks. None of these can give the user any guarantee of completeness. The new method is scientifically derived as a method, presented, explained and applied to several interesting topics in the field of health care information systems. Some simple mathematical formulae can be introduced.

1. Background

The evaluation of security in information systems technology is presently evolving into a secure field of expertise. Several methods to quantify risks are even made commercially available, or are being developed by universities[1],[2].
Little or no literature seems to exist as to the foudations of these methods and no formal proof of the completeness of the approach is given. Many of them simply start out from a checklist type of statement, specifying all the risks that are interesting enough to appear in the paper at hand. How can one be sure at that point that no elements of the lists are missing?. The topic 'security' itself ought to make one uneasy about this question and its presumed answer. Elements that could be forgotten that can very well be of subtle but nevertheless fundamental importance. Those methods neither give clues about how to proceed with the checklist type of reasoning when dramatic technology changes are at hand.
The number of different aspects in the field of security is large. And there is more to that: there are many different types of elements that at first glance have no greater correlations with one-another than that they appear on the same check list (Database integrity rules;Data modelling; Closed shop data centres; Fire protection; Privacy legislation; dial back modems;Program testing;end user procedures, etc.
A method that aims to unify these topics in a consistent way must conform to a number of tests that any scientific theory should fulfill:

1. The previously known facts must still be explained at the usual level;
2. The theory must preferable be simple and elegant;
3. The theory must shed a new light on old facts, or even better, predict new phenomena.

---

[1]   Email HVP@DAUT.AZM.NL

Theoretical physics is well known for its firm foundations in axiomatic theory. Being a theoretically trained scientist myself, I prefer to have as little elements as possible in the theory that have been put into it in order to obtain nice results. These theories are usually called **semi-empirical** theories versus the **first-principles** class of theories that I prefer. This does not imply that in my opinion all semi-empirical methods are therefore useless!

Furthermore, as information systems deal with reality, i.e. claim to be a true representation of reality, one might hope that they themselves obey to some degree the laws of reality, i.e. the laws of elementary physics. *As I hope to show, the application of laws of physics to secure information systems, can in fact produce the aforementioned checklists in any desired level of detail.* In addition the statements about secure systems can be put in an elegant mathematical form.

No expectations should be held about a mathematical proof of secureness of information systems. Supposed that were possible at all, the proof of the inverse case might be more economically looked for, as to prove systems *insecure.* Firstly there is always the human element in it, that probably will defy putting security completely into mathematics. Secondly , being able to prove a system secure is one thing to be really happy with. Most likely a system is secure until its insecureness is being proven. That can be related to Poppers falsification remarks.

2 The Method

The method I propose consists of three steps. These are sufficient to define a state in which security within the system is defined.

1. **Identification** : Define the subjects that one is interested in. In principle one could chose to identify a field of interest completely, however this may prove to be cumbersome;
2. **Outer product**: Create a matrix form the selected elements, such as to have an enumeration of subjects both on rows and columns;
3. **Judgement**: Apply the quality operator.

New in this approach is the use of a mathematical, or symbolical operator. Operators are quite useful things. They are virtual instruments that act upon the objects they are defined for to work on. One might think 'multiplication by 3' as an operator that acts upon numbers. Or 'Create a laboratory request' as an operator that works in the space of empty lab requests. In this case the quality operator is a judgement of quality, it separates the good from the bad. Simple, though it may seem, we need no more than that to create the definition of a secure system.

The quality operator to be applied here is the judgement of good and bad to the relation in which the entities from within the matrix elements can be placed. At present it is hard to give a strict form of the operator, but its meaning will become clear when we discuss an example.
The general act of the operator is to separate the occurrences within a matrix element into subclasses of good and bad. The resulting form of the element is hence a subdivision in four

parts: Good-good, good-bad, bad-good and bad-bad. (GG,GB,BG and BB respectively)

In this table we can exactly identify the relevant security structure for the items at hand. Because of their properties for our discussion we now add qualifying names to the elements:

Table 1: The fundamental structure of the quality operator

	GOOD	BAD
GOOD	GG= Structured area	GB= Closedness area
BAD	BG = Impenetrability Area	BB = Chaos area

Of course GG is the desired state of security. Bad items should not affect the items is the Good area, and conversely, Good items should not leave into the bad outer world.

The task for a security manager is hence to specify :
I   What the structure is of the field of interest;
II   When a Good item turns into a Bad item;
III When a Bad item is known to remain outside the field of security interest
IV   When time permits, ponder upon the nature of chaos.

If one uses mathematical terminology the formulation can be compactly written down.[2] See appendix A.

3 Application

3.1 Identification

First let us take a distant view at an information system. One can identify as belonging to it: End Users (U), Workstations (W), Network components (N), Host computers (H), Databases(D), Tables (T) and Attributes (A). These are the components that one can more or less see. Two components should be added that one almost takes for granted, namely the physical space (R) the components occupy, and Time (Θ). The latter being the only 'invisible' item. This completes the first step of the method.

---

[11]

The notation in this formalism must not be taken to deal with numerical operations, but rather symbolical actions.

3.2 Create outer product

Applying the second rule of the method leads to the following 9x9 matrix:

	U	W	N	H	D	T	A	R	Θ
U									
W									
N									
H									
D									
T									
A									
R									
Θ									

Here both horizontally and vertically, the items of interest are labelled, just in order to make reading and identifying the matrix elements more easy. This matrix fully describes the field of interest for security, and is able to generate all of the security classes seen in regular textbooks. The maximum number of relevant distinct classes thus is 81. Further in this paper some of the elements will be discussed in more detail.

3.3 Interpretation of the effect of the quality operator

Let us now, for the sake of illustration, apply the Q operator to some of the matrix elements. In doing so we specifically reproduce the shortlist of the introduction of this paper. The notation that is used, will be

GG = structure area, GB = closedness area, BG = impenetrability area, BB = Chaos area

Except for the end user procedures we will not need to use the Time invariance argument to its fullest extent.

- **Database integrity rules;**   *GG* of tables versus databases
- **Data modelling;**   *GG* of tables versus tables
- **Closed shop data centres;**   *BG* of users versus room
- **Fire protection;**   *GG* of both room and users versus Time
- **Privacy legislation;**   *BG* and *GB* of users versus tables
- **dial back modems;**   *GG* of network components versus users
- **Program testing;**   *GG* of database and tables versus Time. Here to be interpreted as the demand for transition in time from one correct state to another.
- **end user procedures, etc.**   Time invariance of the secure information system.

So far we have in the analysis only covered part of the matrix. Other matrix elements can be identified as useful security topics.

3.4 A step further

One of the aims of this study is to create additional awareness of security on fields not previously covered. Let's take two examples: one of the health care industry: the use of smart cards, and one from Networking environments.

Healthcare:In Europe many providers of cost reimbursements, provide their clients with smart card in order to identify the natural person. This creates the microcosm PERSON/CARD.

	Person	Card	
Person		Correct card for person	Wrong card for Ensured person
		Valid card for un-ensured person	Invalid card for wrong person
Card			

Networking : Diving a bit further into the computer hardware, we can identify the well known problem in network technology, that of address mimicking, in which a hacker replaces the correct network addresses of a legitimate addressee by the ones of himself.
We have as items: PC, Ethernet card(-address) and Cable, from which we form a matrix.
This matrix has been simplified in order to stress the relevant points:

		Ethernet card (address)		Cable	
		Own	Alien	Own	Alien
Ethernet card (address)	Own	Legal *sender- receiver* relation	Address substitution		
	Alien	Server mimic			
Cable	Own			Cabling totplogy	Eavesdropping
	Alien			Cross talk (sending)	

In the relevant matrix elements those items have been filled in that make the hacker problem identifiable. Please note that the proper Ethernet address int this approximation does not necessarily the proper PC in case of the use of network adapters that plug into e.g. a parallel port of a portable computer.

References

[1]   E.g. see the CRAMM methodology that is being used within the SEISMED program.

[2]   B. Barber *et al.*: *Data Security for Health Care*, vol I- III, IOS press 1996

Medical Informatics Europe '97
C. Pappas et al. (Eds.)
IOS Press, 1997

FOIN : a Nominative Information Occultation Function

Gilles Trouessin[1], François-André Allaert[2]

[1] CEN/TC251/WG6 Expert CESSI–CNAMTS 14, place St-Etienne
31000 Toulouse – France *Tel.: +33 562.269.139 E.mail:cessi@mipnet.fr*

[2] EFMI/WG2 Chairman CEN BIOTECH Bourgogne CHRU du Bocage
21000 Dijon – France *Tel.: +33 380.293.431 E-mail:aallaert@u-bourgogne.fr*

Abstract:

This article is intended to show that a great amount of work has to (and will) be done in terms of security for the healthcare information system community. Some very promising results have already been obtained in France, especially at CNAMTS, for providing the required security and privacy of nominative information in the context of futur electronic exchanges between private/public hospital and CNAMTS, the french biggest mandatory healthcare insurance. FOIN, a robust anonymisation function, is just an example of such recent progress that traduces the french national engagement towards more flexible interconnection between various authorised healthcare information systems in close conjunction with more and more reliable and secure procedural and technical requirements. Firstly, the legal and medical needs for so strong anonymisation functions are described; secondly, the most important security requirements of these sensible functions are detailed and, lastly, the main security and implementation features of FOIN are globally indicated.

Keywords: Legal obligations, Security, of medical data, Secure Hash Functions.

1. Needs for strong anonymisation

1.1. Medico administrative needs

According to new governmental rules of April 96 to control more strictly health expenses, all medical practitioners will have the duty to send the personal administrative information but also the medical ones of all the patients they are curing to the national healthcare insurance provider. This information will be sent by telematics on the public telecommunication network. Therefore, it requires a high level of protection to insure its confidentiality and its integrity during transmission and storage.

This transmission will use the personal number (NIR) devoted by the state to each citizen, which is a perfect identifier of the person and will allow the healthcare provider to gather medical information of a same person treated simultaneously or successively in different public or private hospitals or in ambulatory care. However, the use of this personal number worries the medical community but also a large audience because it may represent a first step towards its wide use in other field which will threaten personal freedom and privacy. By exception, an authorization has been given to the use of this number under condition that a strong anonymisation will be provided during transmission and storage.

1.2. Legal aspects

According to the french law on data privacy "informatique et libertés" of January 6th, 1978, the use of the personal number of each citizen is strictly submitted to the authorization of the highest French administrative Court, the State Council, and published in the official journal of the French Republic. An agreement has been given by the court the 12th of september 1996 in order to allow the healthcare insurance provider to certificate the link between each patient and the health insurance system and to provide a better control of medical goods and services delivered to the patient.

The main problem is now to conciliate the need for identity of the Health Insurance provider and the right to confidentiality of the patient. The setting up of the personal medical data transmission on a network and the storage of all information on a unique place represent a real danger and compel to use cryptographic methods to prevent attacks from hackers. In case of a breach of confidentiality, the healthcare insurance provider will be found liable according to the Penal Code and a very wide political embarrassment will appear in this very sensitive field.

2. Main security requirements for anonymisation

The french Ministery of Business and Social Affairs dealing with national Healthcare Information Systems problems asked recently CESSI (CNAMTS department dedicated to security aspects) to develop a system that garantees **strong occultation** of such sensible information as NIR number (i.e., access key to electronic nominative information).

Strong occultation means **robustness** w.r.t. *anonymisation, collisions* and *access control*.

2.1. A robust anonymisation function

Anonymisation *"robustness"* means it doesn't exist any direct and/or indirect method allowing to find which nominative identifier is hidden behind any anonymous identifier.

2.1.1. Direct robustness

A robust anonymisation function must satisfy the *direct robustness requirement*; it is recommended to be based on a *one way fonction*, a well-known security concept; and security can protect against attacks that directly reverse the anonymisation process.

A *one way function* is a mathematical function for which calculation is only possible in the direct way:

- *direct way*: $y = f(x)$ means that the result y can be obtained when applying function f to the data x;

- *reverse way*: $x = f^{1}(y)$ means that the data x could be re-obtained by applying function f^{1} to y, f^{1} being the reverse function corresponding to f;

- *one way function*: in the case of a *one way function* H, its reverse function H^{1} does not exist so that it mathematically impossible to obtain x from y.

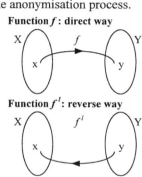

Function f: direct way

Function f^{1}: reverse way

2.1.2. Indirect robustness of an anonymisation function

A robust anonymisation means also indirectly robust.

If the anonymisation function is publicly known, there is then a possibility of indirect attack:

- *pre-calculation:* it is possible to precalculate $y_i=f(x_i)$;
- *x − y correspondance:* it is then easy to establish a link between x_i (nominative) and y_i (anonymous) ;
- *indirect attack:* for an intruder possessing these correspondances, each anonymous identifier y_k can be seen equivalent to its corresponding x_k.

Pre-calucations:

x − y correspondance table:

nominative id.	anonymous id.
x_i	y_i
x_j	y_j
x_k	y_k
...	...

Taking into account security requirements that protect against this type of attacks will ensure that nobody can indirectly reverse the anonymisation process.

2.2. A robust collision-free function

"Robustness" for a collision-free functions means that there is a very high probability, for two distinct nominative identifiers, to correspond to distinct anonymous identifiers.

In other words, a robust collision-free function means that after the anonymisation of two distinct nominative identifiers corresponding to two distinct patient identities, thus obtaining the corresponding anonymous identifiers, there is no possible ambiguity between these two anonymous identifiers.

This was precisely the very first need of the french Ministry of Business and Social Affairs and CNAMTS: having anonymous but unambiguous identifiers so that statistics and data processing treatments can still be done in order to follow healthcare behaviors.

A *one way function* is not the same mathematical concept as a *collision-free function*:

- *collision-free function:* there is, for any couple x and x' of distinct nominative identifiers, a high probability that their corresponding anonymous identifiers $y = f(x)$ and $y' = f(x')$ are non equal;

- *non collision-free function:* there are couples of distinct nominative identifiers x and x' for which there is not a sufficiently high probability that their corresponding anonymous identifiers y and y' are non equal.

A collision-free function:

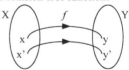

A non collision-free function:

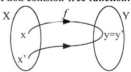

Taking into account this security requirement ensures that:
- data integrity is also maintained for the treatment of anonymous information, i.e. on the only basis of anonymous identifiers;
- responsibility of CNAMTS, which has to produce statistics on healthcare behaviors, will not be engaged for having produced, accidentally or even intentionally, wrong data or statistics due to the choice of a non collision-free anonymisation.

2.3. A robust access control function

A robust access control function is required if there is a possibility for the anonymisation function to be more or less partially publicly known.

A robust access control policy [1] [2] can be implemented in multiple, but complementary, ways such as:

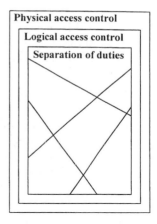

- *physical access control*: authorised persons/authorities, only, must have physical access to data processing devices allowed to execute the anonymisation function;

- *logical access control*: authorised persons/authorities, only, must have logical access (i.e., by software access control) to the data processing devices that are allowed to execute the anonymisation function;

- *separation of duties*: a precise conjunction of various persons/authorities, only, must be authorized, in order to obtain a required consensus needed for the execution of the very sensible anonymisation function.

Taking into account these three security policy requirements ensures that the anonymisation process will only be executed in conformance with all the conditions within which it has been specified and authorized to be executed.

3. Main features of F.O.I.N. and FUTUR applications

3.1. Main features of F.O.I.N.

In response to the *direct robustness requirement*, FOIN[3] has been specified on the basis of a powerfull one way function (i.e., SHA/SHS[4] Secure Hash Algorithm/Standard) which has been first specified by NIST (i.e., the USA National Institut for Standards and Technologies) and is currently recommanded by SCSSI (i.e., the french national agency: Service Central de la Sécurité des Systèmes d'Information) for such demanding usages as strong anonymisation.

In response to the *indirect robustness requirement*, FOIN[3] has been specified on the basis of new fundamental concepts implemented in the work done by CESSI/CNAMTS:

- the *authenticity concept* which consists in using a secret input when applying FOIN[3], so that anonymous identifiers can only be obtained in an authentic way, i.e. by the authorised and authentic owner(s) of this secret input;

- the *double-anonymisation concept* which consists in applying anonymisation twice:
  - firstly by the sender: *FOIN-Sender* is applied with a secret input, *Secret_Sender*, so that first-level anonymous identifiers are obtained from nominative identifiers,
  - secondly by the receiver: *FOIN-Receiver* is applied with another secret input, *Secret_Receiver*, so that second-level anonymous identifiers are obtained form the previous first-level anonymous identifiers.

The combination of the *authenticity* and *double-anonymisation* concepts ensures that no useful correspondance table can be built either at the sender stage or at the receiver stage, because a potential intruder could never obtain both secret inputs (i.e. the *Secret_Sender* and the *Secret_Receiver*).

Lastly, in reponse to the *access control robustness* requirement, FOIN[3] has been specified as follows:

- first, in response to the *physical access control* requirement, we have specified FOIN[3] to be implemented on an separated and isolated data processing device;
- second, in response to the *logical access control* requirement, we have specified that FOIN[3] should be only executed if the authorisation policy has been implemented on the basis of chipcard strong authentication;
- third, in response to the *separation of duty* requirement, we have specified the authorisation policy for the execution of FOIN[3] on the basis of Shamir's threshold scheme[5]: this means, in short terms, that the secret inputs, the *Sercet_Sender* input at the sender level and also the *Sercet_Receiver* input at the receiver level, have each been shared among a given number of authorised persons, or authorities if delegation is possible, that altogether have globally the responsibility to either authorise (if the threshold is reached) or refuse (if not reached) the execution of this sensitive function.

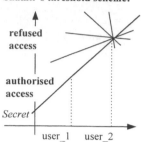

Shamir's threshold scheme:

3.2. Future applications of F.O.I.N.

Many future applications and usages of this function can be planed, since it is based on:
- the state of the art of security technologies (one way function, threshold scheme),
- a clear separation of duties (with robust logical access control facilities),
- legal authorisations from CNIL (i.e., french Commission Nationale de l'Informatique et des Libertés) which is at the origin of the demand for the elaboration of such a robust FOIN function and for its evaluation,
- government acceptation (i.e., the french Ministry of Social Affairs was involved in the specification process of FOIN and SCSSI has been involved in the evaluation process),
- healthcare professionals acceptation (private/public hospitals are/will be recommended to use FOIN because it is integrated in a national software of medico-administrative information transmission to mandatory healthcare insurer).

The final version of FOIN has been completed and a validation (by CNAMTS) and evaluation (by SCSSI) process has been completed on the basis of the final specification and implementation features of FOIN, so that more details on FOIN and the secret sharing technique will be soon publicly available. In any case, due to its robustness, this function must already be seen as a basic solution for a first serious approach of a future standardisation of the concept of *robust anonymisation function*.

4. References

[1] *Security in Opens Systems - A Security Framework*, ECMA TR/46, European Computer Manufacturers Association, July 1988.

[2] *Information Technology Security Evaluation Criteria*, Harmonized Criteria of France–Germany–the Netherlands–the United Kingdom, ISBN 92-826-3004-8, June 1991.

[3] *FOIN: Fonction d'Occultation d'Informations Nominatives*, CESSI/CNAMTS, Mai 1996.

[4] *Secure Hash Algorithm/Secure Hash Standard*, ISO/IEC CD10118-3 Information technology- Security techniques-Hash-Functions Part3: Dedicated hash-functions, ISO/IEC JTC1/SC27, April 15, 1995.

[5] *"How to share a secret"*, A.Shamir, Comm. of the ACM, vol. 22, n° 11, Nov. 1978, pp. 612-613.

Medical Informatics Europe '97
C. Pappas et al. (Eds.)
IOS Press, 1997

The Chernobyl Accident: predicting cardio-vascular disease in the ex-workers

B Richards, Department of Medical Informatics, UMIST, Manchester, UK
T. Lugovkina, Regional Centre of Radiation Medicine, Katrinsburgh, Russia

Abstract. This paper describes a computer package that has been used to predict the likelihood of the onset of cardiovascular diseases in these patients who were former workers (liquidators) on the Chernobyl site in the Ukraine, Chernobyl being the place where the Nuclear Power Station was destroyed when the atomic reactor got out of control and spread radiation over a very wide area both on the ground and into the atmosphere. The programme predicts the future morbidity in those patients with an accuracy of 90%.

1. Introduction

There was an accident at the Chernobyl Nuclear Power Station in 1990. Many of the people who were previously workers on the site have begun to show the effects of radiation. The work described below was an investigation into the effects of that radiation and the building of a computer software package to evaluate the risks.

Non- fatal doses of radiation can produce different reactions in the human being, the result depending on the individual features and on the strength and time-scale of the dose [1, 2]. One well known effect of radiation is the increase in cardio-vascular pathology. It has been already documented that atherosclerosis is a rather common occurrence amongst those exposed to radiation. [2]

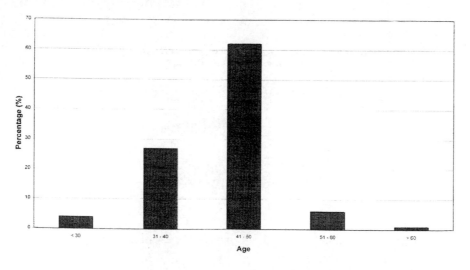

Figure 1. The current age structure of the Chernobyl workers

The N2 Regional Hospital in Katrinsburgh was chosen as an appropriate place to set up the Regional Centre for Radiation Medicine. This occurred in 1990 and since then more than 4000 workers from Chernobyl have become patients. Of these patients, approximately 90% of them are now in the age range 30 to S0 years old. Figure 1 shows the total distribution against age.

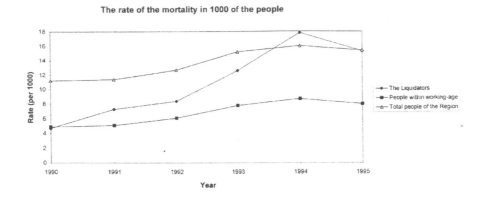

Figure 2. Mortality rates per 1000 of the population

As one monitored the incidence of coronary and cerebral circulation disorders among the workers, it became clear that there was a distinct increase in pathology from one year to the next. This was in contrast with a control cohort from the same city population [3]. Figure 2 shows the mortality rate, per 1000 people, for three different cohorts over the five year period from 1990 to 1995. It will be seen that, whereas the cohort representing the people of normal working age (20-60 years) shows only a slight increase, (from 4.9% to 8%), the increase in the ex-Chernobyl workers increases dramatically from 4.7% to 15.3%, an increase of at least a factor of three. The figure also shows that the incidence of mortality amongst the general population remains almost steady at approximately twice that of the working age-group.

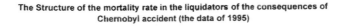

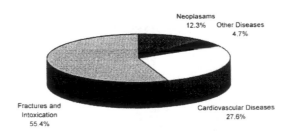

Figure 3. Major causes of death amongst the Chernobyl workers

When one analyses the mortality amongst the workers in 1995, three major causes of death were identified. There were Trauma (including suicides) and Intoxication (55.4%), Cardiovascular Diseases (27.6%), and Neoplasms (cancers) (12.3%). This distribution is shown in Figure 3. Thus one can see that cardiovascular diseases play a significant role in the mortality of this population.

In the light of the above it was decided to attempt to predict the individual risks for workers who, whilst having only functional disorders, were nevertheless patients at the hospitals and were therefore also candidates for cardiovascular problems [4].

The main aim of this research was to attempt to predict the risks to individuals by the use of mathematical methods, and then to embark on programmes of preventive therapy.

2. Methodology

It is no secret that the cause of cardiovascular disease is multi-factorial, and because the patients attending the Centre have had high levels of radiation and are now exhibiting psychological stress, the method of solution to the prediction problem seemed to be more attainable by the use of Pattern Recognition [5].

Each individual will have a list of attributes and, in any one individual, the values taken by these attributes will form a pattern or "alphabet". One will expect those patients with similar alphabets to cluster together in n-dimensional space, (where n is the number of attributes/parameters, generally less than 50). A discriminant function needs to be determined using these patients whose medical state at time t=0 is known and whose state at time t = 1, 2, 3, years is also known. It should then become possible to use the coefficient so determined in order to predict, for a new patient, the likely state of that patient in the years ahead.

The list of parameters (attributes) considered included the patients' age, sex, clinical symptoms observed whilst working in Chernobyl, the length of time spent in Chernobyl exposed to the radiation after the accident, the type of work done on the site and the closeness of the radiation source, the blood biochemistry and haematology results, the ECG analysis, etc.

3. The Package KVAZAR

The computer package KVAZAR was developed by Dr Kazantsev working in the Institute of Mathematics of the Urals Branch of the Academy of Science of Russia under the direction of Professor Mazurov, the Head of Department. [5]

This package KVAZAR is intended to be used for forecasting and classification. It uses pattern recognition and multivariate statistics. It has already demonstrated its success in several fields including geology, biology, medicine, and technology, [6]. It is thus a useful tool for discriminant analysis, and cluster analysis.

Figure 4 shows the Main Menu from the KVAZAR program, and Figure 5 shows the selection of a particular module.

This programme runs on an IBM compatible PC. Of course there are limitations on the programme. It can only cater for 40,000 elements: thus it can deal with 40 attributes on 1000 patients or 50 attributes on 800 patients.

```
┌─────────────────────────────────────────────────────────┐
│                      MAIN MENU                          │
│                                                         │
│   1. Computing of statistics of processing data         │
│   2. Regression analysis                                │
│   3. Analysis of separation of vector from given set    │
│   4. Taxonomy (cluster-analysis) of vectors             │
│   5. Taxonomy (cluster-analysis) of features            │
│   6. Discriminant analysis                              │
│   7. End of package processing                          │
│                                                         │
└─────────────────────────────────────────────────────────┘
```

Fl - Help F3 - Time ENTER - Execution ESC - Exit

Figure 4. The main menu in the KVAZAR program

```
┌─────────────────────────────────────────────────────────────────┐
│                        SELECT                                   │
│                                                                 │
│   1. To begin the  solving "Training by tutor" problem          │
│   2. To continue the solving of "Training by tutor" problem     │
│   3. To recognise the vectors by early constructed decision rules│
│   4. To analyse the allocation of the features in the groups of vectors│
│   5. To exit to main "menu" of the package                      │
│                                                                 │
└─────────────────────────────────────────────────────────────────┘
```

Fl - Help F3 - Time ENTER - Execution ESC - Exit

Figure 5. The menu to select a particular module in the KVAZAR program

4. The results

A total of 100 patients were used in the training set to determine the coefficients in the discriminant analysis. These coefficients were then used on a further set of 100 patients, whose outcomes were known, in order to test the effectiveness of the predictions. An accuracy of 90% was obtained. The most Significant variables contributing to accurate predictions were the blood triglycerides, lipoproteins, thrombocytes, alcohol consumption, and the number of cigarettes smoked. These latter two being of the greatest statistical significance.

The programme is now being tested on a much larger number of patients. The coefficients will be refined on a larger training set and further test sets will be used.

5. Conclusion

This programme is a most valuable tool for the determination of a likely prognosis and hence as a vehicle for advocating the most efficacious forms of treatment for these patients. The system is working well and is highly regarded.

6. References

1. Gofman J.W. Radiation and Health, Sierra Club Books
San Francisco, USA, 1981

2. Moskalev J.l., Djuravlev V.F., The risk in different conditions of radiation influence. Energoatomizdat,
Moscow 1983

3. Sharnerin V.M., Shalnova S.A., Kukushin S.K. et al
Cardio-vascular diseases and their risk factors in liquidators of the Chernobyl accident based on screening
researches 1993-95, Cardiology No 3, p44-46, 1996

4. Oganov R. G. Prophylatic cardiology: successes, failures, perspectives. Cardiology No 3, p4-8, 1996

5. Mazurov V.D., Kazantsev V.S., Beletsky N.G., The package of application programs for Pattern
Recognition, KVAZAR, Sverdlovsk, 1979.

6. Lugovkina T. Richards B., et al. Pattern recognition for the evaluation of the risk of
cholelithiasis. Healthcare Computing 1996, Harrogate p206 - 211, BJHC Ltd. Weybridge UK 1996

Medical Informatics Europe '97
C. Pappas et al. (Eds.)
IOS Press, 1997

Hepatocellular Carcinoma: the Virtual Hospitalization in Day-Hospital

Riccardo MACERATINI [1], Maurizio RAFANELLI [2], Fabrizio L. RICCI [3]

[1] Centro Interdipart. di Ricerca per L'Analisi dei Modelli e dell'Informazione nei Sistemi Biomedici, Univ. La Sapienza, Corso Vitt. Emanuele 244, 00185 Roma
[2] Ist. di Analisi dei Sistemi ed Informatica, CNR, Viale Manzoni 30, 00185 Roma
[3] Ist. di Studi e Ricerche sulla Doc. Scient., CNR, Via De Lollis 12, 00185 Roma

Abstract. The virtual hospitalization can be considered as the telematic evolution of the Day-Hospital, implementing the integration between hospital care and home care and predefining an hospital system which "goes to the patient home". In this paper the authors describe characteristics, motivations and advantages of this proposal, as well as the interaction model. Then the medical problem is illustred: the liver tumors, which are the more frequent malignant neoplasms, and, in particular, the epatocellular carcinomas, which represent about the 50% of these tumors. The Organization Model, the Information System and the Modalities of Telemonitoring for Hepatocellular Carcinoma are still illustrated and a brief cunclusion is given.

1. Introduction

In all the technologically advanced countries the cost of the health care is strongly increased. Two are the possible ways which are in front of the politicians (and of the health care managers). The former is the reduction of the public assistance, the latter is the optimization of the cost/benefit ratio redicing the wastes and optimizing the human and material resource use. In particular, by the business reengineering it is possible to emprove the care quality, decreasing the service waiting and execution times and, then, to reduce the service costs. The new organization system will be based on a new information system, which will use new informatics technologies and methodologies, which will allow to reduce the number of accesses to public specialistic structures and to optimize their use, assisting with continuity the patient everywhere he will be, allowing the control of the active diagnosys and care process on the patient and using, by teleconsulting, the medical expertise, distributed on the territory, in the different specialized medical centers.

A way to define these models is the redefinition of the existing ones, considering the present development of the telematic technology.

The virtual hospitalization can be considered as the telematic evolution of the Day-Hospital (DH), implementing the integration between hospital care and home care and predefining an hospital system which "goes to the patient home".

In this first phase of design and implementation of a new organization and information hospital system the authors refer only to the DH case, because its dimention is small but its social impact is strong (facility to accede to high tecnology services) with a substantial reduction of the costs (for example, the decrease of the hospitalizations). The business reengineering applied to the DH generates the virtual hospitalization, and, by the telemedicine system use, guarantees the syncronization, the integration and the optimization of the diagnostic, therapeutic and reabilitative interventions.

2. The Virtual Hospitalization: Characteristics, Motivations, Advantages

The virtual hospitalization is a reality at present technologically implementable by the use of the telematics.

It presents different *characteristics* [1]:
- the DH service acts on the patient also if he is physically present in the hospital only for very limited periods (the strictly necessary ones);
- the patient results "present in the hospital" also if he is in his home and continues to do his daily activities;
- the physician has an up-to-date situation of his health status and of the already made or in progress or to carry out actions (diagnostic examinations, therapeutic protocols, rehabilitative protocols, etc.) and, moreover, he knows the structures involved in such operations;
- the physician use all the health care structures which are on the territory to intervene on the patient (primary health care structures, laboratories, car hospitals, etc.), minimizing the moving of the patient on the territory and the waiting time and maximizing the information flow;
- in chronical situations, the patient can be monitored "at his home".

The implementation of the virtual hospitalization allows to verify the applicability of the business reengineering to the hospital sector with the advantages offered by the telemedicine systems which the technology develops and the market offers. It is important because has as priority the incentive of the health care service development by criteria of "distributed telematics". It is note that the medicine is essentially "Hospital Oriented" and the evolution of the DH towards the virtual hospitalization can have a relevant social impact.

The hospitalization presents three basic faults: the cost of the hospital charge, the cost deriving from the working activity not made and the psyco-affective problems depending on the hospitalization. The diffusion of the DH (useful in oncology, in the minimal surgical act and in the serious chronical diseases) allows the cost reduction, such as the "hotel" cost, and, on the other hand, the possibility to continue the working activity as well as the stay in own family. The telemonitoring at home reduces the period of hospitalization and emproves the life quality, integrating itself with the assistance post-hospitalization at home. Part of these hospitalizations made in DH can be implemented "virtually" nursing telematically the patient at his home or at his working place. Such a solution allows to improve the quality of the health care because it assures the continuity of the care also when the patient cannot go to the hospital, and decreases the social cost both for the hospital, and for the patient and his relatives (that often have to accompany him), reducing the troubles deriving from the moving of the sick and/or disabled people.

The *advantages* offered by the virtual hospitalization are briefly reported in the following:
- a better use of the different competences and of the health care resources;
- availability in real time of specialistic advices for minor health care centers;
- a better assistance to the communities which are territorially distributed;
- a capability to support different pressures deriving from demographical changes;
- a possibility to carry out in a better way the new diagnostical, therapeutical and adjuvant protocols;
- a reduction of the hospitalization times of the patient and of the home-hospital moving;
- a reduction of the public and private cost regarding the health care assistance;
- adaptation of the health care assistance to the variation of population.

3. The Interaction Model

The health care carries out during the virtual hospitalization involves the following "actors":
- the patient (object of the health care);
- the responsible of the health care (a physician, a team of physicians) that follows all the process of diagnosis and care relative to the patient;
- the supplier of the health care (the responsible of the health care, a specialist, a nurse, the same patient, a relative of the patient) that carries out the diagnostic, therapeutic and rehabilitative activities;
- the specialist (a physician, a team of physicians) that offers consultation in the evaluation of the data regarding the diagnostic examinations, in the definition of the diagnostic and therapeutic protocol.

Depending on the disease and on the type of activity to carry out on the patient, this last can be identified as the supplier of the health care (for example, for the taking of some biological parameters, such as the temperature, or of the giving of some drug by oral way, etc.). The intervention of medical and nursing staff as health care supplier can, in every case, obtain a more direct relationship between this staff and the patient because this last is even more aware of the therapeutical and diagnostical phases to which he is subjected.

The exchange of information among the different actors can happen both directly and by the access to the information which are in the medical folder of the patient. This information are supplied by all the actors according to well defined procedures of privacy and protection of the data. A further possibility of interaction between the health care responsible and the specialist consists of the teleconsulting which allows the discussion at distance of the results regarding diagnostic analyses and the definition of the following therapeutic interventations.

Contrary to the classic hospitalization, in the virtual hospitalization the patient is sometimes "physically" distant from the responsible of the health care. In order to guarantee the continuity and the quality of the clinical process, it is necessary that the responsible of the health care has always the up-to-date situation of the patient. This fact is obtained by the clinical folder which consists of both the clinical information and of managing information for the work organization and for the interaction among the different health care structures involved.

The clinical folder has to have both the clinical information and the list of the clinical activities suggested, planned and carried out (clinical protocol), as well as the execution state of the single activity (managing procedures) and of the information flows among the structures involved in this activity. This means that in it is stored also the clinical protocol which the responsible intends to follow in order to assure the coherence of the clinical acts.

In this context it is necessary to manage in a federate way among all the health care services involved in the virtual hospitalization the medical folder. It will guarantee also the storing and the trasmission of the biomedical images at high definition. Respecting the single autonome organization of the structures involved, the advantage of a federate management consists of the immediate availability of the medical folder of a given patient on all the territory, reducing the moving of the patient, of the medical and nursing staff, avoiding the repeating of already made diagnostic procedures.

4. The Medical Problem

The liver tumors are the more frequent malignant neoplasms, with over une million of new cases/year in the world. The epatocellular carcinomas (HCC) represent about the 50% of these tumors, with a ratio M/F of 4:1. The incidence is low in the USA (1.9 deaths per 100000 inhabitants/year), medium in Europe and South Africa (4,9 - 20), high in Cina, Korea and Mozambique (23,1 - 150), with a mortality at 5 years of the 80%. In the last ten years this incidence in Europe and in Japan is strongly increased, as well as the epatitis C, which at present has to be considered as the main etiopathogenetic factor (or co-factor), in case is high the synthesis of DNA [2], and the chronic active epatitis B (relative risk = 10-21.3%, risk that can be attributed = 31.1-56.3%, risk which is 98 times higher respect to patients HbsAg negative).

The recent progesses in the non invasive diagnostic by imagines have brought a changing of scenario: the ultraeterography (which allows an easier discrimination between HCC nodule and regeneration nodule with cirrhosis in progress), the echo-color-doppler, the computerized tomography (spiral, porto-TC) and the new method for the NMR with epato-specific means of contrast and evaluation of the enanchement curves allow at present to carry out a early diagnosis and a careful staging. Essential complements to the minimal criteria of standard staging (TNM) with regard to the therapeutical planning, are the vascolarization, the istologic type [3] and the human epato-specific alpha-phetoprotein dosage (HAFP-mRNA) [4] in the peripheral blood, correlated ($p < 0.001$) to the presence of the intra-epatic microdiffusion, portal thrombosis and metastases.

The liver neoplasms which are not treated have a survival less then three years in the 87% of the cases. Their association with the chronic epatitis can contra-indicate an invasive surgical approach and can vice versa suggests miniinvasive acts which, associated to a constant monitoring of associated diseases, obtain results of life expectancy and quality which are equivalent or superior to those of the resection or of the transplant.

The epatic percutaneous ethanol injection (max three modules, Child A-B, max volume 3 cm) presents the 98% of survival at one year and the 48-56% at five years [5]. The consequence of this fact is that the number of patients with primitive cancer of the liver that have a longer life expectancy and, then, need a continue monitoring and specialistic and multidisciplinary cares is in a strong increase. The solution to the high costs of the abovementioned situation is the virtual hospitalization which reduces such costs improving the life quality. The DH allows the virtual hospitalization by the management of the Medical Record of the patient by therapeutical and diagnostical telemonitoring.

5. The Organization Model, the Information System and the Modalities of Telemonitoring for Hepatocellular Carcinoma

The system architecture consists of the following integrated units: Medical Epatology Service, Surgical and Oncological Epatology Service, Day Hospital (DH, Surgical and Oncological), Listening Center, Hospitalization Department. The Operative Unit of Medical Epatology (OUME) carries out the screening of the new cases and, if there is the suspect of HCC, the patient is sent to the Operative Unit of Epatic Oncology which chooses among three different procedures: a) periodical controls in cooperation with the OUME; b) ultraeterography with biopsy; c) hospitalization in the DH.

If the HCC is strongly probable or istologically confirmed, all the procedures for the final confirmation of the disease or for the staging and the evaluation of the therapeutical options regarding the state, the operative risk and the associated diseases. In case of indication to the resection in DH, a neoadjuvant chemio-therapy and then the patient is sent to the surgical department for a regular hospitalization. The palliative treatments are made in the DH with associated the virtual hospitalization. When the patient is accepted, his Medical Folder is open. This Medical Folder is based on a Minimum Basic Data Set which is common to all the the operative units. The analyses of laboratory are carried out or verified, as well as the liver ecography, the thorax radiography, the electrocardiogram with cardiological examination, the spyrometry with pneumologic consultation (optional), the anestesiologic examination (optional); in case of necessity of other examinations, another "hospitalization" is planned. In general, within 2-7 days all the results of the diagnostic procedures are available, so that the following five situations can happen: 1) the surgical act is confirmed and the patient plans the hospitalization date (as conventional hospitalization); 2) the surgical act is not confirmed (high operative risk, presence of other more serious diseases, etc.); other mini-invasive procedures are activated (PEI); 3) the surgical act is confirmed, but it is necessary to put off it and to carry out a particular therapeutic protocol in order to reduce the operative risk; 4) there is an indication for palliative chemiotherapic procedures; 5) the indications are only palliative (advanced disease).

In the third case a monitoring and a therapy is proposed. This one will be carried out at home of the patient or across other health care structures on the territory, which will be controlled by telemedicine tools.

At the dismission from the DH (second hospitalization) the patient will be equiped with a cellular phone and/or a small suitcase of "telemedicine" which are connected to the Listening Center. He will have also the prescription of his therapy and a set of instructions for the correct use of the telematic system. The cellular phone (or a textual teledrin) is useful to communicate with the patient in every moment and everywhere he is. The small suitcase of "telemedicine" contains the instrumentation for the monitoring at distance, by telephone network, of the patient (for example, "cardiobip", or teleECG, etc.). The Listening Center, working 24 hours a day, consists of the same operators that work at the DH, and carries out by telematic way all the planned interventions (periodical verify of the patient conditions, suggestions to the patient and relative control, reservation of other controls, definition of the surgical act date, storing in real time of the information on the patient in his medical record, emergency management, etc.). In this way the patient will be accepted in the hospital for the surgical act only a few of hours before it (all the information is already available) and can be precociously dismissed because he will be continuously in contact with the Listening Center which will guarantee urgent assistance actions at home or a new hospitalization. The patient, in such a way, will do only a few of accesses to the DH (some controls reserved telematically). Only when the patient will give back the small suitcase of "telemedicine", he will be considered "dismissed" from the hospital.

The virtual hospitalization manages also the *emergencies*, which can be a consequence of a complicance depending on medical or surgical therapy, on mini-invasive procedures (PEI, etc), which can enter in the possible unforeseen complication; non classified a priori emergencies are those depending on unknown pre-existent or sopraggiunte diseases. The change of scenario when new diseases appear, or for the progression of neoplasms or of associated diseases (hepatitis, etc). In acute new problems or in emergency due to complications, the patient calls the physician. Different answers can be given: a) the probem is solved by phone (complications of low entity which the patient, assisted by phone, cas solve by himself); b) nursing staff is sent to the home of the patient to take physiologic parameters which cannot be tele-transmitted or for necessity of infusional therapies or other home cares; c) if the situation presents a problem, a physician is sent; d) in case of strong gravity or for necessity of urgent diagnostic laboratory or instrumental procedures, the DH (or conventional) hospitalization is carried out

A design methodology proposed and followed by the authors for the implementation of the first phase of this sperimentation consists of the definition of the different phases of this design, which are briefly listed in the following:
1) the clinical protocols
and, in particular, the role of the *distance*
2) the evolutive scenaros of the disease
and, in particular, the role of the *vital parametrers*
3) the clinical-managing funtionalities
and, in particular, the role of the *medical examination "at the bed"* of the *pazient* and of the *emergencies*
4) the organizing-information model
and, in particular, the role of the *Listening Center*
5) the systems and the technologies of the telemedicine
and, in particular, the role of the *integration*

6. Conclusions

The telemedicine systems which support the virtual hospitalization has to be seen as particular applications of telematic technologies for the medical assistance. This study has an high innovative paradigm, both for the health care and for the production environment. With regard to the medical assistance, it gives a contribution to improve its quality and effectiveness, to increase its accessibility and to reduce its costs. A recent study has quantified in 950 million of Euros/year the saving in Italy regarding the hospital cost if this services (DH and virtual hospitalization) was active on all the national territory.

References

[1] Maceratini R., Rafanelli M., Ricci F.L. Virtual hospitalization: reality or utopia? 8th World Congr. on Med. Inf., Medinfo '95, Vancouver, July 23-27, 1482-1486, 1995
[2] Tarao K, Ohkawa S, Shimizu A. et al. Significance of hepatocellular proliferation in the development of hepatocellular carcinoma from anti-hepatitis C virus-positive cirrhotic patients *Cancer*, 73, 1149-54, 1993.
[3] Yamashita Y, Matsukawa T, Arakawa A. et Al; US-guided liver biopsy: predicting the effect of interventional treatment of hepatocellular carcinoma. *Radiology*, 196, 799-804, 1995.
[4] Komeda T, Fukuda Y, Sando T et Al. Sensitive detection of circulating hepatocellular carcinoma cells in periferal venous blood. *Cancer*, 75, 2214-9, 1995.
[5] Ebara M, Kita K., Sugiura N. et Al.: Therapeutic effect of percutaneous injection on small hepatocellular carcinoma: evaluation with CT. *Radiology*, 195:371-7, 1995.

Medical Informatics Europe '97
C. Pappas et al. (Eds.)
IOS Press, 1997

A Sentinel Network Of General Practitioners For Epidemiologic Surveillance In Italy

Capozzi C*, Buonomo E°, Fusiello S*, Lucchetti G*, Mariotti S+, Noce A°, Palombi L°.
+Epidemiology and Biostatistics Lab, Istituto Superiore di Sanita', Rome
°Dep. of Public Health, Epidemiology Lab, Tor Vergata Univ., Rome
*Informedica, Janssen-Cilag s.p.a., Rome

Summary

A Computer Network of General Practitioners (GP's) has been established connecting 110 general practitioners representing a statistically selected national sample, homogeneously distributed all over Italy. The purpose of the network is to increase the epidemiologic surveillance on the health status of the Italian community, to collect useful data on the routine activity of the GP's, to promote computer use among them, and to organize some "ad hoc" investigations on specific subjects (case-control studies). To this purpose, a specific software was developed both to meet the requirements of epidemiological research and to manage general practitioners' clinical files. A working prototype of health card using micro-computer technology is also being experimented on a subset of the GP's.

Introduction

Data collected by general practitioners on their patients and on the diseases they observe during their activity are a valuable source of information, which is difficult to make use of because of lack of common protocols. The wide-spreading familiarization of GP's with programs for managing clinical files on personal computers on one hand, and the increased availability of telecommunication resources on the other hand, has considerably improved the possibility of collecting homogeneous data in view of an epidemiologic approach, and of implementing a "sentinel network" on the territory, to constantly monitor the trends of the most important pathologies in the population.

An information network including general practitioners (GP's) using the same clinical record software, willing to partecipate in public health surveys and to contribute yielding clinical information about their patients, was implemented with two major purposes: a) to collect suitable data from GP's, for monitoring the health status of the Italian population; b) to promote computer's usage among GP's [1].

Other more specific purposes of this network are: 1) to study the behavior of GP's in terms of diagnoses and prescriptions; 2) to investigate drugs' consumption corresponding to different diseases; 3) to study the disease incidences of the most common diseases clinically evaluated by GP's.

Methods

For the realization of the project, a group of monitoring doctors has been selected among 8.000 GP's distributed throughout Italy, who were encouraged by Janssen-Cilag to use computer applications in medicine since 1985. The first level of the network, including at the moment 110 doctors linked up in tele-processing with a mainframe computer in order to collect data and exchange information has been operative since June 1994. The GP's who participate in this level of the network are selected in such a way that their patients constitute a suitable geographical sample of the whole Italian population.. A new clinical record software program has been designed specifically to meet both the requirements of epidemiologic research and the basical needs of GP's: while allowing a user-friendly approach and operational speed, it guarantees data completeness and reliability, through the definition of a Minimum Data Set (MDS) of comparable clinical information collected by standardized methods. The information belonging to the MDS, coded according to international scientific standards by means of tables of pre-defined codes, is requested for all patients. The data gathered through the network are used by epidemiologists and Health planners belonging to the National Institute of Health, to the Department of Epidemiology of the second University of Rome, and to the National Research Council, which is the main sponsor of the Project.

Results

As a first example of epidemiologic use of the network, a survey on hypertension treatment was conducted, in which all 110 GP's were asked to measure the systolic and diastolic blood pressure of all patients entering their ambulatory in a week of November, 1994, and record the measurements in the clinical record, in addition to normal anamnestic findings and prescriptions. Data collected by 50 doctors were gathered through the network and centrally analyzed. No anti-hypertensive prescriptions were given to many patients with abnormal pressure levels, and an abnormal proportion of prescriptions of "heavy" drugs, which might potentially have strong side-effects, was found. The GP's were asked to participate to round tables on hypertension in one of four Italian cities (the nearest to residence). Advise on the most recent trends in hypertension treatment was given by a well-known cardiology teacher of the University of Rome. Free discussions took place among participants. The detailed results of the survey are available [2-4]. A second survey involving the same 50 doctors was scheduled for November, 1995, to monitor eventual changes in prescription habits, following the panels. Data about this second round show that after participation to round tables, the monitoring of hypertension was both more frequent and more accurate, and the subministration of different types of anti-hypertensive drugs more balanced.

A second level of the network with the purpose of validating a model of health card using CP-8 micro-computing technology was started at the end of 1995. Purpose of this level of the network is to explore the possibility of including in the network different levels of care providers such as specialists, hospital departments, clinical laboratories, and of experimenting with the transfer of patients' health information from the GP's archives to central health structures. This network level was implemented in two small geographic areas, one in Northern Italy and the other in the South, including overall 16 GP's equipped with a CP-8 smart card reader, driven by the same software program used in the first network level. About 6000 smart cards were distributed to selected patients with higher health care needs by the participating 16 GP's. Several health structures in the two areas were similarly equipped with work-stations running the same software, among them the pediatric and general medicine departments of local hospitals, and emergency units. Smart card use in these structures is monitored by specially trained personnel.

Discussion

Sentinel networks are very important for monitoring the health status of a country. Network of this type are known to be fully functional in a few European countries, the first TP network being probably the one in France, which was originally based on the MINITEL. Other information networks are being operated in England, Northern Ireland, Denmark, Holland and Switzerland, although some of these use paper reports rather than teleprocessing for collecting data from the GP's. A review of European sentinel networks in Public Health was published in 1995 [5].

The GP's sentinel network here presented, as far as we know, is the only one which is spread all over Italy, encompassing different regional health conditions.

The General Practitioners included in the network showed a good attitude in recording their visits using a clinical record software, and demonstrated willingness to participate in public health projects for monitoring the health status of the population. The participation to panels in which the results of a survey on hypertension treatment were examined was high, and a subsequent survey showed that they had learned from the discussions. The experimentation with the smart card prototype was also successful, although up to now, due to the limited number of patients (6000) to whom the cards have been distributed, the interaction with the health facilities equipped with the card readers has been somehow limited.

Aknowledgements
Part of this work was made possible by a grantof the National Research Council (CNR)- Targeted Project "Prevention and Control Disease Factors"; Sub-project: "Community Medicine"; Research Line: Informatization of General Practitioners". Research Contract N. 95.01290.41.

References

[1] Mariotti S, Buonomo E, Lucchetti G, Palombi L, Panfilo M, Fusiello S: An experimental network of General Practitioners for purpose of Epidemiologic surveillance in Italy. Abstract of presentation at the Medinfo '95 Conference (Vancouver): Proceedings of Medinfo 1995, pp.1553-4., 1995.

[2] Palombi L., Buonomo E, Mariotti S, Panfilo M, Fusiello S, Lucchetti G, Panà A. Attività assistenziale di medicina generale: una indagine realizzata su una rete informativa di medici di Base. Recenti Progressi in Medicina, v. 86, n. 2, pp. 48-52, 1995.

[3] Palombi L, Panfilo M, Mariotti S, Fusiello S, Buonomo E, Lucchetti G, Panà A: Informatizzazione del medico di base. Atti del convegno "Informatica e Telematica nei servizi sanitari", Univ. Tor Vergata 1995. Medicina e Informatica , Suppl 1, 1995.

[4[Capozzi C: Utilizzo di una rete informatizzata di medici di base a scopi epidemiologici e formativi: Risultati di una prima indagine sperimentale. Igiene e Sanità Pubblica 6/1996; L11: 627-36.

[5] Boydell L:"The Epidemiological Bridge": Role of telematics in the collection of epidemiological data from general practice. In: Telematics in Primary Care in Europe. J. DeMaeseneer and L. Beolchi, Eds, IOS Press, 1995.

Medical Informatics Europe '97
C. Pappas et al. (Eds.)
IOS Press, 1997

215

An Access Interface Platform for
Health/Social Information Services:
HealthGate

P. Angelidis, G. Anogianakis, S. Maglavera

BIOTRAST S.A., Thessaloniki, Greece

1. Introduction

This work presents a generic solution to access Health/Social Information Services, by means of an access interface platform which is here described in general terms. This access platform has been named HealthGate and has been designed within project *Infocare* under the Health Telematics EU co-funded programme.

The platform comprises:
1. a set of generic services or modules that can be easily assembled to build specific applications
2. a development environment that allows the design of common solutions to scenarios with different access technologies available and user needs (user types, tasks to perform and usage environment)

2. Health/Social Information Services

Health Information Services aim to supply the appropriate information to a wide range of user groups: citizens in general, healthcare purchasers, third party payers, administrators and providers of resources, health/social professionals and researchers [1]; all of them demanding such a variety of information services that it is easy to envisage the health sector as one of the most demanding in the Information Society. InfoCARE is concerned with a significant spectrum of health and social information services:

1) services oriented to provide information to the citizens or the professionals, to facilitate them the access to the knowledge about the available health/social resources and services offered in the area/region; help them to make the most appropriate choice to their individual problem; and to arrange the appointment of specific services and the recommendation on how to access to the service;
2) services designed to support health prevention campaigns ;
3) services to provide the access of the user (citizens or professionals) to information concerning a specific health, social or related problem to support consultation sessions. This class of services will be only considered in the project at a very preliminary level.

Apart from the common features and their trend which characterises any kind of information service, in the case of health/social applications some constraints need to be taken specially into account in the design and specifications stages of Health Information Services:

a) High multimedia predominance to make the service attractive must be supported.
b) Security and data confidentiality is critical and must be assured.
c) Access control through authentication and access priorities protocols are mandatory.
d) Different user experience, social and educational levels must be accommodated.
e) Feedback service evaluation and user characterisation must be provided to optimise performance, usability and service cost-efficiency.

f) Unlimited database accessibility and sharing, regardless of the location and structure, must be supported.

g) Enough bandwidth and transmission resources must be assured.

The generic scenario of the health/social information service we are considering is shown in Fig. 1, which presents the main elements involved, together with the information flow between them:

a) The service provider centre, responsible for editing, delivering, maintaining and processing the information both to citizens and professionals, and monitoring service quality;

b) The networks, that conforms the telematic environment to bridge users and providers;

c) The citizens both at home and/or public access points (i.e. kiosks,..) at health centres, community pharmacies,..;

d) The professionals both in a health centre and/or his/her public/private consultation office.

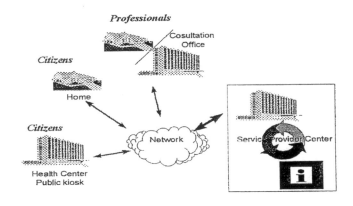

Fig. 1   Basic scenario of Health Information Services

3. Access interface approach proposed

To provide an efficient solution to the specificities of the Health Information Services stated above a platform is proposed to drive the definition of the functional specifications of the InfoCARE Demonstrators. The solution proposed rely on a generic computer and telephony platform concept, suitable to the health information services, that has been named *HealthGate*.

The main objective of this computer and telephony platform is to provide a standard interface for the users to access health services. It consists of a client/server architecture, based on a remote object invocation model [2] and database remote/local management, to assure terminal platform portability, world-wide availability, an efficient environment for services design, while providing transparent connections to integrate most terminals available: PC's, public kiosks, mobile laptop, Network PC's.

HealthGate proposes and interface independent of the access device (Phone, Web), offering the same dialogue interface to the user either by a Computer/Internet-terminal or by a Call Centre agent. This property, called *consistency*, fits naturally the interface concept that citizens demand, providing a mixed *Human/Computer* interface [3].

Consistency allows an easy vehicle for users to migrate to Internet-world or other access mechanisms with a lower cost and higher performance, providing a powerful Information Society educational tool for citizens.

Finally, it is clear that this universal access, available through advanced technology has to include another important constituent: any change required to include new services as they become available has to be easily integrated without much extra-effort, allowing user groups to quickly benefit of new and future services and dialogue environments. To cope with this HealthGate includes a well defined developing guidelines and tools for Health/Social Information Services

4. Description

HealthGate access interface for information services consists of a generic platform to fulfil most needs of a wide variety of user groups, both citizens asking for health/social care and professional carers, without depending on special technology knowledge and with a world-wide availability. It has been structured, as shown in Figure 2, following the Computer and Telephony Integration (CTI) conceptual guidelines, as a combination of Call Centre and Internet technologies, involving different agents: user groups (citizens and professionals) and communicating entities showed in the picture.

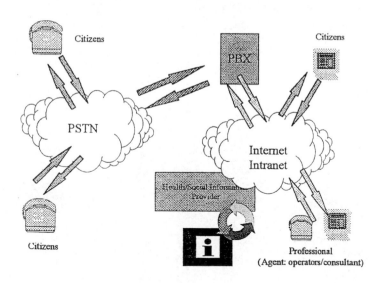

Figure 2   Computer and Telephony Integrated structure

HealthGate allows that call centres and computer resources living together in a seamless system. CTI is based on client/server structures into a LAN/WAN environment where agents, switch boards (PBX) and computers, are sharing resources. With CTI, some capabilities are improved: hardware devices and system design costs are reduced, integration of voice and keypad recognition devices, etc.

5. Service Access Interface

Generally speaking, Information Services can be considered composed by two clear cut and independent elements: the Information Service Interface (ISI) and the Information Service Procedure (ISP).

- ISI is responsible for the user interaction/event management, providing tools to enhance man-machine, or man-information interface.
- ISP is responsible for the specific processing of the information retrieved by ISI, running as a background procedure.

For example, an appointment service can be mapped into ISI and ISP elements as follows: ISI is the user interface to navigate across the different GP's and timetables available, and to introduce the final selection into the database; ISP will process this information to arrange the appointment, reporting the result to ISI.

As commented before, this platform is **only** an interface between users and Health Care Centre's database systems. A generic scheme of the platform is showed in Figure 3, where is clearly depicted the specific role that HealthGate plays into a Health Information Service environment. For the rest of this document, the term *Access Interface* will be used to name the ISI module of a service.

The platform manages user accesses, either by phone or by computer, by interfacing tasks between the service background procedures and the user interactions. The local database is a shared resource that provides communication between the interface and the procedures through the data records. Although, no background procedure developing tools are initially available in the platform, communication links (call-back procedures) will be supplied to connect ISI and ISP layers.

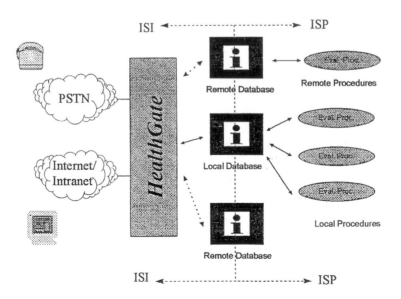

Figure 3   Generic platform access environment

HealthGate will also supply mechanisms to access and back-up remote databases in a transparent way during Health Information Service's design stages, providing easy data distribution, sharing world-wide available data, and avoiding complex database tasks to developers.

6. Access levels

The levels of access of the platform are :
1.   Master :
Supervisor and Access Interface designer are within this category. This access level allows them to modify, consult system variables, and finally design/validate/shutdown specific Health/Social Information Services.
2.   Agents:
Any personnel who is attending Call Centre functions. HealthGate considers two kind of agents, depending on their role in the health model: operators and consultants.
   • Operators : Trained persons to dispatch common consultations or manage prevention campaigns.
   • Consultant : Specialised professionals supplying high value information that agents are not authorised to deliver.
3.   Intranet kiosks:
Professional/citizens accessing the service through any public Web-based terminal: touch-screen systems, Network Computers, laptop, etc. Different data access authentication protocol will be supplied to manage confidentiality and security.
4.   Internet Home Terminals:
Similar to kiosk but with the intrinsic constrains of access performance and Internet.

7. Access and design consistency

The Access Interface of the service is designed in such a way that consistency between accesses is preserved, i.e., voice and agent interactions are similar to an usual Internet navigation. Phone calls are routed to the PBX of the Health Information Provider, responsible for switching and priority managing; optionally, allowing interactions via voice recognition or DTMF. Once a call is attended by an agent, the user accesses the service using the same facilities as Internet user does, through a "human" interface. Three possible devices are available for both communication directions, depending on either the user or the Health Centre initiated the contact: PBX with Voice Recognition Module, Internet-based Terminal, PBX only.
The layered structure of the whole system is depicted in figure 4:

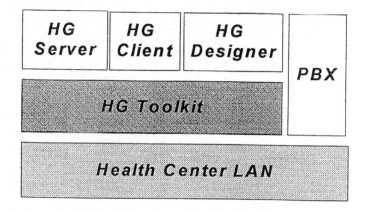

Figure 4   Full system layer structure

Over the Health Centre's LAN, a library, the HealthGate Toolkit, contains all the client/server functionalities, remote object skeletons and stubs, and database remote/local management tools. This library will provide all the software resources to fulfil the requirements of any application, and also, will assure PBX and VRU (optional) accessibility. On top of the middle layer, the HealthGate Toolkit (HG Toolkit), a set of applications are developed: the HealthGate Server, the HealthGate Client and the HealthGate Designer. Hardware devices PBX and Voice Recognition Units (VRU) will be integrated into and connected to the Health Centre LAN (Intranet) through CTI-Link specific mechanisms.

8. References

[1] EC-DG XIII. Work-Programme: "Telematics Applications Programme (1994-1998).

[2] James Rumbaugh, Michael Blaha, Willian Premerlani, Frederick Eddy, Willian Lorensen. "Object-Oriented Modeling and Design". Prentice Hall Int. De. 1991

[3] Alan Dix, Janet Finlay, Gregory Abowd, Rossell Beale. "Human Computer Interaction". Prentice Hall Int. De., 1993

[4] EC-DG XIII Telematics Application Programme Project:HC-1054 InfoCARE D4.1 «FUNCTIONAL SPECIFICATIONS», Sept. 1996

Medical Informatics Europe '97
C. Pappas et al. (Eds.)
IOS Press, 1997

Cardiomedia: A Multimedia Portable Medical Record on Optical Memory Card

D. Delamarre[1], S. Croci[3], A Baskurt[4]Dr M. Bedossa[2], Dr H. Le Breton[2],
M. Decaix[5], Pr JC Pony[2], Pr P. Le Beux[1]

[1]Département d'Information Médicale CHU de Rennes, 2 rue H. Le Guillou 35033 Rennes
[2]Service d'Hémodynamique CHU de Rennes, 2 rue de l'Hôtel Dieu 35033 Rennes Cédex
[4]U.R.A. 1216 Creatis (CNRS), 20 av. A. Einstein, 69621 Villeurbanne Cédex
[3]CERIUM Laboratoire Signaux et Images en Médecine, 2 av. Léon Bernard, 35043 Rennes
[5]CANON France S.A., Centre d'affaires Paris-Nord 93154 Le Blanc-Mesnil Cédex

Abstract. The main objective of the CARDIOMEDIA project is to produce and evaluate a coronarian multimedia data record stored on an optical card. The experimentation concerns patients treated by angioplasty at university hospital of Rennes. Often patients treated in the Regional University Hospital are followed up by another Health structure closer to their home. The patient leaves hospital with his card, which is directly available elsewhere for emergency or for consultation. This will optimize the number of examinations and offer a better patient follow-up. The CARDIOMEDIA card is a specialized record which includes various data type : text, image, image sequence of coronarography and ECG signal. For this purpose optical card with its large memory size is very convenient. For medical imaging, we use in this project the DICOM format for image exchange and management, it is combined with a CARDIOMEDIA specific compressing software. For multimedia record, the HTML format and web intranet method are chosen, this allows intuitive interface which can combine various data type and helpers like DICOM image viewer.

1. Introduction

In the medical information system, medical data necessary for the patient follow-up are physically and logically dispatched through various particular information system, public or private, which store the medical patient history. Despite the advance in networks technology, useful and necessary information for the physician are not available at a given time and a given place. Another main feature is the large form and type of data in the medical area. Today, there are textual data with numeric data, signal, image and video in the patient medical record. In this context the optical memory card, with its large memory space, can be a good candidate for a portable medical record to provide a better information communication between medical actors.

The main objective of the CARDIOMEDIA project is to produce and evaluate a coronarian multimedia data record stored on optical card. This project concerns patients treated by angioplasty. The Epidemiological Data show that one patient out of three hospitalized is affected by a coronarian pathology. Often patients treated at Regional

University Hospital of Rennes are followed up by another health structure closer to their home. For this purpose, it seems to be better to store images and coronarographical results on non erasable supports for next consultation and or for a potential new hospitalization. This will optimize the number of these examinations and offer a better patient follow-up.

2. Materials and methods

2.1. Memory card technology

Memory card is a normalized information support in its size and form, but from a technology view point there are various system used. Today two of them are relevant for the medical domain. The first one is the smart card, which has computing capability but a limited memory capacity. The second one, the optical memory card is a passive support but with a large memory size, 4 to 6 Mbytes. The chip card applications fields are holder identification, with data which can be updated. Optical card can be used for application which need large memory space. If a smart card can store typically 2 text pages, 2000 pages can be stored onto the optical support. Therefore, the data type can be more complex and includes images, sounds and other numeric signals [1].

In regards to medical data, it is necessary to have secure and confidential support. On this topic, smart card have an active control with personal identification number (PIN) [2]. The Canon optical card implement an access control to data partition by password which must be set before the first write access. Another way to confidentiality is the encryption method, there is standards in this domain like the Data Encryption Standard (DES) and the Rivest, Shamir and Adelman algorithm (RSA) [3]. Furthermore, the WORM technology of optical card ensure that data are physically not updated from their first writing.

2.2. Health field application

In the medical area, there are three target applications [4, 5], we can consider the card as (i) the insurance card, (ii) the health professionals card or (iii) the patient card. The smart card is relevant for the two first ones. The third application view the card as a portable medical record, the amount of data is potentially high and in this case the optical card is relevant. There are multiple advantages for the card owner which has always personal information on a normalized support. The CARDIOMEDIA project is an example of a specialized cardiologic record which focus on the third type of application.

2.3. Information system and user interface

The client-server web model, as a intra-web system has been experimented in private hospital network [6,7]. On server side, we can have multiple location for information and servers on the local network, specific developments are added to provide new services. For the CARDIOMEDIA application, the optical card becomes a complementary data source as an import export device of the information system. On client side, it is a user friendly interface with hypertext and multimedia capabilities which can display multimedia document. Client software exists for many platforms.

3. Implementation and results

3.1. Medical description of the CARDIOMEDIA medical record

The CARDIOMEDIA medical record is designed for coronarian patient who have been treated by angioplasty. The main data elements are described in the following. In the operating room, physicians describes the coronary artery state by using two images before and after dilatation procedure. They also need one image sequence cycle to show heart flow from a dynamic point of view. The record includes also the ECG signal after the procedure. Textual information typed by the secretary from the local information system are added to the patient data card, this is administrative data and the patient discharge summary (Fig 1).

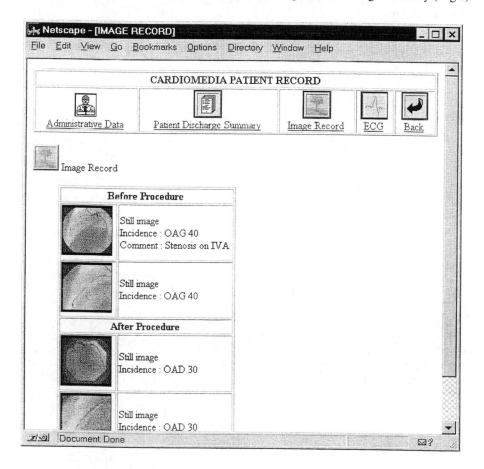

Figure 1: Web user interface: Users access to patient record elements through an hypermedia web interface on intra-web system.

3.2. Description of the CARDIOMEDIA prototype

The CARDIOMEDIA system can be further divided in two main functions. The first one is the acquisition system, in compliance with existing records databases and radioangiography materials, which permits to conceive a portable patient card and store it on optical card. The second one is the system for processing the multimedia data card with the record viewer. The technical characteristics are described in table 1.

3.3. Technical characteristics

Table 1: CARDIOMEDIA station characteristics

Image size	512 x 512 x 8 bits
Multimedia integration	HTML intranet WEB
Image format	DICOM GIF DCM
Compress ratio	12
CARDIOMEDIA record size	11 000 Kb
Compressed CARDIOMEDIA record size	840 Kb
Optical memory card capacity (with EEC)	4 890 Kb
Writing time for a record (compressed)	113 s (7.4 Kb/s)
Reading time for a record (compressed)	46 s (18 Kb/s)
Compress/decompress time for image	3s / 2s
Computer	PC pentium / 32 Mb RAM
Optical card device	Canon optical card reader/writer RW-50

Imaging : Images are recovered from existing radioangiography materials, the time necessary for physicians selection is low and evaluated as 5 min at the end of the procedure. From the control video image and sequence are captured and stored into the DICOM format [8]. This format is adapted for medical use and allows a progressive solution in regards to new version of image processing equipment which can produce numeric data directly in this exchange format.

Compressing : The CARDIOMEDIA compressing module is a specific one, and is the result of research works in the medical domain area [9]. The acceptable average compression ratio is up to 12, therefore a full CARDIOMEDIA record having a size of about 11 Mb before compressing, can be stored in only 0.8 Mb after compressing.

Optical Card : All access to the optical card are submitted to access control, this is done by an indirect manner. First a password is set by the creating system when cards have no data recorded, this is a functionality provided by the Canon optical card library. Secondly, there is a record viewer which control users and release card password.

Viewing : The consultation module is based on the intranet-Web technology [10]. All textual and image documents are embedded in multimedia HTML document. Image and sequence can be viewed on the web client or on a specific DICOM viewer .

Integration in a clinical information system : CARDIOMEDIA includes a PC intranet Web server, with specific Common Gateway Interface (CGI) which supplies a single interface for write or read an optical card, and viewing a record under access control. Furthermore, the intra-web feature provides integration ability, the card object is directly integrated in a local information system.

4. Discussion and conclusion

Building a portable medical record is related to a storage technology for sensitive information which must be compliant with some constraints. It must have a sufficient memory size capacity, a reliability and durability of information, a quick access.[1]. If the first objective is to offer a better information communication, access control must be also effective. The CARDIOMEDIA project with its optical memory card can be used as a candidate for this applicative domain. Such a portable medical record has multiple implications on various health system actors, users and providers. The project aim is to use such a card to focus and targeting the following objectives. For the patient itself, the card offers a better security in emergency situation and follow-up. Furthermore it becomes an active communication agent with the freedom to carry and give his card to the physicians for consultation. For Cardiologists, it will answer to their request in terms of information communication and information quality related to continuity of care. For hospital and medical information department, this project answers the need to establish some model which includes such a portable information support in the hospital information system, the intra-web model can be a suitable integration platform. From the health expenses point of view, a card can reduce the number of film duplication and unnecessary examinations for diagnosis and associated drug medication. Finally for Industrials, this project is an occasion to elaborate an application with a real portable multimedia medical record, adapted to the users needs and in fact to the market, from a concrete experiment. The same system could be used for other pathologies, such as chronic diseases, obstetrics, urology and for periodic examinations like mammography.

Acknowledgments : *This Project is partially financed by the Council for Hospital and Health Informatics (CIHS project 005)*

References

[1] Guibert-H; Gamache-A. Optical memory card applicability for implementing a portable medical record. *Med-Inf-Lond.* 1993 Jul-Sep; 18(3): 271-8.

[2] Beuscart R., Grave C., George P. Carte à mémoire et accès sécurisé. *Technologie Santé* : 14 : pp. 106-110 (1993).

[3] Engelbretcht R., Hidebrand C. and Jung E. The smart card: An ideal tool for a computer based patient record. *In : MEDINFO 95 proceedings.* R.A. Greenes et al (Eds) IMIA 1995, pp 344-348 (1995).

[4] Fedi P. Les professionnels de la santé et la carte à mémoire. *Gestions hospitalières* : 317, pp. 479-482 (1992)

[5] Lindley R. A. and Pacheco F. Smart Practice: Smart card design considerations in health care. *In : MEDINFO 95 proceedings.* R.A. Greenes et al (editors) IMIA 1995, pp 349-353 (1995).

[6] Bouaud J., Seroussi B., Zweigenbaum P. An experiment towards a document-centered hypertextual computerised patient record. *In MIE 96 proceedings,* J Brender & al (Eds), IOS Press, pp 453-457 (1996).

[7] Willard K.E, Hallgren J.H., Sielaff B., Connelly D.P. The deployment of a world wide web (W3) based medical information system. *In : SCAMC 95 proceedings,* R.M. Gardner (Ed), AMIA, pp 771-775 (1995).

[8] Jensch P. & al. DICOM V3.0 - The CEN trial implementation. *SPIE vol 2165 PACS Design and Evaluation* (1994).

[9] Benoit-Cattin H., Baskurt A., Prost R. 3D medical image coding using separable 3D wavelet decomposition and lattice vector quantization. *Signal Processing Special Issue on Medical Image Compression,* Dec 96, 18 pages (In press).

[10] Bernes-Lee T., Connolly D. Hypertext Markup Language, *Internet Draft IIIR Working Group.*

Medical Informatics Europe '97
C. Pappas et al. (Eds.)
IOS Press, 1997

Telematics and Smart Cards in Integrated Health Information System

Sicurello F., Nicolosi A.

Institute of Advanced Biomedical Technologies, National Research Council, Milano (Italy)

Abstract

Telematics and information technology are the base on which it will be possible to build an integrated health information system to support population and improve their quality of life. This system should be based on record linkage of all data based on the interactions of the patients with the health structures, such as general practitioners, specialists, health institutes and hospitals , pharmacies, etc.

The record linkage can provide the connection and integration of various records, thanks to the use of telematic technology (either urban or geographical local networks, such as the Internet) and electronic data cards.

Particular emphasis should be placed on the introduction of smart cards, such as portable health cards, which will contain a standardized data set and will be sufficient to access different databases found in various health services . The inter-operability of the social-health records (including multimedia types) and the smart cards (which are one of the most important prerequisites for the homogenization and wide diffusion of these cards at an European level) should be strongly taken into consideration.

In this framework a project is going to be developed aiming towards the integration of various data bases distributed territorially, from the reading of the software and the updating of the smart cards to the complete management of the patients' evaluation records, to the quality of the services offered and to the health planning. The applications developed will support epidemiological investigation software and data analysis. The inter-connection of all the databases of the various structures involved will take place through a coordination center, the most important system of which we will call "record linkage" or "integrated database".

Smart cards will be distributed to a sample group of possible users and the necessary smart card management tools will be installed in all the structures involved. All the final users (the patients) in the whole network of services involved will be monitored for the duration of the project.

The system users will also include general practitioners, social workers, physicians, health operators, pharmacists, laboratory workers and administrative personnel of the municipality and of the health structures concerned.

1. Medical Records and Electronic Data Cards

"Electronic Record is an essential technology for health care". With this assertion the Institute of Medicine (IOM) of the American National Academy of Science, in 1991, recommended a wide diffusion within the end of this century.

The social-health record is the collection of all the information about a person collected during his interaction with social health structures (social services, specialized ambulatories, hospitals, labs, home care, General Practitioners, etc.) (1). This record represents a bridge between the user and the social health structures in the different services, and it is the core element of the social and health databases (2) (3).

The possibility of using suitable hw/sw technologies allows the management of the available kinds of information (numerical, textual, eidetic data) even in the social health record: we can speak of multimedia records and databases.

In the social/health record we can consider some essential parts of information:
- administrative data;
- emergency data;
- social security and insurance data;
- health care data.

The health care data should permit a complete evaluation of the patient for an up-to-date treatment based on an appropriate evaluation scale.

By the term Electronic Data Card we mean a way of storing personal data, having a standard format of credit card easily usable and portable by any people (4) (5) A smart card can be considered a portable electronic record. Smart Cards support a microprocessor and data are stored on ROM or EPROM, and the Optical Cards or Laser Cards operate mainly in the WORM modality (write once-read many times). At the European level workgroups exist on the harmonization and homogenization of cards in the Social-health field (as the Concerted Action "Eurocards on Patient Data Cards") (6), where some criteria have been setup regarding the identification of the following basic components of a social-health card:
- administration and identification information
- a set of common attributes (manufacturer company, emission and expiry data), name of the subject with possible additional ID information
- medical emergency data
-data related to particular pathologies and/or pathologies involved in card experimentation (diabetes, dialysis, etc.):
- additional social-health information.

The cards are in the users' hands and their technology guarantees a high grade of privacy, ensuring data integrity through different security methods (cryptography, digital encoding, etc.). As a result of the mobility of people, it is necessary to provide access to social and health services throughout the countries.

The use of the Electronic Data Cards on a wide scale will determine a common effort of change and homogenization among the operators.

One important aspect in using social-health records and cards as a personal record is the interoperability of these device inside of the various information systems. This concept is essential because the smart card is the link between the databases and it can be used in emergency situations , where a standardization of data is needed . Interoperability increases the number of organizations that may have access to the data.

However, this also means that the security procedures of the members of the interoperability agreement must be reviewed, ensuring that the agreement cannot be circumvented and that access to cards should be restricted in an appropriate way.

2. Databases technology and multimedia

The possibility of using appropriate hw/sw technologies allows the management of the heterogeneous available information (data, texts, images) even in the social-health record (7)(8). We can speak of multimedia records and of multimedia database systems.

Complete health information is meant as multimedia. It is hoped that diagnosis images and biosignals could be available for every patient, but conveying such kinds of information presupposes an advanced telematics technology.

The concept of the social-health workstation is to provide a single user friendly access to the electronic record for the operators. With the recent advances in desktop computing in user-friendliness and cost-effectiveness and the more widespread availability of industry standard mechanisms for accessing various databases, the concept is very close to reality. In this way the operators will be able to access data in a consistent manner although it may contain information from various sources in a number of different formats and will be therefore Multi-media in nature, e.g. textual, images, graphical, voice, etc.(9).

The workstation based on multimedia social-health record can integrate documents and image scanning technologies to ensure a comprehensive approach to accessing and archiving information in a multi-site environment (10)(11).

3. Record Linkage and telematic networks

The Record Linkage allows the link of the social-health data from different sources (social services, entertainment centers, hospitals, etc.) resident on different databases or information systems and related to the same individual (12)(13). The implementation of record-linkage methods allows for a quick disposal of the complete and updated social-health situation of every subject: it is possible to know his whole administrative and social/health history, even if fragmented into different archives. The benefits of this technology are manifold in the field of preventive medicine, in epidemiology and in social-health scheduling.

The Record Linkage is applied in different ways in many countries on population groups at a social-health district level. The linkage using communication technologies and/or the use of smart cards including information about all the interactions of the subject with the social-health structure will allow the use of specialized resources allocated in different places for different purposes (clinical , statistical, epidemiological, health planning and scheduling, etc.). The integration effort by networks and/or smart cards must ensure a full inter-operability between records, in order to guarantee readability and comparability between records from different sources (14)(15).

In this context a main role will be played not only by the full connectivity of the suitable hardware supports (modem, local and geographical networks), but also by the standardization and coding methodologies. Moreover, the circulation and exchange of social-health information, as well as the possibility of connection to data banks, databases and remote information services for consultation or access to services, require a definition of international standards in order to guarantee data privacy and security. (The data access must be controlled by means of protection methods based on different keywords and levels, for example depending on the kind of operator who is asking for access).

The use of local and geographic networks is spreading more and more thanks to the development of the telecommunication technology (telematics). We plan to use a mix of different communication technologies to build up our networking infrastructure:
- Dial Up Analog line.
- Dial Up ISDN line.
- Local, Metropolitan, Wide Area Networks (LAN/MAN/WAN)

Local Area Networks based on a common protocol (e.g. TCP/IP) will be used to connect PC terminals in the same building. For the external connections on a metropolitan scale, ISDN and leased lines will be used (packet network, frame-relay). For the connections over a wide area and with the European partners, Internet will be used, possibly in conjunction with Euro-ISDN.

Internet represents the most well-controlled and widespread method for large-scale connections. Its capillary presence in nearly all the European and worldwide countries, joined to a high number access points on the territory, managed by several Internet Service public and private providers guarantee reliability and low-cost access.

The problem of the access security and control, fundamental in many sectors but in particular in the social-health field, can be faced by arranging in the connected computers suitable "firewalls" that could prevent non authorized computers to access.

Euro-ISDN is the set of the European ISDN networks. It can be used jointly with Internet in the connections between partners , if needed, in order to achieve a better grade of security and interoperability.

4. The Integrated Social-Health Information System

A project concerning the above issues is starting and it is aimed to develop an integrated information system model of social-health care. Data collected on the chart of the patients' evaluation group are integrated with other information from social-administrative-health services by providing a complete on-line computerized record, thereby improving information sharing among all members of the social-health care team. Part of this information will be on the portable social-health record supported by the electronic smart card.

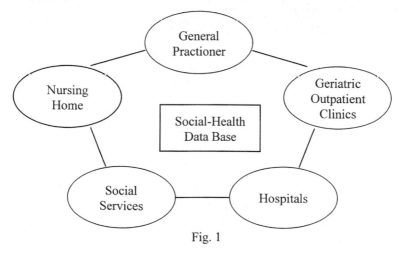

Fig. 1

Linking social centers, physicians office, outpatients' clinics and hospitals can be facilitated by the model of the multimedia and integrated workstation, covering an integration and a cooperation of service groups. At the center of this representation of the system there is the   social-health record stored also in the card and in the various Databases accessed through telematics networks (see fig. 1).

5. Conclusions

State of the art telematics and information technology are able to provide an integrated social-health information system whose objective is to create direct communications links, based on common standards, joining General Practitioners, hospitals and social centres on a European scale. The communication can be performed by means of telematics networks and smart cards.

A project with these features is starting in Milano and in other sites, with the following objectives:
- realize a quick interconnection among all the different network nodes of the involved services
- increase the quality of life of elderly and disabled people on a preventive (social and health) level; on a territorial level (integrated home social-health care) and institutional (in a perspective of care and rehabilitation medicine)
- improve the mobility of the risk people, thanks to the integration of the different service networks present in the project
- achieve a full communication among the network nodes, avoiding waiting lists, reducing the answering times both in the data collection and in the distribution of the data results among the operators (e.g. general practitioners) and improving the services effectiveness and the technical quality perceived by the final users.
- reduce the institutionalization trends through an effective monitoring on the territory.
- improve the home stay of the elderly and disabled people in conditions of countinous safety and care from the social-health services
- manage a precise mapping of the autonomy levels of the elderly and the disabled people on the territory , foreseeing the possible social -health difficulties encountered by elderly and disabled.
- supply an information basis for the measurement of the daily activity of the elderly and disabled people , the different levels of their physical and psychical autonomy and the related health and social requirements.

References

[1] Jones R., McGhee S., Hedley A., Murray K., Patient Access to Information, Current Perspectives in Health Computing, 1988, pp. 206-12.
[2] Barlow, R. , Developing Functional Solutions for Long-Term Care , HC&CC 3rd quarter 95.
[3] Abbott W., ed., Information technology in health care, The institute of Health services Managements, Longman 1992.
[4] Russell I., Jones V., Evaluation of Patient Data Card System: Project Description. Report PHC/002, Health Services research Unit Un. of Aberdeen.
[5] C. O. Kohler, O. Reinhoff, O.P. Schaeffer (Eds): Health cards '95. Proceedings, IOS Press 1995.

[6] A. Pernice, H. Doare, O. Reinhoff (Eds): Health Care Card System. Eurocards Concerted Action, results and recommendations, IOS Press, 1995.

[7]Dick R. S., Steen E. B. "The Computer-Based Patient Record: An Essential Technology for Health Care", Institute of Medicine Washington DC, National Academy Press, 1991.

[8] Barnett G. O. "The application of computer-based medical record systems in ambulatory practice", N. Engl. J. Med. 310 (1984) 1643-1650

[9] Sicurello F. "Towards Standardized and Integrated Medical Records", Proceed. of the Fifth Global Congress on Patient Cards and Computerization of Health Records, Venezia June 1993, ed. by C. Peter Waegemann, Medical Record Institute.

[10] Sicurello F. "Clinical Record Management and MUMPS", Journal of Clinical Computing vol. XVII, number 4, 1989, E. R. Gabrieli ed., pagg.105-110.

[11] Kurland L. T., Molgaard C. "The patient record in epidemiology", Scientific American, 1981; 245: 54-63.

[12] Newcombe H. B. "Record Linking: the design of efficient systems for linking records into individual and family history"; American Journal of Human Genetics, 1967; 19:335-359.

[13] Gill L. E., Baldwin J. A. "Methods and technology of record linkage: some pratical considerations" ; Baldwin JA, Acheson ED, Graham WJ (eds), Textbook of medical record linkage. Oxford University Press 1987: 39-54.

[14] Acheson E. D. "Medical Record Linkage", Oxford University Press, 1967.

[15]Nicolosi A., Sicurello F., Fornara A., Villa M. "Record-Linkage in Health Informations System: Experimentation in a Italian Local Health District", Proceed. of the seventh international congress MIE '87 - Medical Informatics Europe, 21-25 settembre 1987, pagg. 893-898.

Medical Informatics Europe '97
C. Pappas et al. (Eds.)
IOS Press, 1997

Introducing cards into Slovenian health insurance and health care

Marjan Sušelj, dr. Stanislav Čuber, Marija Zevnik
Health Insurance Institute of Slovenia, Miklošičeva 24, 1507 Ljubljana, Slovenija

Abstract

This paper presents an outline of the Slovenian project of introducing card systems into health insurance and health care: bases for its launching, scope, system design, development phases, benefits, and issues of interoperability with the other card systems.

The card system will induce distinct simplifications of the procedures now performed in the health care system, improve the quality of medical administrative services to the patients.

The introduction of the card technology is under way in several European countries. With the Health insurance card system project, Slovenia is joining the EU projects, and can either test in practice and implement the concepts, as well as contributes particular original solutions.

1. Introduction

The Health Insurance Institute of Slovenia (HIIS) is, by the statute, the exclusive provider of the "compulsory health insurance", and also provides "voluntary health insurance". In this role, the Institute is a significant component of the national health care service system, and, in conjunction with other subjects, is responsible for controlling and containing the health care costs, for the efficiency of the system operation, and for its organisation.

2. The Slovenian Health Insurance Card Project

2.1. Background and objectives

In the day-to-day operation of the Slovenian health care service, administrative tasks are virtually completely computer-supported with all the system actors, ranging from the medical service providers to the HIIS services. The present system weak spot, however, is the patient identification and transfer of frequently required administrative data, which is based on the health insurance booklet.

In order to overcome this "manual data entry" involved at the insured person's entrance to the system, the project of replacing the booklet by a new electronic health insurance card, was launched. In the project strategic plan [1], HIIS set up the following objectives:

☐ improvement of the quality of medical and administrative services to the health care system customers - patients, both by the HIIS and the health care service providers;

- facilitation and improvement of the communication between the HIIS, doctors and health care institutions;
- reduction of the (excessive) volume of procedures involved presently in the insured person's asserting its rights;
- improvement of the personal data security within the information systems;
- reduction of administrative tasks, and in this way, improvement of the operation efficiency both with the HIIS and the health care service providers;
- based on reasonable financial inputs, long-term economic benefits at the macroeconomic level.

2.2. The project phases

2.2.1. Analysis

The project analysis phase covered the following issues:

- comparative analysis of projects of introduction of cards in health care systems in Europe and in the world [3, 4, 5];
- determination of the card technology significance for the modernisation of the health insurance and health care information systems [2];
- analysis of the potential functions and data set of the health insurance card [2];
- analysis of the relevant legal framework and organisational options of introducing the project in Slovenia;
- analysis of the legal aspects concerning data security and protection;
- analysis of the information technology infrastructure available the Slovenian health care and health insurance services;
- examination of the quality of relevant data bases and data protection systems;
- analysis of the available card technologies.

Based on the results of the listed analyses, the HIIS harmonised, with the political and professional bodies and institutions, responsible for the planning and strategic development of the health care system, the card system with the following components:

Checked options
Identification of insured person with relevant insurance data
Documentation of selected physicians
Electronic prescription
Documentation of medication consumption
Medical emergency card
Forwarding patients to specialists and hospitals
Documentation of health status and data on medical care

Figure 1. Checked options for card application

Health Insurance Card (HIC)

In the first project phase, this card has two functions:

- An identification document of the insured person and its legal and business relation to the health insurance system;
- Registration of the selected personal physicians

In the second project phase (which is already in the process of conception), some other functions will be added:

- Digital prescription;
- Information on organs and tissues donnorship.

Health Professional Card (HPC)

The security of the access to data is technically ensured by the introduction of the health professional cards. This card, issued by the HIIS, serves to regulate the access (reading or writing) by individual health professionals to the data stored on the health insurance card and in other forms.

In the first project phase, the professional card has two functions:
- ☐ Identification of the card holder;
- ☐ Determination of the holder's access rights.

In the second project phase, it will be augmented by the function of:
- ☐ Digital signature

The network of self service terminals

The HIC is planned to have a limited term of validity. It will have to be prolonged regularly by the card holders themselves. To support the checking and updating of the health insurance cards by the insured persons, a network of self service terminals will be set up, to read the data from the card, compare with the central database, and updated. The terminal application will be user-friendly and simple as much as practicable, and the terminals will be located at all health care institutions with high frequency of patient visits.

2.2.2. System and element design

The design of the whole system and of its elements was outlined in the subsequent project phase. The main task was to recognise problems and develop solutions on the logical level:
- ☐ what data and functions should the card carry [5, 7];
- ☐ how to integrate its application into administrative structures, that is how to further develop the rules and regulations concerning the insurance company, insured persons, the employer, the physicians and the hospitals;
- ☐ how to ensure the implementation of these rules and regulations in data processing applications within the health insurance company and the medical institutions.

Next, the system elements were specified. The specification of the application software were carried out in cooperation with Slovenia's two leading software companies. The expansion of the communication networks for the operation of self-service terminals was conceived in cooperation with the field health care institutions, and based on analytical data on frequency of visits etc.

The logistics of the entire implementation process were also detailed.

Extensive attention was dedicated to solving the technologic problems [6]:

application / data section	access right	HIIS official + SST (type 1)	voluntary insurance + SST (type 2)	physician with contract, to be selected (type 3)	physician with contract, not to be selected (type 4)	physician without contract (type 5)	other health professional with contract (type 5)
identification	read	X	X	X	X	X	X
ident. insured person	write	X					
employer data	read	X		X	X	X	X
	write	X					
compulsory insurance	read	X	X	X	X	X	X
	write	X					
voluntary insurance	read		X	X	X	X	X
	write		X				
documentation	read	X		X	X		
selected physician	write	X		X			
electronic prescription	download	X					

Fig. 2: HIC access rights

The functions of the health insurance card call for a relatively differentiated regulation of *access rights* to its data elements. Figure 2 shows the data groups and professional groups which are entitled to different access to the data groups.

The various groups of health professionals *authenticate* themselves for the health insurance card with a Health Professional Card. The mutual authentication of the two cards is done by way of a symmetric challenge-response procedure using the DES-3 algorithm.

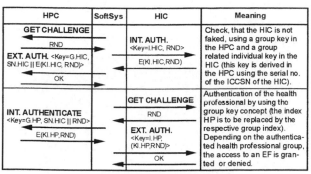

HPC	SoftSys	HIC	Meaning
GET CHALLENGE			Check, that the HIC is not
RND		INT. AUTH. <Key=I.HIC, RND>	faked, using a group key in the HPC and a group
EXT. AUTH. <Key=G.HIC, SN.HIC ‖ E(KI.HIC, RND)>		E(KI.HIC,RND)	related individual key in the HIC (this key is derived in the HPC using the serial no.
OK			of the ICCSN of the HIC).
		GET CHALLENGE	Authentication of the health professional by using the
INT. AUTHENTICATE <Key=G.HP, SN.HIC ‖ RND>		RND	group key concept (the index HP is to be replaced by the respective group index).
E(KI.HP,RND)		EXT. AUTH. <Key=I.HP, (KI.HP,RND)>	Depending on the authenticated health professional group,
		OK	the access to an EF is granted or denied.

Fig. 3: HIC working phase

The group key for every group of health professionals is stored in the Health Professional Card. The health insurance cards each receive their own individual keys. They are derived from the serial number (ICCSN) of the health insurance card by applying the DES-3 algorithm to the ICCSN. This results in

the procedure in the interworking phases of communication as seen in figure 3.

The functions of the *Health Professional Card* have been under discussion for a few years in several projects. Work on the EU TrustHealth Project has good prospects, since an internationally applicable solution will be worked out.

In order to avoid a project-specific solution incompatible with future European concepts, and to be able to carry our project on even if the European concept is not yet finished, we have opted for a subset of the HPC functions under discussion. At first a HPC with just symmetric authentication will be issued. The introduction of the electronic prescription by the Slovene health system will require an HPC with a digital signature. Physicians' HPCs will then be exchanged. We believe that stable specifications on the EU level will be in place by then in order for us to implement a basically compatible solution.

Regarding the *card terminals*, we applied the MCT concept and the suggestions by the Franco-German Agreement [9]. Each terminal is to be fitted with a contact unit for the HIC and the HPC and to have a PIN pad and display for activating the HPC with a PIN number.

In order to facilitate the incorporation of the card technology into the existing application software, we are developing a uniform *application programming interface*.

2.2.3. *Future project phases*

☐ Call for tenders for the system and application elements

☐ Introduction of the card application in a test region (second semester 1997)

☐ Country-wide introduction of the card application by regions (1998);

☐ Test of the electronic prescription in the test region (1998);

☐ Country-wide introduction of the electronic prescription (1998/99).

3. Cost benefit analysis

The project involves considerably high financial investments, however, also its financial benefits are high. The benefits are envisaged to arise predominantly from the decrease of time spent for administrative operations by the health care service providers, as well as by the employers and the insured persons themselves, in regulating the health insurance. The cost benefit analysis [8], however, does not take into account such effects as the

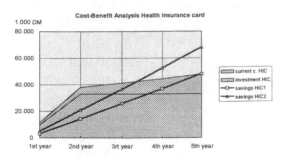

Fig. 4: Cost-benefit analysis of administrative
functions for a five-year period (in DM)

improvement of the data quality, the health insurance institute image, and development potential accompanying the introduction of the system.

Break even point of the cost benefit analysis is reached at the beginning of the fourth project year.

In the first project phase, the system applications will be administrative, thus predominantly the administrative staff and the nurses will deal with the cards. This means they will be relieved of the time consuming menial tasks which presently prevent them from devoting their time to professional tasks, for which they are educated and trained.

4. Conclusions

The international experiences indicate that it is not sensible to rush with the extent of data stored on the cards. In the first project phase, the card is to contain predominantly the data necessary for the identification of the insured person and the selected personal physicians, and to verify the status of the insurance. However, the organisation of the card data structure provides the potential for additional applications to be added in the future (digital prescription, patient file, donation, telemedicine, etc.)

The development of smart card technology is very dynamic and also unpredictable. The above listed orientations are therefore of even greater importance for the project. To ensure the project feasibility, we base the project on proven and tested technologic solutions.

Since the card system will provide the prerequisites for the introduction of the telemedicine, a further benefit will be the development of professional horizons of the health care professionals.

The introduction of the card technology is under way in several European countries. With the Health insurance card system project, Slovenia is joining the EU projects, and can either test in practice and implement the agreed concepts, as well as contributes particular original solutions.

5. References

[1] Projektna naloga ZZZS :Kartica zdravstvenega zavarovanja, 1996
[2] A. Pernice, H. Doare, O. Rienhoff: Healthcare Card Systems. IOS Press, 1995
[3] C.O. Köhler, O. Rienhoff, O.P. Schaeffer (eds.): Health Cards '95. IOS Press, 1995
[4] A. Pernice, H. Doare: Int. Harmonisation of Health Cards EU and G-7 Initiatives, 1996
[5] D. Markwell: EU/G7 Healthcards - WG7, Interoperability of Healthcard Systems, Part 2 - Achieving Interoperability. The Clinical Information Consultancy, 1996
[6] Proc. 11th Int. forum for Plastic Card Technologies and Applications. CNIT, Paris, 1996
[7] D. Markwell: Slovenian health insurance card project - Independent international review. The Clinical Information Consultancy, 1996
[8] HIIS: Slovenian health insurance card project - Cost benefit analysis. November 1996
[9] Franco-German Specification of Common interface of CT Manager APIs, Draft, 1996

Medical Informatics Europe '97
C. *Pappas et al. (Eds.)*
IOS Press, 1997

Computer-Based Patient Records and Mathematical Processing: Brain-Unicard System Experience

Shamil Kh. Gizatullin and Anvar Kh. Amirov*

Burdenko Main Military Clinical Hospital, Moscow, Russia
E-mail: gizat@sha.mks.ru
*Institute for High Temperatures, Russian Academy of Sciences,
Moscow, Russia, E-mail: ravil@amirov.msk.ru

Abstract. The ways of usage of the data from Brain-UniCard Computer-based Patient Records in biomedical and statistical studies is discussed. Mathematical procedures used in computer program are presented. Problems of data presentation for advanced biomedical studies are discussed with the examples of studies of patients with brain traumas and deseases.

Data use from the computer medical systems in biomedical studies is one of the main problems of systems development. The Brain-UniCard is system of electronic medical records for the brain diseases and traumas [1]. From the very beginning of it development Brain-UniCard system was directed to the possibility of fulfillment of biomedical and statistical investigations.

Developing Brain-UniCard system we chose two levels of mathematical methods usage in solution of the practical problems. The first level is level of a practical doctor, the second — level of researcher of specific biomedical problems. These two levels could be divided by the degree of actuality and accuracy of the problem formulation. The first level in common case is could defined by clear and actual formulation of the problem of the receipt of concrete information. Here fast processing of information (especially in case of an acute state of patient) and its clear presentation is important. The second case is determined by more common approach when some problem is transforming into a set of tasks and working hypothesis are based on obtained data from computer medical records.

Usually computer-based medical records include free text and structured data also[1]. It is well known that free texts hardly could be processed in statistics and other mathematical studies. So it was the main reason that in Brain-UniCard system we use structured description of the patient state [2].

We use the scheme when set of parameters and structured set of variants of these parameters are assembled in special files[2]. This scheme allows to make changes in the set of parameters of patient description easily (as well as to make changes in structured set of answers). Such a structure is the base of biomedical and statistical studies, it supports the identity between data input procedure and procedure of processing.

Along with structured data there are many parameters that have so called "free spectra". For example, they are time of analysis, blood pressure, etc. Structured parameters with rigid set of

---

[1] Structure data have a rigid set of variants of patient state description.

[2] It was used tree-like structure for data storage in these files for the quick access and special procedure of data storage.

answers we will call parameters with "bound spectra" (for example, state of conscious has prea
signed number of descriptions: coma, sopor, etc.)

In the case of studies of practical doctor the main problem is presentation of time depen
ence for both kind of parameters. Brain-UniCard system include special subsystem for the prese
tation "free spectra" data in the form of a chart. The main shortage of data presentation in Brai
UniCard system is the absence of indication on medical treatment of patient. Chart with time d
pendence of some parameter have to include indications on the main treatment procedures such
surgery, medication, etc. On our opinion program of presentation of parameters of patient sta
must include special submenu for the choice of events to be represented on a chart[3].

In the case of "practical doctor" presentation of parameter time dependencies inside
CPR must include simplest statistical procedures of data processing. They include line regressio
cubic spline, non-parametric regression. Two of them were realized in Brain-UniCard system.

Time dependence for the structured (non-numeric) data could be presented in the form
histograms. But one more moment should be taken into account in this case. Some variants of p
rameter of patient state could be combined (see below). Direct use of histograms is difficult in su
cases and special solution is needed for each parameter.

Next principal problem is opportunity of investigation of mutual dependencies of vario
parameters of the patient state. Methods that could be applied for these studies depend on the ty
of data: 1) both parameters have "free spectra"; 2) one parameter has "free spectra" and the seco
— "bound spectra"; 3) both parameters have "bound spectra".

The most of biomedical studies (at the level of a practical doctor or at the level of inves
gator) begin with the problem of sampling data from the CPR by some criteria. At the level of
practical doctor this criteria usually very simple. At the level of a investigator samplings are carri
out by multifactor criteria. At the same time our experience shows that in the cases when criteria
not combination of conditions (i.e. condition1 AND condition2 AND condition3 etc.) even inv
tigators with the great experience are at a loss to put more than three logical conditions. Th
biomedical studies are usually multifactor[4] on our opinion sampling system in CPR should be st
like. It means that next sampling is produced from the previous sampling. Such a system is chara
terized by the improper time optimization (this factor is essential for the great assemble of data).

Another important moment of the CPR construction is necessity to provide investigation
specific moment of time from some registration point (for example, a few hours after surge
trauma, specific medication, etc.).

For such studies CPR must allow to make samplings by two conditions: 1) presence of
sired registration point (surgery, trauma, etc.); 2) opportunity to chose desired parameter of
tient state at the moment $T=T0+t$. The first condition simply means the sampling of the set of
tients with desired registration point. But such system of sampling means presence of special set
registration points in CPR, that means registration of some events with special status. Sampling
the second condition brings to the problem of sampling for some time range. This probl
emerges because the low possibility of presence of desired parameter value at the exact time t a
registration point. It means that some procedure of calculation value of desired parameter for

---

[3] Such a problem is very complex. For example, in the case of medication it should
taken into account various ways medication usage — continuos or discrete, their combination, e

[4] In biomedical studies it is important to separate "clear" group of patients or to carry
studies on the great number of patients for reduction of an influence of outside factors.

missible time range is necessary in CPR. It is clear that range of admissible time interval depends on patient state and of the parameter significance.

All the variety of modern statistical and mathematical methods [3] are applicable for data with "free spectra". Algorithms of Brain-UniCard system include two methods: investigation of the mutual dependence of parameters and correlation analysis.

Mutual dependence of parameters are presented in the form of charts and line regression procedure could be applied for such dependencies in Brain-UniCard system. Brain-UniCard system allows to study dependencies for parameters from different physiological systems. Various methods of averaging and approximation of such dependencies are desirable in CPR. On our opinion non-parametric methods could be very useful in biomedical studies [4]. "Phase diagrams" (i.e. time trajectories of mutual dependencies) could be very interesting in this case. In common case patient state could be described as some trajectory in n-dimensional space (here n — is the number of parameters of patient state). In some cases it is possible and useful to simplify such trajectory to 2-dimensional curve. Special points and "behavior" of trajectory could contain essential information about patient state.

Very essential problem in the biomedical studies is association of the various parameters of the patient state in time. In common case probes of the parameters of patient state are carried out in different time and with different frequencies. Also there are many ways of medication. Even in simplest statistical procedures researcher encounter the problem association of parameters in time. For example, in acute states after neurosurgery frequency of blood probes is high, but frequency of biochemical analysis of blood is low. To associate such probes there is special time-averaging procedure in Brain-UniCrad system. Ranges of averaging are equal to 6, 12 and 24 hours. Researcher must pay special attention to range of averaging: in acute states the change of parameters could be very fast and with the high attitude. These factors make averaged values not representative. Approximation procedure could become alternative to averaging procedure. But approximation implicitly means some knowledge of time dependence of parameter.

Brain-UniCard system allows to investigate not only data with the "free spectra" but structured data with "bound spectra" also. Brain-UniCard system include procedure for calculation of frequencies for each variant of parameter's values. Calculation of frequencies is available both for the whole list of patients (for example, distribution of patients upon localization of trauma) and for some sampling (for example, distribution of patients upon localization of trauma for patients in grave condition).

We want to note one more essential point using the example with trauma localization. In common case trauma at right hemisphere of brain could be combined with the traumas with other localization. Thus in Brain-UniCard system there is opportunity to make sampling both for unique (in our case only the right hemisphere localization) and for combined localization (the right hemisphere localization and probable other localization).

Advanced statistical methods of hypothesis verification as well as mathematical models of pathological processes are very complicated procedures. Sometimes the task of primary data preparation is difficult problem that demand special mathematical education. So on our opinion their inclusion into CPR is not advisable. Special programs and computer statistical software must be used for efficient solution of the complex biomedical problems. CPR must to include special modules for conversion data into specific software formats such as ASCII files, dBase files, Exel files, etc.

[1] Gizatullin Sh.Kh., Amirov A.Kh., Osipov I.S. In: Medical Information Europe '96 / Ed J.Brender, J.P.Christensen, J.-R.Scherrer, P.McNair. (IOS Press. 1996) — PP.466–469

[2] Ball M.J., Collen M.F. (eds.) Aspects of the Computer-based Patient Record. (N.Y.: Springe Verlag, 1992).

[3] Handbook of Applicable Mathematics. Vol. VI: Statistics. Part A&B. / Ed. by E.Lloyd ar W.Ledermann. (John Wiley & Sons. 1984).

[4] Hardle W. Applied Nonparametric Regression. (Cambridge University Press. 1990).

Medical Informatics Europe '97
C. Pappas et al. (Eds.)
IOS Press, 1997

Rubrics to Dissections to GRAIL to Classifications

JE Rogers[1] WD Solomon[1] AL Rector[1] P Pole[1] P Zanstra[2] E van der Haring[2]
1) *Medical Informatics Group, Department of Computer Science, University of Manchester, UK*
2) *Medical Informatics Group, Catholic University of Nijmegen, Netherlands*
http://www.cs.man.ac.uk/mig/galen/ or e-mail galen@cs.man.ac.uk

Abstract. This paper summarises the process in the GALEN-IN-USE project by which rubrics from traditional medical coding schemes are analysed into an intermediate, relatively informal conceptual representation which is then automatically translated into the GRAIL formalism and its Common Reference Model.

1. Introduction

GALEN-IN-USE is an EU funded project, a major goal of which is the development of tools and methods to assist in the collaborative construction and maintenance of surgical procedure classifications. Techniques and tools developed in the previous GALEN project [1,2,3,4,5,6] will support this task. Taking part in the initial phase are four national coding and classification centres: WCC (Netherlands), SPRI (Sweden), CNR (Italy) and University of Ste. Etienne (France). The goal is to author, using the GRAIL formalism [6], conceptual representations of individual surgical procedures, with each centre covering roughly one quarter of the total surgical domain. A combined total of 15-20,000 individual representations will be authored by the end of the project. The resulting GRAIL representations will be integrated into the existing GALEN Common Reference Model (CRM) [1,3,4,5]. This will allow:

- an initial classification of the represented procedures to be automatically derived, based on the knowledge explicitly authored in the analyses and the knowledge already in the reference model;
- machine generation of natural language expressions for all representations, in five European languages;
- refinement, extension and reorganisation of the classification using new classification management tools.

More than 20 individual clinicians have been recruited to analyse original code rubrics into conceptual representations, but most have little or no prior experience of the GRAIL formalism or of the particular ontology and modelling style of the Common Reference Model (CRM). This presented a significant challenge to the project: how to reduce the need for training to occur in the complexities of GRAIL and the CRM before any work could begin.

2. An Intermediate Representation

The solution proposed to the training problem was to begin work using a simpler, intermediate conceptual representation [7]. This was originally conceived as a migration step towards eventually authoring directly in GRAIL. The representation was designed in such a way that conceptual representations authored using it might then be automatically, or semi-automatically, expanded into GRAIL. The representation also allows the authors to capture some concepts which the GRAIL formalism in its present form is unable to handle. Finally, the representation serves as the preferred format in which the centres examine and validate their own, and each other's work. The intermediate representation is broadly similar to those used by the CANON group or MEDS [8,9,10,11]. It is characterised by:

- a relatively small set of semantic links (ACTS_ON, IS_PART_OF), compared to the CRM;
- a two-tier domain ontology (known as the 'descriptor list') specific to the surgical domain. Descriptors (leg, excising, tumour) are explicitly typed by one of a small number of classes (e.g. anatomy, deed, lesion);
- a set of constraints, declaring which links may be used with which descriptor classes;
- a grammar defining a layout, or 'template', for well-formed representations.

   Domain experts in the centres work using existing local coding schemes (WCC, NCSP etc.) to scope their task. The rubrics (text) and associated codes, but not the original hierarchy, are extracted from the scheme. Working on sections of a few hundred related rubrics at one time, each rubric is manually analysed to author a conceptual representation of its meaning, using the intermediate representation. The immediate result of this analysis and authoring is called a 'dissection' of the rubric.

   The four centres produced more than 1200 'dissections' in the first four months. Figure 1 shows four completed dissections. Each has a header section, containing information about the original rubric and coding scheme, followed by the conceptual representation itself, introduced by the MAIN keyword. The semantic links are capitalised. Descriptors appear in lower case, preceded by their descriptor class. Initially, authoring involved directly editing an ASCII text file. Any convenience and familiarity which this afforded to the authors was, however, outweighed by the numerous spelling and formatting errors which resulted, preventing satisfactory parsing of the interchange file into the GRAIL expansion environment. Subsequent analyses will be authored using a purpose-built tool, the Surgical Procedure Editing Tool (SPET).

Figure 1.

| RUBRIC "operations on papillary muscle"
CODE "35.31"
MAIN deed:surgical deed
   ACTS_ON anatomy:papillary muscle
   HAS_OTHER_FEATURE method VALUE induced arrest of heart | RUBRIC "reattachment of papillary muscle"
CODE "35.31.i2"
MAIN deed:repairing
   ACTS_ON anatomy:papillary muscle
   BY_TECHNIQUE deed:reattaching
   ACTS_ON anatomy:papillary muscle
   HAS_OTHER_FEATURE method VALUE induced arrest of heart |
| RUBRIC "dividing of papillary muscle"
CODE "35.31.i1"
MAIN deed:dividing
   ACTS_ON anatomy:papillary muscle
   HAS_OTHER_FEATURE method VALUE induced arrest of heart | RUBRIC "repair of papillary muscle"
CODE "35.31.i3"
MAIN deed:repairing
   ACTS_ON anatomy:papillary muscle
   HAS_OTHER_FEATURE method VALUE induced arrest of heart |

3. Expanding dissections into GRAIL

Dissections authored in the intermediate representation are subsequently imported into an environment (TIGGER) built to manage the process of converting them into GRAIL, simultaneously translating them into both the ontology and the style of the CRM. Imported dissections are first parsed for syntax and for whether they comply with certain agreed modelling conventions (such as that all deeds must ACTS_ON something, a convention taken from CEN [12]). The final GRAIL produced is generally more complex than the dissection from which it comes - sometimes very much more so. The translation process is known as 'expanding' and the GRAIL produced from a single dissection as its GRAIL 'expansion'.

   Figure 2 shows a dissection (left) and an automatically generated expansion (right). An expansion comprises a GRAIL representation of the concept at hand, and a series of statements attaching incidental, non-classificatory information to that GRAIL concept, such as the text of the original rubric or the name of the original source file. TIGGER automatically generates, in batches or individually, a GRAIL expansion for each original dissection. However, automatic expansions can only be considered candidate GRAIL conceptual representations of the original rubrics: some may be rejected as invalid when presented to a terminology server. This may occur, for example, if there is a cardinality conflict between CRM semantic links used in the expansion. Rejection may indicate a problem which requires alterations to the original dissection, or to the CRM. A few dissections whose expansions are rejected may require their GRAIL representation to be done manually, bypassing the intermediate representation completely.

Figure 2.

Original Dissection	Generated GRAIL expansion

RUBRIC "dividing of papillary muscle"
CODE "35.31.i1"
MAIN deed:dividing
  ACTS_ON anatomy:papillary muscle
  HAS_OTHER_FEATURE method VALUE induced arrest of heart
	(SurgicalDeed which
	  isCharacterisedBy (performance whichG
	    isEnactmentOf (Dividing whichG <
	      playsClinicalRole SurgicalRole
	      actsSpecificallyOn PapillaryMuscle
	      hasSubprocess InducedCardiacArrest>)))
	  extrinsically hasRubric 'dividing of papillary muscle';
	  extrinsically hasCode '35.31.i1';
	  extrinsically hasPhysicalSource 'cnr.txt'.

Sets of automatic expansions produced in this way are presented to the terminology server for classification. The resulting hierarchy of valid expansions may be browsed in a number of ways. The screenshot (figure 3) shows the automatic classification which is derived for the four dissections given in figure 1. The classification of 'operations on the papillary muscle' as a kind of 'operation on the cardiovascular system' occurs because the CRM 'knows' that the papillary muscle is part of the heart which is, in turn, a component of the cardiovascular system. The GRAIL refinement operation [4] is used to declare that actions on part of something are subsumed by actions on the whole. By contrast, the classification of 'reattachment of papillary muscle' as a child of 'repair of papillary muscle' instead of a sibling (as in the original coding scheme) comes from the knowledge explicitly authored in the intermediate representation.

Figure 3.

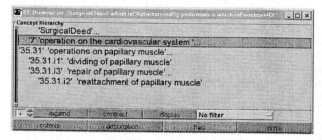

To do the automatic expansion of dissections, however, the TIGGER first requires explicit CRM mappings to be declared for both the descriptors and the links used in a given dissection.

3.1 Mapping the descriptors

This task of declaring mappings for descriptors is performed by modellers already familiar with the GRAIL formalism and the CRM ontology and style. Once declared, a mapping is presumed valid for all subsequent occurrences of the descriptor in any batch of dissections. As more dissections are processed, the list of already mapped descriptors grows. The accumulated, mapped descriptor list is made available via the SPET to all collaborating authors as a suggested core ontology for use in the next round of authoring dissections.

This approach has the advantage that the ontology with which the dissection authors must become familiar is initially quite small. Further, its growth is owned by the authors themselves but can be guided by those familiar with the GALEN ontology. This contrasts with the already large and complex ontology in the CRM, with which the authors would need to be familiar to author directly in GRAIL. Because the process of getting from dissections to GRAIL is planned to be unidirectional, this methodology also permits some redundancy or duplication of descriptors, as many descriptors can be mapped to the same CRM concept.

Mapping a given descriptor to the CRM is informed by inspection, using TIGGER, of all the dissections which employ it - either in the current batch or in all batches processed so far. Such inspection may provide clarification of what is meant by a descriptor, but may also reveal that one descriptor has been used with very different intentions by different authors. A mechanism exists for rejecting such ambiguous descriptors and their associated dissections at this stage, to invite re-authoring.

3.2 Mapping the Links

The links available to dissection authors were chosen such that each is equivalent in intention to the common parent of a range of more expressive links already present in the CRM. Figure 4, for example, shows the CRM links which are to be considered by TIGGER as possible default mappings for the dissection link IS_PART_OF. The mappings from dissection links to the CRM are, therefore, necessarily one-to-many and are declared by the same team of modellers undertaking the descriptor mapping.

To expand a dissection link, TIGGER must determine which, if any, of its candidate CRM link mappings is most appropriate. To achieve this, TIGGER 'translates' the descriptors either side of a dissection link into their declared CRM entity mappings. The candidate CRM link mappings are then tested in list order: the first one permitted to be used in the CRM between the two entities is chosen. Thus, the dissection fragment:

Figure 4.

Dissection Link	Default possible CRM mappings
IS_PART_OF	isSolidRegionOf
	isSpecificStructuralComponentOf
	isStructuralComponentOf
	isSpecificSolidDivisionOf
	isSolidDivisionOf
	isSpecificLinearDivisionOf
	isLinearDivisionOf
	isSpecificSurfaceDivisionOf
	isSurfaceDivisionOf
	isSpecificLayerOf
	isLayerOf

    segment IS_PART_OF intestine

is expanded into the GRAIL:

    Segment which isSpecificLinearDivisionOf Intestine.

because the CRM includes the constraint:

    Segment sensibly isSpecificLinearDivisionOf TubularBodyStructure.

This mechanism can also be used to detect dissections which, whilst considered 'well formed' within the limited dissection grammar, are still semantically incorrect. For example:

    MAIN excising
        ACTS_ON tumour
        IS_PART_OF liver

...can not be expanded: none of the candidate mappings of IS_PART_OF is permitted to be used in the CRM between [Excising], a process, and [Liver], a structure. In future, some semantically incorrect dissections may be rejected at the authoring stage - the SPET will use both the dissection grammar and a limited constraint mechanism to prevent certain link-descriptor pairings being entered at all.

4. Limitations and Future extensions

Coding scheme rubrics frequently contain disjunctions (Excision of tumour or cyst) or conjunctions (Drainage and marsupialisation of cyst). To make the intermediate representation simple, bracketing was omitted from its syntax. As a result, it can only support relatively simple conjunctions or disjunctions. Rubrics with more complex relationships (e.g. partial or complete excision of tibia and fibula, with prosthesis) must be manually enumerated in all their logically and semantically correct conceptual forms. True negation also remains unsupported at present by the GRAIL formalism. However, most of the rubrics which might at first appear to require negation are exclusion or exception criteria. The intermediate representation includes mechanisms for identifying such criteria, which may then be handled within GRAIL by various modelling workarounds or future extensions to the formalism itself.

The relatively relaxed approach to building the descriptor list, with its rudimentary and *ad hoc* class hierarchy, risks it growing to unmanageable and un-navigable proportions. Imposing a more formal organisation would be to some extent to re-invent GRAIL. This may be obviated by offering navigation of the set of mapped descriptors via the hierarchy of their corresponding CRM conceptual mappings.

Both the descriptor list, and the CRM itself, are presently authored in English. This is not the first language of many dissection authors. The generation of natural language expressions for the final GRAIL concepts requires annotations in the destination languages for each CRM primitive. A mechanism to address both of the these problems is being studied: dissections will be authored in the local languages, using a local language descriptor list. Each authoring centre will separately maintain a many-to-one translation table from the local terms to a common, English descriptor list shared between all centres. The various translation tables, and the explicit English descriptor to CRM mappings, may be read backwards to derive a list of possible linguistic annotations.

5. Discussion and Conclusion

Although originally conceived as a migration step towards full GRAIL authoring, the intermediate representation and automated expansion process have proved effective in their own right. A high proportion of rubrics can be represented and reliably expanded automatically, and it may be more efficient to author the small remainder directly in GRAIL than to make further enhancements. The success of the intermediate representation is such that, whilst it remains the intention of the project to export CRM modelling expertise from its current localised base, this is no longer on the critical path for the immediate task of building a surgical procedure classification. Further, adding an intermediate layer between knowledge authors and the final representation serves to insulate them from changes in the CRM, and allows those changes to take place more easily and with less disruption.

We are confident that much of the surgical procedure domain can continue to be captured using the intermediate representation, facilitating the involvement of many domain experts by deferring indefinitely any need for them to become familiar with GRAIL or the CRM. A useful by-product of the process is that the act of declaring link and descriptor mappings is building a partial meta-model description of the CRM ontology and style. This will form an important resource for the exporting of CORE modelling expertise, when that occurs.

With thanks to the centres involved in dissection authoring, and others in the GALEN-IN-USE consortium

GALEN-IN-USE is funded as part Framework IV of the EC Healthcare Telematics research program.

6. References

1. Rector, A. (1994). Compositional models of medical concepts: towards re-usable application-independent medical terminologies. in Knowledge and Decisions in Health Telematics P. Barahona and J. Christensen (ed). IOS Press. 133-142.

2. Rector, A., W. Solomon, W. Nowlan and T. Rush (1995). A Terminology Server for Medical Language and Medical Information Systems. Methods of Information in Medicine, Vol. 34, 147-157

3. Rector, A., A. Gangemi, E. Galeazzi, A. Glowinski and A. Rossi-Mori (1994). The GALEN CORE Model Schemata for Anatomy: Towards a re-usable application-independent model of medical concepts. Twelfth International Congress of the European Federation for Medical Informatics, MIE-94, Lisbon, Portugal, 229-233.

4. Rector, A. (1995). Coordinating taxonomies: Key to re-usable concept representations. Fifth conference on Artificial Intelligence in Medicine Europe (AIME '95), Pavia, Italy, Springer. 17-28.

5. Rector, A., JE. Rogers, P. Pole (1996) The GALEN High Level Ontology. Fourteenth International Congress of the European Federation for Medical Informatics, MIE-96, Copenhagen, Denmark

6. Rector, A. and W.A. Nowlan (1993). The GALEN Representation and Integration Language (GRAIL) Kernel, Version 1. The GALEN Consortium for the EC AIM Programme. (Available from Medical Informatics Group, University of Manchester).

7. Gaines BR, Shaw ML and Woodward JB (1993). Modelling as Framework for Knowledge Acquisition Methodologies and Tools. International Journal of Intelligent Systems 8(2): 155-168.

8. Campbell KE, Das AK and Musen MA (1994). A logical foundation for representation of clinical data. JAMIA 1(3): 218-232.

9. Cimino J (1994). Controlled Medical Vocabulary Construction: Methods from the Canon Group. Journal of the American Medical Informatics Association 1(3): 296-197.

10. Evans D (1988). Pragmatically-structured, lexical-semantic knowledge bases for unified medical language systems. Proceedings of the Twelfth Annual Symposium on Computer Applications in Medical Care, Washington DC, IEEE Computer Society Press: 169-173.

11. Huff S and Warner H (1990). A comparison of Meta-1 and HELP terms: implications for clinical data. Fourteenth Annual Symposium on Computer Applciations in Medical Care (SCAMC-90), Washington DC, iEEE Computer Society Press: 166-169.

12. CEN PT 251:ENV 1828 Surgical Procedure Modelling

Medical Informatics Europe '97
C. Pappas et al. (Eds.)
IOS Press, 1997

Flexible electronic patient record:
first results from a dutch hospital

I. van der Lubbe[1], R.P. van der Loo[1], and J. Burgerhout[2]

[1]Care for Care bv, Zaagmolenlaan 4, 3447 GS Woerden

[2]Hewlett Packard Nederland bv., Amstelveen

Abstract: This paper covers a pilot project that has been done at a dutch general hospital. They searched for the feasibility of a flexible patient record based on intranet technology and a system integrator (CAI). Based on an extended analysis of the organisation (i.c. hospital and pilot specialism), information and communication, the specifications for the interfaces are defined. Furthermore the structure and number of data to be stored in the Patient Data & Result Server are defined. Finally, a prototype of the flexible patient record has been developed. This prototype is not yet in routine use. However, experiences of the clinicians have learned that the web technology in combination with a system integrator could be a major step in the "wide" acceptation of the electronic patient record.

1. Introduction

The Electronic Patient Record (EPR) needs to be a special point of attention in the changing world of healthcare. This is stipulated by conclusions of dutch government [1;2]. The EPR has to support different functionalities of medical data and nursing data; i.e.: patientcare, quality control, policy and management and research.

An important publication in the field of EPR's is done by the Institute of Medicine (IOM) and is called: "The Computer-based Patient Record: an essential technology for healthcare" [3]. In this report the (dis)advantages of a paper-based record are compared to the EPR. The conclusion is that the paper-based record offers various disadvantages compared to the functionality of the EPR. Also research done in Europe confirms these results [4;5]. However, nowadays most clinicians are still working with the paper record, without being convinced that the EPR offers more advantages. At this moment there are still a number of problems to be solved, before the EPR can be introduced on a large scale. A lot of research has been done on the structure of EPR [6,7,8], the visualisation/presentation of the EPR [9,10] and the possibilities of structured data-entry [11, 12]. In studies of Moorman et al. [13] and Rector et al. [14] the possibilities of structuring freeformat text is investigated. Multimedia information has to be an 'integral' part of the EPR [15]. The EPR not only has to offer access to text and structured data, but also to graphic information, signals, X-rays etc. These data are usually generated and distributed by different legacy systems. Goal of the EPR is the integration of those data. Usually the client-server concept is seen as the solution.

Many dutch hospitals are generally in the phase of renewing the information infrastructure to more functional and connective systems, that are mutually connected in a client-server network. An important issue to solve is the storage of data: central (data repository) or local. Furthermore privacy issue have to solved. For example: who is (can be) authorized to retrieve specific patientinformation. Care for Care and Hewlett Packard offer an information architecture and components with which it is possible to integrate already existing information systems and to present existing infor-mation at a flexible and userfriendly way: the flexible elec-tronic patient record. We expect that this information architecture will contribute to a wider implementation of the EPR. In a dutch general hospital a pilot project has been carried out to search the feasibility of the 'flexible electronic patient record'. In this paper the components of the Flexible EPR are discussed and first results of the pilot-project are presented.

2. Components of the Flexible EPR

2.1 Introduction

An important requirement in the concept of Care for Care and HP is the use of a Patient Data & Result server (PDR). Sometimes the already existing HIS makes use of a PDR. The PDR server is a relational database system in which all relevant patient data and research data are stored. These data come from different (sub)systems (i.e.

laboratory system, radiology system). The connection between the subsystems and the integration and storage of relevant patient data in the PDR server is taken care for by the Integration and Communication-server (CAI server). The information will be presented on a flexible and userfriendly way via the Patient Data Viewer (PDV). The PDV is based on intranet technology. Dynamic HTML pages are automatically generated by CAI. These HTML pages are made available by an internal web server that makes it possible to show the client the relevant pages at their PC, with help of a standard web browser (i.e. Netscape or Internet Explorer). Figure 1 shows the components. The most important aspects of the above mentioned Flexible EPR are "integration and communication" and "Intranet technology" as the basis for visualisation.

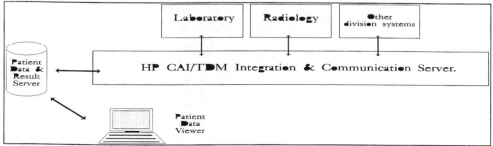

Figure 1: Components of the information architecture

2.2 Integration and communication

The integration toolset (CAI) offers users to create an integrated information environment without the necessity to invest in existing hard- and software of currently installed systems (i.e. laboratory-, radiology system). CAI consist of several components:

- A Transaction Distribution Manager (TDM) which integrates several applications and synchronise the information exchange between these systems. CAI supports besides HL-7 messages, EDIFACT and DICOM formatted massages.
- A system which enables users to access all relevant applications in different information systems that occur in the network in a transparent manner,
- A single logon facility usually existing within the entrance system where users log in and where of the security is organised.

2.3 Intranet and visualisation EPR

Important (technical) conditions for wide acceptance of the EPR are e.g.; the use of a userfriendly graphical userinterface, hardware portability, proprietary operating systems, access to information stored in other information systems and integration with several medical applications [16]. The World Wide Web, a system consisting of local internet browsers and internet-based Hypertext servers, is an elegant way to solve above mentioned problems [17]. Nowadays webbrowsers are available for the most popular hardware and operating systems and offer access to a large amount of servers on the internet. These browsers use standard user interfaces which can pre-sent text, images, video and sound. Besides that, browers support the possibility to switch to other resources on the internet by using links within Hypertext documents.

Internet already supports several medical applications [18]. Many authors state that the WWW seems to be an interesting environment to develop easy access to the multitude of information. Untill now the focus was on the application of electronic libraries and medical education [20, 21, 22]. Many researchers predict that within a short period of time the internet and WWW will be used by health providers and patients to get insight in the EPR and even for medical consultation [23, 24, 25]

3. Setting of the pilot-project

3.1 Background

The hospital makes use of the 'old-fashioned' WANG HIS. The HIS is connected to some departmental systems, like PALGA (pathology) and PACELAB (laboratory). The hospital wants to migrate to a flexible and userfriendly IT solution *based on their current HIS*. The EPR will be the center of the system. In Figure 2 the current and expected future information architecture are shown. Patient related data from the existing HIS and the departmental systems will be available, by means of dynamic HTML-pages, for client PC's; using CAI and an internal web server.

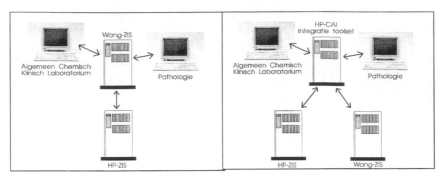

Figuur 2A: Current IT solution.   *Figuur 2B: Planned IT-solution*

The main aims of the pilot project are to evaluate the (technical) feasibility of the flexible EPR and to get an insight in the (dis)advantages of an EPR based upon WWW-technology. An important issue is the(network) security. The pilot is carried out for the ear, nose and throat specialism. On the one side because the specialism has a positive attitude towards the EPR and IT more in general. On the other hand because of the fact that the ear-nose and throat specialism is 'easy' to formalise and already a lot of research for this specialism has been carried out related to the EPR. The scope of this project is narrowed to the presentation of results of laboratory and pathology.

3.2 Approach

After a thorough literature search the information needs of the users were investigated (May-August '96). The information needs were investigated by use of ISAC-A and FCO-IM. Recently a prototype based upon this analysis has been round off. This prototype has been developed with continuous feedback and participation of users (i.e. clinicians, nurses). In the next phase of the pilot the data-basemodel will be implemented. Next the flexible EPR will be tested in routine use.

4. Results

4.1The prototype

Using the Web brower Internet Explorer, the "Home-page" of the application can be accessed via the client PC. The "Home-page" offers several possibilities to select a patient. (i.e. via the spe-cialism, department or the name of the patient). When a patient has been selected a short relevant medical history is displayed (figure 3). The contents of the medical history are tailored to the requirements of the user(s). Aspects of the medical history are for example: (admission)diagnoses, patient history, medication, report(s) of surgery and the latest medical correspondence.

At the top of the screen a photo of the patient and overall patient data are displayed. These data will be in top of the screen during the use of the EPR. At the left side of the screen a graphic structure of the contents of the patient record is visible. By a simple mouse click the user can easily 'jump' from one place (i.e. radiology-report) to another (i.e. pathology results) place in the patient record. An item is only shown if results are available (eg. Labresults) and the user is authorized.

By use of four icons on the left side of the screen, the user has easy access to ; e-mail func-tionality, CD-ROMS's accessible by the network, selection of new patients and literature databases (i.e. MEDLINE). Right now we are working at a connection with a patient education system and a quality control system (by use of protocols).

By using the hierarchical contents of the medical record on the left side of the screen it is easy to control patient results or medical correspondence. When selecting a laboratory result from a survey, the concerning results will be displayed. Besides general patient data, also characteristic laboratory results will be displayed at the top of the screen like laboratory number, name of the applied doctor and report date. From this report one can decide to display some laboratory results in time (figure 4) Using VBScript, Java applets and ActiveX components a graph can immediately be drawn. At the same time it is possible to call in and edit laboratory results in MS-Excel

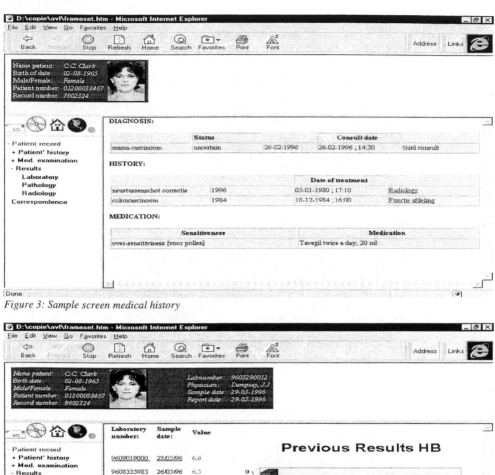

Figure 3: Sample screen medical history

Figure 4: Example of laboratory results

When a user wants to access a pathology report while reading laboratory results, he easily clicks within the structure of the medical record on the item pathology. From the next survey he'll select a pathology result. Also at the pathology result/report some characteristic data will be displayed (like pathology number, applied clinician, material etc). Besides text also images can be shown of a pathology report (figure 5). Also voice reports and videos are directly accessible.

4.2 User experiences

The prototype has been developed by continuous interaction with clinicians and nurses. The users were very pleased by this working method. One of the great advantages using Intranet technology indicated by users is the familiar user interface and the intelligent and intuitive navigation through the medical record. The users indi-ated that easy navigation through multi-media applications and direct access of literature databases is an important requirement for further dissemination of the EPR,

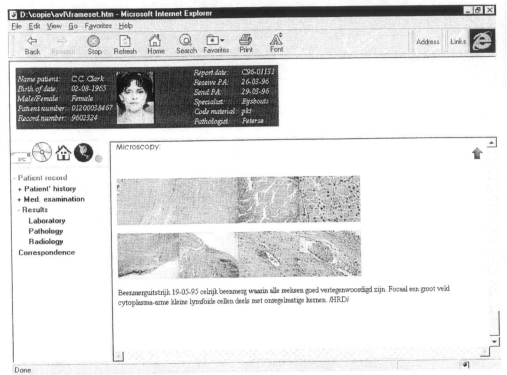

Figure 5: Sample screen of a miscroscopic report

5. Discussion

Our experiences developing the prototype flexible EPR indicate that Web-technology in combination with CAI as system integrator can be an important step in "wide" acceptance of the Electronic Patient Record. CAI takes care of the important connection between the (extern) subsystems. Intranet-technology not only offers the great advantages of the electronic highway, but certainly the advantages of a user friendly and intuitive user interface. We expect to implement the flexible EPR for the ear, nose and throat specialism in routine use on short notice.

Healthcare is an information intensive sector. Healthcare exists of many autonomous and diverse practitioners which all are responsible for an effective and efficient 'shared care'. Taking into account the increasing complexity of healthcare and the growing needs, it is not imaginable that the goals of the dutch government (efficient, accessible and qualitative good care) can be realised without an electronic infrastructure in healthcare. Dutch government already expressed their belief in internet as an electronic highway [1;2].

Nowadays a growing number of people is searching the internet for useful information. Several health care institutions already have their own web-site [26]. A good example of the fact that also dutch healthcare is exploring the advantages of the internet, is the "digital hospital" [27]. An even so interesting development is the web site "KNMG artsennet" [28]. This is an initiative of various dutch associations of clinicians.

Besides the many advantages of the use of intranet-technology there are still some disadvantages. There is a possibility that "undesired users" try to log into the computer system via the internet. However there are some methods to code the information, through which privacy can be guaranteed. The growing number of inter-net users slows down retrieval times. Current technological developments (eg. Distribution via cableTV) will provide a solution. Furthermore it should be say that intranet is surely not confronted with above mentioned problems.

In the pilot hospital the results will be translated into a roll-out plan. Possibly the flexible EPR, based upon internet-technology, will be developed in close cooperation with other hospitals. In the development much attention will be paid to the structure and navigation of the EPR, privacy guarantees and tuning with (dutch) legal aspects (like the WGBO, BIGG and quality laws)

References

1. Ministerie van Welzijn en Sport. Informatietechnologie zorgsector: feiten en opinies, 1995 (in dutch)
2. Ministerie van Welzijn en Sport. Beleidsnotitie Informatietechnologie in de zorg, 1995 (in dutch)
3. Dick RS, Steen EB. The computer based patient record. An essential technology for healthcare, 1991. Washington DC: National Academy Press
4. Tange HJ. The paper-based patient record: is it really so bad ? Comp Meth Prog Biomed. 1995; 48: 127-131.
5. Berger SD, Hilderink HGM. The medical doctor and the clinical information system: a feasibility study. Proceedings AMICE, 1995; 15-23
6. Weed LL. Medical Records, medical education and patient care: the problem oriented medical record as a basic tool, 1971, Cleveland
7. Fries JF. Alternatives in medical record formats. Medical Care. 1974; 12: 871-881.
8. Tange HJ. How to approach the structuring of the medical record. Proceedings of the 8th European Health Records Conference
9. Williams JG, Morgan JM, Severs MP, Howlett PJ. Let there be light. British Journal of Health Care Computing. 1993;10:30-32.
10. Buckland R. The language of health. British Medical Journal. 1993;306:287-288
11. Sittig DF. Computer-based physician order entry: the state of the art. J Am Med Informatics Assoc. 1993;1:108-123.
12. Lee F. et al. Implementation of physician order entry: user satisfaction and self-reported usage patterns. JAMIA. 1996; 3: 42-55
13. Moorman et al. A model for structured data entry based on explicit descriptional knowledge. Methods Inf Med, 1994; 33: 454-463
14. Rector AL. Foundations for an electronic record. Methods Inf Med, 1991; 30: 179-186
15. Cimino JJ, Socratous SA, Clayton, PD. Internet as clinical Information System: application development using the World Wide Web. JAMA; 1995, 2, 273-284.
16. Hammond WE. The role of standards in creating a health information infrastructure. Int J Biomed Comput. 1994; 34: 185-194.
17. Schatz BR, Hardin JB. NSCA Mosaic and the World Wide Web: global hypermedia protocols for the Internet. Science. 1994; 265:895-901.
18. Kleeberg P. Medical uses of the Internet. J Med Syst. 1993; 17(6): 363-366.
19. McKinney WP, Wagner JM, Bunton G, Kirk LM. A guide to Mosaic an the World Wide Web for physicians. MD Comput. 1995; 12(2): 109-114.
20. Metcalf ES et al. Academic Networks: Mosaic and the World Wide Web. Acad Med. 1994; 69(4): 270-273.
21. Kahn RM, Molholt P, Zucker J. CPMCnet: an integrated information and Internet resource. In: Ozbolt JG, ed. Proceedings of the 18th SCAMC. JAMIA. 1994 Supplement: 98-102.
22. Kruper JA et al. Building Internet accesible medical education software using the World Wide Web. In: Ozbolt JG. Proceedings of the 18th SCAMC: JAMIA. 1994 Supplement: 32-36.
23. Kassirer JP. The next transformation in the delivery of healthcare. N Engl J Med. 1995;332(1): 52-54.
24. Galvin JR et al. The virtual hospital: a new paradigm for lifelong learning in radiology. Radiographics. 1994;14;875-879.
25. Rizollo MA, Dubois K. Developing AJN network: transformating information to meet the needs of the future. In: Ozbolt JG. Proceedings 18th SCAMC: JAMIA. 1994 Supplement: 27-31.
26. Lowe HJ, Lomax EC, Polonkey SE. The World Wide Web: A review of an emerging Internet-based Technology for the Distribution of Biomedical Information. Journal of the American Medical Informatics Association. 1996;3:1-14.
27. Digitale ziekenhuis, Internet: http://www.ziekenhuis.nl
28. Lanphen J. De KNMG en haar leden op Internet. Medisch Contact. 1996;51:1130

Medical Informatics Europe '97
C. Pappas et al. (Eds.)
IOS Press, 1997

Development of a standardized format for archiving and exchange of electronic patient records in Sweden

Ted Wigefeldt [1,3], Sten Larnholt [2], Hans Peterson [1]
[1] SPRI (The Swedish Institute for Health Services Development), Box 70487, S-10726 Stockholm, Sweden
[2] Sahlgrenska University Hospital, Östra, Department of Geriatrics, S-41133 Göteborg, Sweden
[3] Genisys Software AB, Box 2401 S-40316 Göteborg, Sweden

Abstract. This paper describes an effort to standardize the long term archiving format of the electronic patient record. A format is given in SGML (Standard Generalized Markup Language) and also tested as a prototype in a production system.

1   Introduction

During the last decade 85 % of the primary health care units and about 15 % of the hospital care units in Sweden started to use electronic patient record systems. These systems generate a large amount of information that is stored on data media.

In many regions in Sweden there are regulations that medical records should be available for a very long period of time. The medical information that is stored on data media must be readable on any technical platform and by any electronic patient record system. The Swedish National Archives' approved archive methods are today microfilm and paper. One of the disadvantages with this form of long term information storage is that it is practically impossible to sort out information on research a perspective. Structured information in electronic patient record systems is easily handled for the purpose of statistic use and research.

To solve the problems with long time storage of medical information that is stored in different electronic patient record systems SPRI (The Swedish Institute for Health Services Development) in collaboration with Sahlgrenska University Hospital created the project DEJAVU.

The purpose of this project is to develop a general format, which will enable storage of medical information on a long time basis. The format, technology and the test system are described in this paper.

2   Background

Within an application the medical information will probably be divided into two types of archives - a primary archive and a secondary archive.

The primary archive's physical division of the elements into items and item complexes will follow the proposed standard of CEN TC251 Env 12265 (EHCRA). The main benefit in the direct mirroring of the elements into the database. Searches and handling of this database will be efficient in extracting individual objects. The drawback is the high degree of references and associations to maintain. One must also have access to a unique tool to interpret the information.

The secondary archive will accommodate information stored in a format more suitable for long term storing. The structure must be as flat as possible and referenced information must be stored in one unit together with the referring element. The format must also be robust and readable without specialized tools.

3   Problem definition

3.1   *Different types of medical records*
The most common model will in the future be the *object oriented* medical record. Within this category we will find a dispersed amount of objectorientation. The simplest form consisting of elements categorized by titles to the more advanced virtual medical record. One adaptation to objectorientation is the CEN Env 12265 framework. But the object orientation gives models complicated structures with elements connected in multiple dimensions.

Document oriented records is by nature stored in a single dimension flat format. Each document consists of 3 types of information, *data, structure and format.*

Data could be text, graphics, pictures or multimedia objects as well as video and sound.

The *structure* forms the relations between the document elements. Examples are paragraphs, lists and headlines.

The *format* gives the document an appearance. Examples are fonts, indentation and italics.

3.2   *Our objective*
The main problem to be solved is the translation of the objectoriented medical records multidimensional network structure into the flat structure of the dokument. At the same time most of the information elements and their references must be preserved. We also want to achieve this in an technologically independent and standardized way.

One goal for the project has been to use as much standard tools and methods as possible in describing the format for archiving and transportation. One such description tool is SGML (Standard Generalized Markup Language).

4   Model
The purpose of our work is to find a way to transform structured data into a standardized document format. This format will allow us to transport information between various vendors' applications and operating systems. In this format a document could be considered to have an unlimited lifetime.

A suggestion for such a model can be described in four steps. It is in this environment that the proposed format is set to work.

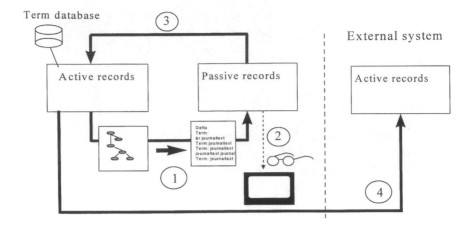

1. The electronic patient record is extracted out of the original structure and then transformed into SGML format. The existing term catalogue is the basis for labeling the information with SGML-tags.
2. An SGML (HTML) viewer is integrated with the available EPR system to make the archived records visible on demand.
3. The system has the power to parse and unpack achieved records or parts thereof to regain as active record elements.
4. The archive format will be tested in transporting record information between two physically separated systems.

4.1   SGML

SGML (Standard Generalized Markup Language, ISO 8879:1986/A1:1988) which is an international standard since 1986, is a declarative language that in a standardized way makes it possible to lay out the structure for electronic dokuments.

The two main parts of SGML is the DTD (Document Type Definition) and the documentation itself. The DTD describes the elements and the structure of every type of document. Within the document text is mixed with markers or tags which are described in the DTD.

5   Result

One outcome of the project is a SGML-DTD suited for term based patient record information. This DTD makes it possible for an objectoriented record to maintain its advanced structural design in the translation from database format to the document format. The DTD describes all the concepts defined in Env 12265.

The object descriptions in the DTD are completed with the DTD for HTML (Hypertext Markup Language) 2.0. In doing so, all archived documents will be viewable with HTML browsers. In this way we apply an established and cost-effective technology, and at the same time we can maintain a structure laid out in Env 12265. All this secured for long time and with the possibilities for additions.

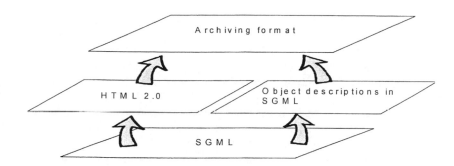

A very simple example showing the combined format will follow below. The only intention here is to show the principle.

In this example we will archive the bloodpressure of a patient. In the medical record the bloodpressure is shown as:

Bloodpressure   120/80

The pure HTML code to show the above pressure and value is:
```
<TABLE>
<TR>
<TD COLSTART="1">
<STRONG>Bloodpressure</STRONG>
</TD>
<TD COLSTART="2">120/80</TD>
</TR>
</TABLE>
```

The pure object format in SGML is expressed as:
```
<ITEM>
<TERM TERMID=1000 TERMNAME=Bloodpressure>Bloodpressure</TERM>
<TERM TERMID=1002 TERMNAME=Systolic>120</TERM>/
<TERM TERMID=1003 TERMNAME=Diastolic>80</TERM>
</ITEM>
```

The combination of HTML and the SGML patient record DTD gives us:
```
<TABLE><TR>
<TD COLSTART="1"><STRONG>
<ITEM>
<TERM TERMID=1000 TERMNAME=Bloodpressure>Bloodpressure
</TERM></STRONG></TD>
<TD>
<TERM TERMID=1002 TERMNAME=Systolic>120</TERM>/
<TERM TERMID=1003TERMNAME=Diastolic>80</TERM></TD>
</ITEM></TR>
</TABLE>
```

6   The prototype

To test if the proposed archiving format is functioning and if it can form a suitable base for a standard, the ability to handle the archives have been added to a modern electronic record system.

The Melior EPR system from Siemens Nixdorf Informationsystems AB adapts to the CEN EHCRA framework. The term catalogue describes the structure and relations between the medical items. The term catalogue has been completed with descriptions of markup tags. The documents can then be built from the descriptions in the term catalogue.

Together with security adaptations a viewer is added to the system, which gives the possibility to show the archived record.

There is also the facility to activate the archived record by move it back into the original database structure. An SGML parser - an interpreter or translator - decodes and unpacks the elements and rebuilds the database structure with all references.

The same method has with success been tested to transport records between physically separated systems.

7   Discussion

If we have a standardized archive format - when is the right time to store ? Will it be after some time, say every year, or will it be every time the information is signed?

How much of the record must be saved in one piece?

Another problem that can be solved with a standardized archive format is taking backups in an uniform way. Today the backup is taken mostly in native format direct from the database. With an archive format a backup can be taken independently of vendor and type of database or record system.

The most common format for exchange of medical information between systems is the EDIFACT and HL7 protocols. A standardized archiving format could probably serve as compliment to ease the exchange of structured medical information, especially if the structure is unknown from the beginning.

8   Conclusion

By development work and through testing we have found SGML suitable as a tool for long term archiving of electronic medical record documents. We have also developed a DTD (Document Type Definition) in SGML, which we consider to be a beginning to a common and standardized format to be used in long term archiving of patient records. Everything seems to indicate that the format can be used as an exchange format when moving records between separate systems. The format is also sufficient flexible to let us store structured records.

9   References

[1] CEN TC251, Env 12265, Medical Informatics - Electronic healthcare record architecture
[2] EJA - Den elektroniskt lagrade patientjournalens datalagring och informations transport. SPRI. Statusrapport Februari 1997.
[3] Eve Maler & Jeanne Andaloussi, Developing SGML DTD's from Text to Model, Prentice Hall 1996
[4] M. Colby & D Jackson, Special Edition Using SGML, Que Corporation 1996
[5] International Standard ISO 8879-1986, Information processing – Standard Generalized Markup Language (SGML), First edition – 1986-10-15.

Medical Informatics Europe '97
C. Pappas et al. (Eds.)
IOS Press, 1997

A hypermedia radiological reporting system

Mariano De Simone[1], Francesco M. Drudi[2], Cecilia Lalle[3],
Raffaella Poggi[2], Fabrizio L.Ricci[3]

1 Medical InformaticsConsultant, Roma, Italy
2 Radiology Ward, Policlinico "UmbertoI", Roma, Italy
3 National ResearchCouncil - ISRDS, Via C .de Lollis,12 - Roma, Italy

Abstract: Report is the main phase of a diagnostic process by images. The product ofthe process is the diagnostic report. We are proposing an hypermediastructure of diagnostic report in radiology, in order to facilitateexchange between radiologist and clinician (specialist in internal medicine or surgeon) on a clinical case, without anymore charge on the side of the radiologist but with an 'off-line'consultation. An hypermedia radiological report software will produce further advantages in many aspects: radiologistand clinician could access patient's data directly from DB on patients;radiologist could check DB on exemplary cases real-time; clinician couldread preliminary and final reports available in network and make requests on-line. The proposed hyper-reportsystem is modular. Starting from the 'report text' writing, edited by theradiologist on the basis of most significative images, it is possible toinsert comments in text, drawing and 'external' images form.

keywords: diagnostic process; diagnostic report; hypermedia;hyper-report; report

1. Introduction

Report is the main phase of a diagnostic process by images. The product ofthe process is the diagnostic report. We are proposing an hypermediastructure of a diagnostic report in radiology, in order to facilitateexchange between radiologist and clinician (specialist in internal medicine or surgeon) on a clinical case, withoutany more charge on the side of the radiologist but with an 'off-line'consultation

What is called 'hypermedia' is a technology integratingmultimedia data and knowledge underlying those data.

The radiological exam is generally realized inmultimedia form, as a set of text, images, and sometimes vocal comments [1]. To realize an hypermedia report (onwards 'hyper-report') we mustimplement a software associating both knowledge and links amongconstituting elements to the intrinsic multimedia essence of radiologicaldata [2]. An hypermedia tool will solve most of the problems arising from the current practise. Actually, to allow acompleat and correct interpretation of the report and to enable theclinician to run across the logical-diagnostic path that lead theradiologist to 'that' diagnosis, it is a must including knowledge underlying the passing 'description --> diagnosis'. Thatknowledge, together with the multimedia essence of the report, is thepivotal element to the production of an 'hyper-report'.

A hypermedia software for the radiological report willhelp:

- radiologist during the report, with specific tools toedit the report, including facilities to the linking of report-text, imagesand knowledge;
- clinician reading the report, with specific tools allowing the access tospecific data and to knowledge undelying the diagnosis.

The goal is to facilitate clinician during the readingof the report without extra specification coming from the radiologist. Atool like this one will meet diagnostic and therapeutical requirements ofthe clinician, mainly in wards as orthopaedy or neurosurgery. Orthopaedic needs careful analysing ofpathological situation by images, while neurosurgeon has to carefully planthe intervention for example to remove a carcinoma. The structure of thereport must compley with two main functions: communication and documentation. To best results we have toimprove both: the communication between radiologist and clinician along thereport process and the information-documentation in writing/reading thereport. Analysing implemented computer-based reportsystems we may conclude that:

- most of the systems is for didactical purposes (e.g.:[3, 4]);
- systems with clinical purposes are under testing (e.g.: [5, 6]).

Our system is not just a tool to writing/reading an hyper-report, but mustbe included in a telematic scenario, foreseeing functionalities involvingradiologist and clinician as ((teleconsultation)), with real-timecommunication of results, extemporary specifications and on-line discussion. Requests for integrations could be sendby e-mail [7].

Direct access is allowed, through external links, todatabases on hyper-reports, exemplary cases and radiological atlas.

2. Telematic systems scenario

Assuming telematic implementation of report process, we may hypothesize ascenario where information flow does not involve the main actors(radiologist and clinician) directly, but through an internal hospitalnetwork (IntraNet) integrated with RIS (Radiological Information System), for the real-time sharing of preliminaryhypermedia report to:

- a database on patients (including EMR's, electronicmedical records');
- a database on hypermedia reports;
- a database on exemplary cases;
- a database on radiological atlas.

More functionalities may derive from IntraNetalong the radiological report process (booking, test performance and reportphases). An IntraNet example is electronic mail. Such a scenario can not exclude direct or paper-basedcommunication; the result is an additional and unessential informationsystem [8].

Benefits of telematic scenario compared with apaper-based one are:

- direct access to patient's data (through DB on patients) both forradiologist and clinician;
- availability, for the radiologist, of a DB onexemplary reports to real-time consultation and comparison;
- on-line availability, for the clinician, of bothpreliminary report (just text or text including pre-images) and finalreport (in hypermedia form), allowing teleconsultation and additionalrequests.

3. System's description

System analysis starts with determination ofelements that compound the radiological report. Report structure is shownin fig.1.

radiological report
    input data
        request
        diagnostic question
        patient's data
    exam description
        performed exam
        technical specifications
    text of report
        report sentences
            signs
            location
            measure
        diagnostic interpretation/result
        notes
    indexing
        ACR code
        keywords

Fig. 1 - Structuring elements of radiological report

Including links with 'internal' (i.e.related to the test itself) images and/or 'external' (i.e. related to previous tests, or included inhyper-reports, exemplary cases or radiological atlas databases) images tothe structure represented in fig.1, we proceed toward the hyper-report [9]. The global hyper-report structure proposed, included correlation links,is reported in fig.2, where we made use of an OMT (Object ModellingTechnique, v. [10]) representation. From that schema, it comes out the followingsemantical deepening links (to the integration of data and knowledge),represented in bold and with evidence of the direction (with arrows):
  - internal to the hyper-report:
        report text sentence <---> image
        <sign> in report text sentence ---> image
        image <---> processed image (zoom, etc.)
        image <---> comment
        report text sentence <---> vocal comment
  - external to the hyper-report:
        comment post-it ---> drawing on radiologicalatlas
        comment post-it ---> exemplary image (from DB exemplary cases)
        comment post-it ---> previous images (same patient; same or differenttools)
There are also compositional links (aggregation,generalisation), and functional links (that can be travelled over specificfunctions of Human Computer Interface) represented with dashed lines.
We have made use of the following structuredrepresentation of sentences of the report:
        <sign> present in **<location>** withsize of **<measure>**

4. Hypermedia report: writing and reading precesses

In writing a report, the radiologist choose themost significative images. Then the report starts: the radiologist locates <signs> on images, semeiotical information, and emphasizes them insidethe <location>, or may emphasize just the <location> (to the lowerdefinition level).
Zoom images on specific areas may be derived from the primitive images, toallow accuracy in reading of <sign>, and coloured contours, selected from amenu or created 'ad-hoc' by the

operator, may be used as outlines for theclinician. They are useful, inthe reading, in individualisation of <sign> and/or <location>. Then, theradiologist may individualise dimensions with arrows, contours or othermarks, if necessary with scales for measurement. In the writing process, <sign> and <measure> excludeeach other; if <measure> is present, its marks are also underliners of<sign> [11].

The radiologist writes, on a 'post-it' called <report sentence> andconnected to each image, section of the text of the report related to theimage itself, with the whole description of <sign>, <location> and<measure>. Sentences are written on a vanishing field. The copy of <report sentence> on the main screen creates a linkbetween final report sentences and corresponding images.

The radiologist inserts then the 'comment post-it',including text, drawings, vocal comments and processing (e.g.: 3D images),'internal' and/or 'external' comparing images.

Finally, analising sequence of report sentences on mainscreen, he proceeds to the final editing, including diagnostic conclusions.Automatically, system generates ACR code; keywords may then be included[12].

In the reading process, the clinician analises report-text, makes use of links withimages (internal and/or external), if necessary processes images (at alower level than radiologist), reads 'comment post-it' with access toprevious or exemplary cases. More possibilities arise by means of the teleconsultation and the electronic-mail.

5. Systemfunctionalities

System functionalities may be structuredmainly in (a) text editing and (b) image processing sections.

a) Text editing

The final text of the report may be generated in asingle phase or through different phases, with generation of singlesentences, linked to corresponding images, concurring to the definition ofthe final report.

> *<Text> editing*: text may be inserted invocal form or by keyboard: in this case, are foreseen typical editingfunctionalities as write, cancel, copy, paste, etc..

> *<Report sentence> 'post-it' editing*: radiologist edits reportsentences on hidden text-fields ('post-it') placed on images; at the end,text is automatically copied on <report-text> screen.

> *<Comment> 'post-it' editing*: radiologist edits comment sentences, useful to clinician, on 'post-it'placed on most significative images. Such a 'post-it' may include text,drawings (from radiological atlas), vocal comments, all kinds of data fromprevious tests or exemplary cases.

> *<Report-text> final editing:* at the end ofthe report-sentences editing, the radiologist goes to the report-textscreen and proceeds to final editing, inserting also diagnostic results andnotes; after the automaticalgeneration of ACR code, fills the keywords field.

b) Images processing

Radiologist may process main images to facilitate'reading', to emphasize part of them, or to address clinician's attentiontowards restricted 'regions of interest' (ROI). Requested functionalitiesmay be grouped as follows.

> *Main images processing*: among the manydifferent kinds of processing there are simple contrast, brightenes andresolution modifications or more compex 3D rebuilding; it will depend onimage processing software available on radiological workstation.

> *Production of zoom images*: the radiologist,starting from an image produced during the test, may realize a zoom imageof the ROI.

Inserting of coloured contours: to emphasize <signs> on images, radiologist may insert coloured contoursover the images, taken from an available menu (circles, ellipsis,rectangles) or created by simple drawing tools. Using two different colorscould make evidence of patological (e.g.: red) or not patological (e.g.: green) signs.

6. Conclusions

Hyper-report building process is modular; it develops since the bookingphase, by insertion of diagnostic request and patient's data. Next phasefacilitates radiologist in writing the so-called hyper-report. Although inwriting phase radiologist will needmore time, it will be fastest and easiest the reading for the clinician.Real-time investigation in analising hyper-report will avoid directconsultation between the two, allowing clinician direct access tohypermedia explanating and deepening comments.

The hyper-report modular building is based on different clinical elements:the diagnostic request (that may be differentiated in diagnostic,((pathological stage)) or therapeutical request), body-part or interestedorgan, pathology and finally test result itself. A negative-result test will need just report-text production. A testaddressed to surgical intervention will need an higly structuredhyper-report, with inserting of many kind of comments.

Hyper-report goal is improving of exchangesbetween radiologist and clinician, allowing radiologist better managementof time during report process and facilitating clinician in planninginterventions.

Prototype is under development by Radiology Ward at Policlinico Umberto Iof Rome, in Macintosh environment. Many clinicians are cooperating tovalidate reading aspects and to verify proposed functionalities.

References

[1]   I. Brolin "I principi fondamentali della refertazione clinica", inChiesa A. et al.: informatica in radiodiagnostica, Libreria GoliardicaParmense, Parma, 1978

[2]   K. Kuhn,T. Zemmler, M. Reichert, D. Rosner, O. Baumiller, H. Knapp "An IntegratedKnowledge-Based System to Guide the Physician During Structured Report", in*Methods of Information in Medicine*, n.33, p.417-422, 1994

[3]   D'D'Alessandro M.P.; Galvin J.R., Erkonen W.E.; Santer D.M., Huntley J.S.,McBurney R.M., Easley G. "An approach to the creation of multimediatextbooks for radiology instruction", in American Journal of Roentgenology(AJR) 161(1) pp.187-91 aa.7/1993

[4]   Shultz E.K. , Brown R. W. ;, Beck J. R. "Hypermedia in Pathology - The DartmouthInteractive medical record Project", *Supplement to :AmericaJournal of Clinical Pathology* 91(4) pp S34-S38 aa.Aprile/ 1989

[5]   Inamoto K., Inamura K., Umeda T. "Oral diagnostic report andsynchronized image filling using magneto-optical disks ", in*Computer Methods and Programs in Biomedicine* 37(4) pp.327-31aa. 5/1992

[6]   Kitanisono T., Kurashita Y., Honda M., Hishida T., Mizuno M., AnzaiM. "The use of multimedia in patient care", in *ComputerMethods and Programs in Biomedicine* 37(4) pp.259-63 aa.5/1992

[7]   F. M.Ferrara "Architecture of Health Information System" inRAYS v. 21 n.2 apr-giug., pp. 152-173, 1996

[8]   F. Consorti, P. Merialdo, G. Sindoni "Transactional WorkFlows,Cooperative WorkFlows and Hypermedia Design Tools in Health-Care ",1996

[9]   C. Bucci, D. Scorretti, F. Floris, G. Capocasa "Sistemi informaticiin radiologia: DREAM. Gestione pazienti", in RAYS, aprile-giugno 1996

[10]   J. Rumbaugh, M. Blama "Object-Oriented Modeling and Design",Prentice Hall, Inc., Englewood Cliffs, New Jersey, USA, 1991

[11]   F.M.Drudi, F. Ferri, R. Minarelli Della Valle, F.L. Ricci "Analisi del refertoradiologico e del processo di refertazione radiologica", CNR-ISRDS,Rapporto Tecnico, Roma, 1994

[12]   M. DeSimone, C. Lalle, F.L. Ricci, A Rossi Mori "Context Tree Methodology forthe Formalisation of Health-Care Activities", Rapporto Tecnico n.17/1996CNR/ISRDS, Roma, 1996

Medical Informatics Europe '97
C. Pappas et al. (Eds.)
IOS Press, 1997

Doctor Friendly Electronic Patient Record

Smiljana SLAVEC[1], Miran REMS[2], Gregor CERKVENIK[3]

(1) INFONET - Engineering of Medical Informatics, Kranj, Slovenia
(2) General Hospital Jesenice, Surgery Unit, Jesenice, Slovenia
(3) University Medical Centre, Department of Surgery, Division of Plastic Surgery & Burns, Ljubljana, Slovenia

Abstract. In this paper we would like to show importance of using modern information technology in implementation and development of health information systems. Our main focus is on doctor's work. Doctors will use computer only if they will see clear advantages. Traditional data gathering and display are not sufficient, so modern software should provide speech interfacing and computer graphics in various applications and enable the use of electronic mail, hand held computers, electronic data interchange, etc. among other *features*. This paper tries to show the needs for applications of those *features*. They are already implemented as part of our hospital information systems.

1. Introduction

In this contribution we wish to define the most important starting points and problems faced with when trying to launch information systems in health care, above all, when we wish to approach the system to the doctor.

In most of 23 Slovene hospitals, information systems containing ELECTRONIC PATIENT RECORDS, have already been implemented, in some of them they have been complemented for several years[1]. Information systems have a great value as they support the simple flow and collection of information in the period of treating each individual patient. The collected data mean quality and fast accessible archives. According to these data many analyses, professional as well as business ones, can be executed[2].

Yet we are not satisfied with the way these data are used by doctors. Very often the input as well as the application of data are indirect. The input of data is carried out by administrative staff; nurses and other staff (lab technicians, pharmacists). The doctor most often checks the written record which he orders and gets prepared by others.

We have been investigating where the reasons for such a state could be. As potential reasons the following can be quoted:

- The doctor wishes to devote most of his time to direct work with patients in which he is expert and sovereign. He is not used to the computer work. He doesn't master it to the same level as his own proffesional work, therefore he prefers to leave it to the others who are more familiar with this system and so the gap widens.
- In the majority of hospitals the complete computer support of the treatment process isn't assured in the whole, the fact being that in some hospitals there isn't a suitable equipment

for all segments. This again leads toward redoubling of certain information flows and irrational solutions and paper consumption

- It is difficult to assure direct access to the computer technology on every single doctor's workplace. The most vital problem here is the access to the data and data input during the patient's visit .

When analyzing, we found out the outstanding updating and quality of administrative and balance data. The users put in data regularly and they often analyze them. The basic reason is probably the direct impact of these data and their application in financial field, respectively, what the institution also gives stimulations for?

The doctor doesn't want to use the computer at his everyday work unless advantages in the process of treatment are evident. Therefore a solution has to be made (for his job) which he will adopt and include into his regular working process.

We have, therefore, tried to establish in which respect the needs of a doctor differ from those of existing information solutions.

If we simplify the process we can say: the doctor talks to the patient, examines him, sends him to check-ups, looks at the lab tests, ultrasound tests, x-ray photographs. He is interested in comparing the results which he got to the others, he observes the trend of each individual observation. In more complicated or unclear cases he wants to consult other specialists who must send him the material.

There is a very simple conclusion. A doctor needs a program which would make a good use of all advantages of the up-to-date technology in order to support such a complex and varied way of work.

It is necessary to enable the use of graphics, display and processing of pictorial material, sound recording and bring Internet and Intranet to his workplace.

The basic goal is to assure PROMPT and SIMPLE access, as well as QUALITY and EFFICIENT data presentation[3].

In the continuation the realized options, above all, have been demonstrated and executed as to reach this objective.

2. Data presentations

Possibility to monitor time series and establishing trends

Laboratory tests

Due to the fact that information systems have been applied in hospitals for several years already, many data have already been collected. The direct transfer of lab tests from analyzators into the system has been enabled which assures a simple and quality input.

The doctor at his work is often interested in comparing the momentary tests with the tests existing in the system. For easier and more accurate decision it is necessary to analyse time series and monitor the value trend. The trend in the process of diagnostics and monitoring the efficiency of therapy is essential, many times it is more important than absolute result[4].

For clear presentation of trend we used the possibility of computer graphics and we offered the doctor a graphic presentation of results. According to the content of the problem it is possible to focus on one examination only, but we can, however select a graphic display of more graphs simultaneously. In this way we realize the second big advantage: possibility to compare trends of various examinations.

To upgrade this, we can also make statistic data processing.

X-Ray photographs, ultrasound diagnostics

The comparision of the results and establishing trends is not reasonable in the case of measured quantities only, but also at other types of examinations. It is reasonable to compare x-ray photographs, too.

Momentarily, we cannot launch a complete system for storing and processing x-ray photographs in our hospitals, because a good enough equipment is not avaliable. But we can, however, assure support to the most vital decision making phases. We include into information system those photographs which are vital for monitoring process at certain patients. With this we can also use a little inferior quality of photographs, enable simple comparison and , of course, allow the possibility of using original material in the archives. Not insignificant is the fact that integrated hospital information system enables reinstatement of well settled and fast accessible archives of x-ray photographs.

Sound

Direct recording of the doctor's findings enables a much more rational link between a doctor as a data creator and momentary mediator - administrative staff. The text input is simpler and more reliable if compared to parallel systems, like dictating machine for instance. The system will be later upgraded by the actual option of Voice Recognition.

Images

More and more often the problem how to document certain activities implemented during the treatment of the patient arises. A tedious text often cannot show the real flow authentically enough. It is above all difficult to describe critical situations in which we had to react fast and where we had to undertake unusual solutions.

Many medical operations are recorded, yet the recordings are stored in remote archives, very often just temporarily, because there of the space problem. (The recordings of laparoscopy operations, endoscopy tests, plastic operations are stored.)

The method of "freeze" of some segments from video recordings which are kept in information system, where they are directly accessible, has proven to be very useful. They can also be used for monitoring of individual patient and as a part of knowledge basis which is used for educational purposes (Fig.1).

3. Telecommunications

In medicine the information and knowledge flow is extremely important. Herewith we distinguish above all possibilities:
- data flow about a defined, individual case
- information and knowledge flow among various environments, not bound to individual cases
- access to literature

- access to knowledge banks

We can offer support to information flow by launching Intranet and Internet.

The possibility of electronic data transfer can be used in order to enable the simplification and faster communication among professionals[5,6]. The documentation is very easy to prepare, enclosures are taken directly from the system and they don't have to be collected separately. The user can take appropriate time to process the sent case and he is not disturbed in his normal work process.

Electronic mail, however, has already been used in hospital information systems, but the professional data don't interchange among the information systems yet. In the first place we plan the exchange among selected doctors in primary care and specialists in hospitals, labs and pharmacies.

The chances given by Internet are known to everybody, it is vital that we have Academic computer network in Slovenia which enables free of charge access to all Slovene doctors. Many of them benefit from this possibility already.

We can find the confirmation of our starting conclusions about the applicability of data from information systems in the field of telecommunications. We can state that there are several solutions launched also in the field of business.

For several years there has been electronic data interchange among health providers and health insurance company. Invoices are sent in EDIFACT standard form. At the moment EDI is run in about a half of public institutions, among private providers there are only few who decided to use it. In the course of last year pilot projects of EDI data for medical care statistics have been gathered. The system will be launched in some regions in 1997.

Smart Card

We expect much from launching smart cards planned by state insurance. The vital advantage will already be on the level of administrative data because it will enable equal identification of patients in all environments. In case that its functions later increase, as the project anticipates, it will mean one of the possibilities of storing and transmitting important data to the electronic patient record (emergency data, electronic prescriptions).

The role of medical informatics in telemedicine is dependent on using the power of the computerized database not to only feed patient specific information to the health care providers, but to use the epidemiological and statistical information in the data base to improve decision making and ultimately care. The computer is also a powerful tool to facilitate standardising and monitoring of care and when applied in continuous quality improvement methodology it can enhance the improvement process well beyond what can be done by hand. The coupling of medical informatics with telemedicine allows sophisticated medical informatics systems to be applied in low population density and remote areas[7].

4. Conclusion

We can assert that software, enabling the stated forms of data display, has been well accepted by doctors. We, therefore, assess that we will substantially increase the information application, moreover, the functioning of the entire system will thus be more universal.

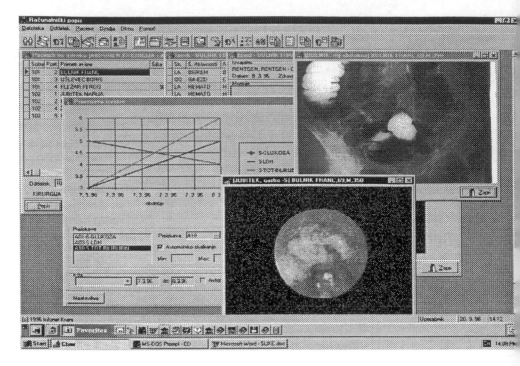

Figure 1: Electronic Patient Record

References

[1] S. Slavec : Elements of Health Information System Uniformity and Development of Software. Medicinska informatika MI-94, Bled,Slovenia,1994, 285-288

[2] R. Neame : Human Issues in the Development of regional (National and Provincial) Health Information. MIE-96, Copenhagen, Dennmark, 1996, 3-7

[3] P. Degoulet, F-C. Jean, C. Safran : Multimedia Workstations: Electronic Assistants for Health-Care Proffesionals. Yearbook of Medical Informatics, 1996, 65-75

[4] M. Bohanec, M. Rems, S. Slavec, B. Urh : Decision Support of Nosocomial Infection Therapy. MIE-96, Copenhagen, Dennmark, 1996, 599-603

[5] B. Frandji, P. Cooper : Seamless Telematics across Regions - *Star*. Evolution and Practical Approach of,Open, Modular, Patient Based Health Care Telematic Solutions. MIE-96, Copenhagen, Dennmark, 1996, 36 - 40

[6] A. Barth, M. Eichelberg, S. Von Gehlen, A. Hewett, P. Jench : Integrating CSCW and Video-Conferencing in Telemedicine. MIE-96, Copenhagen, Dennmark, 1996, 123-127

[7] T.P. Clemmer: The Role of Medical Informatics in Telemedicine. In Yearbook of Medical Informatics 1996, 275-286

Medical Informatics Europe '97
C. Pappas et al. (Eds.)
IOS Press, 1997

Management of Hospital Discharge Data in Belgrade

Saulic A., Jelaca P., Simic S.*
Institute of Public Health of Belgrade, 29. Novembra 54a, 11000 Belgrade,
*Institute of Social medicine, Statistics and Health Research, Medical Faculty Belgrade,
Dr Jovana Subotica 19, 11000 Belgrade, Yugoslavia

Abstract. The paper presents a database on clinically treated patients in
Belgrade, a computerized health-statistics information sub-system. It also
analyses the organisation of report processing related to hospitalisation,
types of indicators on hospital treatment (wich are the result of such a
processing) as well as their further utilisation on different levels of
management within the system of health care in Belgrade.

1. Introduction

Database on clinically treated patients in Belgrade is a part of the health statistics
information system. The data are collected through individual statistical reports -
Hospital Discarge Reports (in accordance with the relevant Regulations). Computerized
processing of those data started in 1979 and has been going on ever since.

The format and contents of Hospital Discharge Reports has not changed significantly
over the years, so that data can be easily compared since the beginning of this program.
All collected and processed data have been kept in the Data Base Management Center
of the Serbian Institute for Health Insurance (the Belgrade branch) and represent a
valid basis for follow up, analysis and evaluation of the use of hospital facilities as well
as the very functioning of this part of health care system in Belgrade.

2. Organisation of Hospital Discharge Reports Processing

An Hospital Discharge Report is a part of legally provisioned medical documentation
related to patients treated in hospitals. Its format and content are equal to the first page
of Patient's History and is filled partly on a patient's admisson to hospital (patient's
personal data, type of health insurance, and the reason for hospital treatment), and
partly on patient's discharge (medical data, data relating to medical services during the
hospital treatment and financial data). Such reports are collected and sent for
processing on a monthly basis , together with a copy of a Discharge Summary. Before
the processing, all data are checked and then coded - a process done by a team of MDs
and nurses. Entering and processing of those data are centralised and performed on
terminals and central unit within the Data Base Management Center of the
aprementioned Serbian Institute for Health Insurance (the Belgrade branch).

After entering the data for one-year period, they are processed by a defined set of
computer programs. The result of this process is a Statistical Bulletin of the Belgrade
Branch of the Serbian Institute for Health Insurance. The data base is then taken by the
Institute of Public Health of Belgrade, which, in its computer center performs all
processing that is furder needed for the creation of the legal health statistical reports, as
well as other relevant reports to be used by a number of further users. Among them

are Serbian and local administrative agencies, institutes for health insurance, other institutes of public health and individual health institutions wich receive feedback information on their work. The annual processig rate is 220,000 - 250,000 Hospital Discharge Reports. Data structure of the report consists of 48 fields of total lenght of 194 characters.

3. Hospital Treatment Data in Belgrade

3.1. Features of Hospital Facilities and Provision of the Population with Hospital care

According to the statistics for 1995, the city of Belgrade had a population of 1,625,000. In 26 hospitals and 2 minor in-patient facilities (wich are the part of out-patient health centers) there were 12,441 beds [1]. Inner organisation of health care institutions and their names have not been standardized. They are not divided to the hospitals wich treat acute and chronic cases. Table 1 shows the existing institutions divided according to the level of specialisation and organisation of work within them.

NUMBER, TYPES AND FACILITIES OF THE BELGRADE HOSPITALS

Table 1.

Type of hospital	Number of hospitals	Number of beds	%
1. The Serbian Clinical Center	1	3,761	30.2
2. Clinics and institutes	9	2,358	19.0
3. Clinical hospitals	4	2,902	23.3
4. Specialized hospitals	8	2,086	16.8
5. Rehabilitation centers	4	1,332	10.7
TOTAL	26	12,441	100.0

The greatest number of those facilities is a higly-specialized type of hospitals, whereas the activities of general hospital are mostly performed by large clinical hospitals. A majority of hospitals is also a teaching facility for students of Medical School of the Belgrade University (ord. number 1-3), so that clinical beds make 72.5% of all hospital beds.

Table 2 shows hospital beds by specialist services provided for the population of Belgrade. The group of pediatrics and child surgery comprises also the beds of all childrens wards in other branches, while the number of beds is calculated for the 0-18 aged population. Beds in obstetrics and gynecology wards are calculated for the female population aged 15 and above. There are 7.6 beds per 1,000 population in Belgrade (5.5 are in teaching hospitals). The average value for Yugoslavia is 5.56 beds per 1,000 population (1.2 in teaching hospitals) [2].

HOSPITAL BEDS ACCORDING TO BRANCHES OF MEDICINE

Table 2.

Branhes	Number of beds	%	Rate per 1,000 population
1. Internal medicine	3,167	25.5	1.9
2. Surgery	3,549	28,5	2.2
3. Pediatrics and child surgery	1,680	13.5	4.1
4. Obstetrics and gynecology	1,289	10.4	1.9
5. Psychiatry	1,171	9.4	0.7
6. Rehabilitation (adults)	1,287	10.3	0.8
7. Emergency medical services	298	2.4	0.2
T O T A L	12,441	100.0	7.6

3.2. Indicators of hospital performance in Belgrade

Data base on clinically treated patients serves as the information source about the performance of hospitals on various levels of their management [3]. Depending on the user demand, hospital performance indicators are calculated for: individual wards, hospitals, groups of hospitals (clustered by geografy or function). Table 3 shows values of basic indicators calculated cumulatively for all hospitals in Belgrade.

INDICATORS OF HOSPITAL PERFORMANCE IN BELGRADE IN 1995

Table 3.

Indicators	
1. Average lenght of hospitalisation (in days)	14.7
2. Average number of patients per one bed annualy	19.4
3. Average number of addmitancies daily	661.6
4. Average annual bed occupancy (in days)	290.5
5. Average rate of bed occupancy (%)	79.6
6. Hospital mortality (%)	3.6

Data base of this type allows the analysis of utilisation of hospital care by population of both sexes and different age, and comparisson with the data in medical literature [4]. Female patients had a greater number of episodes of hospitalisation, greater number of treatment days and longer lenght of stay. Greates number of episodes, treatment days and lenght of stay was registered in the age group of 65 and more (Table 4).

INDICATORS OF UTILISATION OF HOSPITAL CARE IN BELGRADE IN 1995

Table 4.

Indicators	Total	Sex		Age			
		Male	Female	0-19	20-49	50-64	over 64
1. Number of discharges per 1,000 population	148.6	135.3	161.1	109.7	138.1	150.7	284.3
2. Number of days of treatment per 1,000 population	2192.5	1905.2	2461.9	1322.0	1935.0	2495.8	4818.5
3. Average lenght of stay	14.7	14.1	15.3	12.1	14.0	16.6	16.9

A review of hospital morbidity according to the 9th Revision of ICD is given in Table 5.

RATE OF DISCHARGES FROM HOSPITALS IN BELGRADE BY FIRST-LISTED DIAGNOSES, SEX AND AGE, 1995

Table 5.

Category of first-listed diagnosis and ICD-9 code	Total	Sex Male	Female	Age 0-19	20-49	50-64	over 64
1. 001-139	4,174	2,128	2,046	1,144	1,650	744	636
2. 140-239	27,009	12,959	14,050	2,427	8,618	9,265	6,699
3. 240-279	6,702	2,893	3,809	966	2,189	1,923	1,624
4. 280-289	2,189	981	1,208	635	567	405	582
5. 290-319	9,751	5,118	4,633	1,142	5,981	1,821	807
6. 320-389	16,262	8,410	7,852	3,761	4,281	3,930	4,290
7. 390-459	34,656	19,291	15,365	704	6,530	12,119	15,303
8. 460-519	18,673	10,294	8,379	10,593	3,682	2,062	2,336
9. 529-579	20,090	11,339	8,751	3,939	6,366	5,380	4,405
10. 580-629	16,996	5,590	11,406	2,434	8,955	2,804	2,803
11. 630-676	26,802	0	26,802	1,310	25,439	16	37
12. 680-719	3,670	1,772	1,898	827	1,666	712	465
13. 710-739	13,069	5,610	7,458	1,864	5,683	3,489	2,033
14. 740-759	4,741	2,716	2,025	4,153	446	81	61
15. 760-779	2,363	1,138	1,225	2,363	0	0	0
16. 780-799	4,328	2,234	2,094	1,962	984	693	689
17. 800-999	14,747	9,620	5,127	3,387	6,050	2,594	2,716
V01-V82	15,281	4,328	10,953	1,392	9,909	2,650	1,330
T O T A L	241,503	106,422	135,081	45,003	98,996	50,688	46,816

A majority of diagnoses belong to the circulatory diseases (390-495), in wich cardiovascular diseases make 75.7% (26,227 discharges). In the female population most frequent are diagnoses within the complications in pregnancy, delivery and puerperium group (630-676). In this group, normal delivery and other indications for medical care during the delivery (650-659) make 60.3% (16,157), While abortions and ectopic and molar pregnancies are represented by 13.1% (3,502). In the group of neoplasms, malignant neoplasms are represented by 71.2% (19.233).

Among the features, special attention is given to the processing and follow-up of surgeries. These medical procedures have been monitored according to the adopted classification of the Serbian Institute for Health Insurance. Each surgical intervention has a precisely defined number of points (beeing called "complexity factor"), designed as such according to the degree of complexity of the very surgical intervention and the type of resources needed for this intervention. Factors are ranked in ascending order (1-600). A majority of surgeries comes from the complexity factor group of 11-50 (30.5%). Surgeries within the complexity factor above 100 make 19.7% of the total number of performed surgeries. Table 6. gives the number and structure of performed surgeries, grouped according to the complexity factor.

SURGERIES PERFORMED IN SURGICAL UNITS AND HOSPITALS, RANKED CCORDING TO THE COMPLEXITY FACTOR IN BELGRADE IN 1995

Table 6.

Complexity factor	Number of surgery	%
1. 1 - 10	27,053	30.5
2. 11 - 50	28,225	31.9
3. 51 - 100	15,847	17.9
4. 101 - 200	15,315	17.3
5. over 200	2,154	2.4
T O T A L	88,594	100.0

4. Conclusions

Hospital care is the most expensive and greatest sub-system within the system of health care (both in the world and in our country). More than 50% of all health workers are employed within hospitals. Of all financial resourses allocated for health, some 45% are spent for hospital care. Our system is also an irrational one, due to the greatest number of beds aimed at highly specialised medicine and the lack of beds for general purpose, chronic deseases and conditions. It is therefore necessary to develop methods to monitor and analyse the work of such a great sub-system, in order to develop new, restrictive ways of payment for its huge expenses. Data base on hospitalised patients represents, therefore, a valuable source of information to help us resolve all those issues.

Numerous problems related to data scope, accuracy in processing, out-dated maner of performance and equipment amortisation, has resulted in the application of new strategic decisions for this base. A new, distributed processing manner has been allrcady designed. It supports the role of hospitals (in which all the entries and part of data-processing will have been performed). Institute of Public Health of Belgrade will have become a database management center. The new applications use standardised software and are modularly projected, in option of inclusion into the existing hospital information systems. In the facilities that still do not have their own information systems, they will serve as a base for its development.

References

[1] Health Care Statistical Yearbook of Belgrade 1995. Institute of Public Health of Belgrade, Belgrade 1996.

[2] Statistical Yearbook of Yugoslavia 1995. State Institute of Statistics, Belgrade 1996.

[3] E. H. Shortlife and L. E. Perreault, Medical Informatics. In: Computer Applications in Health Care. Addison-Wesley Publishing Company, New York 1990.

[4] E. J. Graves, 1993 Summary: National Hospital Discharge Survey, *Advance Data* **264** (1995) 1-11.

Medical Informatics Europe '97
C. Pappas et al. (Eds.)
IOS Press, 1997

Computer-aided prescription - A prototype system

G Anogianakis[1,2], D. Goulis[3], D. Vakalis[3]

1 BIOTRAST s.a., 111 Mitropoleos Str, GR-54622 Thessaloniki, Greece
2 Department of Physiology, Faculty of Medicine, Aristotle University, Thessaloniki
3 Imperial College School of Medicine, St.Mary's Hospital - The Mint Wing, Unit of
Metabolic Medicine
4 2nd Internal Medicine Clinic, A.H.E.P.A. Hospital, GR-54006 Thessaloniki, Greece

Abstract. This study intends to satisfy two purposes : To prove the necessity of an electronical prescription aid and to propose a structure that can be interpreted into software which will be able to cover that need. The complicated market reality and the disadvantages of the written pharmaceutical directories make the existence of an electronical aid absolutely necessary. The structure of a prescription system should be based upon the drastic substance with its consequences (adverse effects, relative and absolute contraindications. pharmakokinetics and interactions). Every drastic substance will lead to the connection of pharmacology with the market reality and its own consequences (product identification through text and image, trade name, pharmaceutical company, strength, package information). The whole structure constitutes a completed relation - database system that is capable of answering any simple question or query that concerns the field of prescribing. The final production of such an aid is believed to help in a very high degree prescribing in a more precise and correct way, saving financial means for the patient and the health insurance as well as saving the doctor's time.

1. Introduction

Medical prescribing has with plenty of peculiarities. In many cases, the Greek National Health System, demands an inexperienced doctor to prescribe drugs that concern a wide spectrum of clinical medicine. This duty proves to be difficult as knowledge about trade reality, trade name and package information provided by the medical curriculum is considerably limited. The existence of a great number of drugs containing the same drastic substance, as well as, the continuous changes in the market, result in additional difficulties.

In Greece about 5000 products are released containing 1500 drastic substances. Every day 1 new product is released, withdrawn or altered modified. It is obvious, therefor, that the doctor who is obliged to prescribe through a wide spectrum of drugs is to be supplied with specific aids.

2. Electronical prescription

This is satisfied by a series of written pharmaceutical directories. However, the printed pharmaceutical guide (WPG) is inferior to the electronical one (EPG) in many points (table 1). Up-to-dateness is particularly important issue. Supplements to printed material do not seem able to confront this issue. Frequent republication may constitute an accepted solution, but unfortunately, it is not profitable for the limited Greek market and can not be realized. The superiority of the latter WPG is the obvious choice in the fields of the rapid information of discovery finding, of the ability to answer queries (compound questions) and special uses (automatic dosology conversions, prescription printings, product identification section via photographs, ability to keep prescription files). Probably the only disadvantage of the EPG is its handiness and its cost of use. But, if we take into consideration that the places where prescribing takes place allows for the installation of a computer, the constantly decreasing cost of purchase and the existence of portable computers, these drawbacks don't probably prove to be so important and, in any case, are surpassed by the numerous and serious advantages mentioned above.

Properties	EPG		WPG	
up-to-dateness	✓	high	✗	low
	✓	auto classification of drugs	✗	no such capability
	✓	informed by the user	✗	no such capability
fast info searching	✓	high speed	✗	low speed
simple questions & queries	✓	high performance	✗	low performance
easy to use	✗	average	✓	high
	✗	high cost	✓	low cost
special uses	✓	auto search of drug	✗	tables of info
	✓	auto dosage adaptation	✗	no such capability
	✓	auto printing	✗	no such capability

Table 1. Comparison between Electronic Prescription Guide (EPG) and Written Guide (WPG)

3. Prescription system structure

The drastic substance was chosen as the basis of the electronical prescription system since it constitutes the core of every single drug. Generally, the drastic substance is corresponded to the medicine by a multiple-to-multiple relation, as the same drastic substance may be found into numerous drugs, while, simultaneously, a drug may contain various drastic substances. Nevertheless, the former should be selected as a classification base since a drug containing numerous drastic substances simply possesses all its properties. On the contrary, the attempt to use the drug (trade name) as classification base would cause a lot of problems (data repetition without cause, inability to set questions, inability to update). According to the above, the EPS would be constituted by two related databases the drastic substance database and the drug database (figure 1).

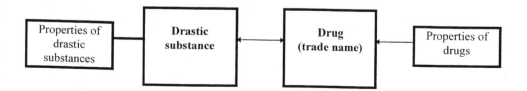

Figure 1. Relation between generic (drastic substance) and trade name (drug)

4. Drastic substance Database

The main database consists of the drastic substance and its main properties (table 2).

Properties of the drastic substance
classification
indication
contraindications - absolute
contraindications - relative
adverse effects
interactions
dose
special information

Table 2. Properties of the drastic substance

- classification: it has to do with a classification tree that ends to the drastic substance (gastrointestinal system medication --> ulcer - healing drug --> H2-receptor antagonist - -> ranitidine). The classification base is multiple: <gastrointestinal system> is an anatomical entity, <peptic ulcer> is a disease and <H2-antaginist> is a pharmacological category. As a matter of fact, it is a rather arbitrary admission (the only one that is embodied into the system) not only for the multiple classification base, but for some simplifications that it adopts, as well : ranitidine also has some more indications apart from peptic ulcer. However, it has been found that it has great practical importance, as it contributes significantly to the friendliness of the system.
- indications: it is about diseases, clinical situations or micro-organisms for which it has been found that the drastic substance helps effectively. The above entities are absolutely defined while the indications have been selected one by one by the Greek National Drug Organization (EOF).
- relative and absolute contra-indications: it is also about diseases or clinical situations where the substance is forbidden to be provided.
- adverse effects : it is about signs, symptoms, clinical entities and diseases that can be caused by the substance. They have all been thoroughly described or they are under intense investigation.
- interactions: it refers to the mechanism of action of a substance (increase or decrease of its efficacy) in the presence of another one.
- dosage : it refers to the quantity of the drastic substance that is recommended to be provided. This piece of information is multiple while the dose is altered according to the indication (we provide a peptic ulcer with a different dose rather than gastro-esophageal reflux), the form of the medicine (sirup, tablets, capsules, ointment) and, of course, the particulars of the case (child, elderly, cardiac, hepatic or renal failure, mild or severe disease, immunosupression). Along with the quantity of the provided drastic substance some more information is also given such as the route (PO, IM, IV), the number of repetitions during the day (three or four times a day) and the time which the drug is given (before or after meals).
- special information: it is about special information of three categories i) pharmacological (pharmacokinetics and pharmacodynamics of the drastic substance), ii) special clinical situations (G6PD - deficiency, pregnancy, lactation) and iii) legal information (characterization of a substance as a narcotic, which needs a special prescription sheet). The information mentioned in category (ii) are described in the

contra-indications, as well. Nevertheless, the frequency and importance of their presence demand special mention. The information in category (iii) constitute the only clues related to the drastic substance that do not remain constant from country to country.

5.   Drug Database

Each drug (trade name) is characterized by a series of main properties (table 3).

Properties of the drug
package
identification

Table 3. Properties of the drug (trade name)

- package: it is about a series of information such as the form of the medicine (tablet, capsule, sirup), the strength of the drastic substance (20 mg) and the number of units per package (20 tablets, 200 ml). It should be noted that a drastic substance can appear under the same name in various forms (150 mg tablets, 300 mg tablets, 300 mg vials).
- product identification: it is about a piece of optical and written information that depicts the package and its content (optical : an image of the package and an image of one tablet, written : small, oval, pink tablets with the inscription "Amoxil 250").

6.   System development

After the production of the two main system databases follows the production of the secondary databases that concern the properties of the generic name and the trade name (generally, 1 database for each property). Consequently, the main database consist of a key-field (ID), the generic or the trade name and a series of code-fields that correspond with the secondary databases. The latter ones, interpret these codes : the database of the adverse effects consists of the adverse effect name field, as well as, its code field that correspond with the field of the main database.

For the EPG development is needed, at first, the completion of the main database of the drastic substance along with its secondary databases. After this, the completion of the drug (trade name) database and its own relating database as long as the two main databases are related, corresponding each trade name to its generic name. Consequently, the trade name, apart from its own properties, inherits, automatically, all the properties of the generic name. If the product contains more of one pharmacological substances, it inherits the total of their properties.

A particular problem that arises due to this structure is the possibility that we desire the drug to inherit fewer properties than the summary of the properties of the pharmacological substance. When we introduce a corticosteroid into the EPG we render it the total of adverse effects and some indicative dosages. When, in a second phase, we introduce eye drops into the EPG, having this corticosteroid as a pharmacological substance, we do not desire it to inherit all its adverse effects, as some of them are impossible to appear using the ear drops. Even more, the doses of the corticosteroid for Addison disease are of no interest to us, except only the doses for allergic conjunctivitis.

This problem can be surmounted if we proceed to a division of the advance effect database into more specific databases that will be called in each situation.

7.   Conversation

The EPG, the theoretical structure of which was developed above, is believed to help effectively a great number of doctors as far as the field of right prescribing is concerned. The EPG will be able to reply to a number of simple questions, queries and orders. The most important of them are the following :
1. finding the prescription properties of a drug, when its trade name is known ("provide me with all the information concerning Zantac)
2. finding a medicine that has a particular clinical situation as indication ("find me a drug that helps with duodenal ulcer or a drug that can be applied to a Staph. aureus infection")
3. ability to trace a drug via the optical identification section ("is the presented white tablet a Zantac tablet ?")

Apart from these, the EPG answers to a great deal of other questions, as well (information about the drastic substance, information regarding the pharmaceutical company, ability to trace a drug by its adverse effects, presentation all of the products containing the same drastic substance). Certainly, the EPG presents all the abilities due to its electronical nature (automatic prescription printing, automatic dosage conversion, sound and optical warnings when a drug is being prescribed, keeping prescription files, presentation statistical data).

If EPG is associated with a computer network system that will connect all the medical offices of Greek providence, it will prove to be an invaluable aid for hundreds of junior doctors who are medically responsible for hundreds of thousands of people, mainly at rural areas. EPG will instantly help them to prescribe easily and fast, to discover the alternative drugs that the present clinical situation dictates, to save a great amount of time, which will be available for medical acts of greater importance and to be always informed about the constantly changing pharmaceutical market. The State will be also very content, as the proper use of drugs will minimize the cost of State Relief, and, also, the use of a computer network system will make the inspection of each doctor's prescription profile much more easier, as well.

Nevertheless, it must be noted that EPG doesn't substitute for the doctor. The doctor always has the final word on any diagnostic or therapeutic action. The EPG simply attempts to give him an effective tool that saves him time, financial means (while the justified use of drugs will minimize the prescribing cost), helps his memory and liberates him from treatment dilemmas ›.

References

1. Goulis DG, Tsimpiris N, Tsaligopoulos MG : Greek Prescription Guide : A computer-aided approach, Proceedings of the 3rd Hellenic Congress of Medical Informatics, Thessaloniki, 1994, p 57
2. Hellenic Drug Organization, unpublished data, Athens, 1995
3. Smith MC, Reynard AM : Information & Learning Resources in Pharmacology. In : Smith MC, Reynard AM : Textbook of Pharmacology, WB Saunders, 1992, 1166-1181
4. Hellenic Drug Organization : National Formulary, Athens, 1987
5. Physicians' Desk Reference, 49th ed., Medical Economics Company, New York, 1995
6. British National Formulary, No 29 (March 1995), British Medical Association & Royal Pharmaceutical Society of Great Britain, 1995

Medical Informatics Europe '97
C. Pappas et al. (Eds.)
IOS Press, 1997

Application of a Fuzzy Model of Making a Decision to Choose a Medicine in the Case of Symptoms Prevailing after the Treatment

Elisabeth RAKUS-ANDERSSON
Hogskolan i Karlskrona, S-37179 Karlskrona, Sweden

Tadeusz GERSTENKORN
Lódz University, Faculty of Mathematics, PL 90 - 238 Lódz

Abstract. Fuzzy set theory has introduced many auxiliary methods into medical problems.One of the attemps was the fixing of the optimal level of the drug action in the case when clinical symptoms retreat completely after the treatment [1,5]. In many morbid processes, however, there occurs problem of symptoms prevailing to some extent after the course of the medication process improving too high or too low indices of the measurable symptom. Different medicines applied have many a time an effect on the same symptoms and it is sometimes difficult to choose uniquely that theraputic remedy which brings the best results in the treatment of all the symptoms typical of the given diagnosis. A fuzzy model of decision making is to make it easier to choose a drug which acts optimally in the case of symptoms not retreating to the full after the treatment.

1. Presentation of the Problem

Assume that the patient's state S is described in the form of a fuzzy set

$$S = \mu_S(x_1)/x_1 + \mu_S(x_2)/x_2 + ... + \mu_S(x_m)/x_m$$

where $\{x_1, x_2,...,x_m\}$ is a set of symptoms belonging to X.

In order to watch the process of taking a decision in the case of problem of drugs presented above, we consider a set $A = \{ a_1, a_2,...,a_m \}$ of drugs which may be treated as decisions $a_1, a_2,...,a_m \in A$ with a view to have an effect on the symptoms representing certain states, characteristic of given morbid unit. Let us assume that each symptom $x_j \in X$ is understood as the result of the treatment of this symptom after the cure with the drugs $a_i \in A$, $i = 1, 2, ...,n$ has been carried out. On the basis of earlier experiments, the physician knows how to define in words the effectiveness of the cure of these symptoms, which we shall describe in terms of the linguistic variable "the effectiveness of the cure of symptom" -- { none, almost none, very little, little, medium, large, very large, almost complete, complete }. Each notion from the list of terms of the linguistic variable is the name of a fuzzy variable. Assume that all the fuzzy variables are defined on the space $Z = [0,1]$ where the intervals of Z essential to these variables can be presented in a table.

Let us define a utility function U as a function $U : A \rightarrow [0, 1]$ such that "a_i is preferred to a_j, $i, j = 1, 2, ..., n$, if and only if $U(a_i) > U(a_j)$". The values of the utility function U are equal to the midpoints of the presented intervals, representing the verbal definitions. If we take a decision $a_i \in A$, $i = 1, 2, ...,n$, concerning states (results) $x_j \in X$,

$j = 1, 2, ..., m,$ then the problem is reduced to the consideration of the triplet (X, A, U). The utility matrix $U = X \times A$ expresses a relationship between the drug (decision) a_i and the effectiveness of the retreat of the symptom x_j. In the matrix U each element u_{ij}, $i = 1, 2, ..., n, j = 1, 2, ..., m,$ is a value of the utility function, defining the utility following from the decision a_i with the result x_j.

The utility of matrix U is built by the physician basing himself on his experience. The matrix U can take, for instance, such a hypothetical form:

$$U = \begin{bmatrix} \text{medium} & \text{very large} & \text{medium} & \text{large} & \text{large} & \text{medium} \\ \text{medium} & \text{very large} & \text{large} & \text{large} & \text{almost complete} & \text{medium} \\ \text{large} & \text{complete} & \text{large} & \text{large} & \text{almost complete} & \text{large} \end{bmatrix}$$

After substituting the numerical representatives, one can write the matrix U down as

$$U = \begin{bmatrix} 0.5 & 0.85 & 0.5 & 0.7 & 0.7 & 0.5 \\ 0.5 & 0.85 & 0.7 & 0.7 & 0.95 & 0.5 \\ 0.7 & 1.0 & 0.7 & 0.7 & 0.95 & 0.7 \end{bmatrix}$$

The fuzzy utility [2,3] for each decision (drug) a_i, $i = 1, 2, ..., n,$ with the patient's fuzzy state $S \in X$ characterized by means of the membership function $\mu_S(x)$ is defined to be the fuzzy set

$$U_i = \mu_S(x_1) / u_{i1} + \mu_S(x_2) / u_{i2} + ... + \mu_S(x_m) / u_{im}, \quad i = 1, 2, ..., n.$$

2. Solution of the Problem

The problem of choosing an optimal decision is solved as follows [2,3]:

1) We form a non-fuzzy set Y which is the sum of the supports of the sets $U_1, ..., U_n$.

2) We choose the maximal element of the set Y.

3) We define the fuzzy sets U_i':

$$U_i' = \mu_{Ui'}(u_{i1}) / u_{i1} + \mu_{Ui'}(u_{i2}) / u_{i2} + ... + \mu_{Ui'}(u_{im}) / u_{im}$$

in which $\mu_{Ui'}(u_{ij}) = u_{ij} / u_{max}$, $i = 1, 2, ..., n;$ $j = 1, 2, ..., m.$

4) The next introduced fuzzy set has the form:

$$U_{i0} = \mu_{Ui0}(u_{i1}) / u_{i1} + \mu_{Ui0}(u_{i2}) / u_{i2} + ... + \mu_{Ui0}(u_{im}) / u_{im}$$

where $i = 1, 2, ..., n,$ and membership degree $\mu_{Ui0}(u_{ij})$ is calculated according to the formula

$$\mu_{Ui0}(u_{ij}) = \min (\mu_{Ui}(u_{ij}), \ \mu_{Ui'}(u_{ij}))$$

5) The fuzzy set $A*$ with the elements $a_1, a_2,...,a_n$ of the supports is assumed to be

$$A* = \mu_{A*}(a_1)/a_1 + \mu_{A*}(a_2)/a_2 + ... + \mu_{A*}(a_n)/a_n$$

where $\mu_{A*}(a_i) = \max(\mu_{U_{i0}}(u_{ij}))$, $i = 1, 2, ..., n$, $j = 1, 2, ..., m$.

Now taking maximum in the set $A*$, we ascertain the optimal decision and, consequently, the application of the determined drug should yield the best effects in the process of the retreating of the symptoms.

References

1. T.Gerstenkorn, E.Rakus, *A method of applications of fuzzy set theory to differentiating the effectiveness of drugs in treatment of inflammation of genital organs*, Fuzzy Sets and Systems 68 (1994), 327-333.
2. R.Jain, *Decision-making in the presence of fuzzy variables*, IEEE Trans.Syst. Man and Cybern. SMC-6 (1976), 698-703.
3. R.Jain, *A procedure for multi-aspect decision-making using fuzzy sets*, Int.J.Syst.Sci.6 (1977), 1-7.
4. E.Rakus, *The application of fuzzy set theory to medical diagnosis and appreciation of drugs (in Polish)*, Doctor's thesis, Medical University, *Lodz*, 1991.

Medical Informatics Europe '97
C. Pappas et al. (Eds.)
IOS Press, 1997

A cooperative methodology to build conceptual models in medicine

Elena Galeazzi, Angelo Rossi Mori, Fabrizio Consorti, Anna Errera, Paolo Merialdo

Dottorato in Informatica Medica, Università La Sapienza, Roma
Reparto Informatica Medica, ITBM-CNR, Roma
IV Clinica Chirurgica, Università La Sapienza, Roma

Abstract. We designed a methodology to perform distribute activities on conceptual modelling among cooperating centers. Our methodology assigns responsibilities and tasks and regulates interactions preserving coherence; it passes through the construction of unambiguous paraphrases to make explicit the context within the original sources, and through their compositional representation in an intermediate language. The process is intrinsically iterative, with continuous feedbacks and refinements, alternating analytic view on details and synthetic view on regularities and structures. Our methodology is based on requirements and experience made in the first GALEN project, and was applied in the GALEN-IN-USE project to coordinate modelling activities of three teams of surgeons in Rome with activities of other partners, during the production of an extensive model of surgical procedures.

1. Introduction

Terminological systems used in healthcare include thesauri, nomenclatures, classifications, local controlled vocabularies, formal models [Rossi Mori 1993]. Diffusion of clinical information systems is shifting application of terminological systems to routine management of patient record with multiple re-uses including health care organization, evaluation and planning [Nowlan 1994; Rector 1995; Rossi Mori 1995]. Advanced methods, as *formal models*, are therefore required, providing adequate representation of terminological phrases within computer systems [Rector 1994, Galeazzi 1996].

The stream of UE-funded projects evolving from *GALEN* (1992-1995) to *GALEN-IN-USE* (1996-1998) is creating an environment for the development of methodologies, skills, formalisms, software and awareness about conceptual modelling in healthcare.

Bulding large concept models is an ambitious and expensive task: effort cannot be afforded by a single institution; it requires a large amount of experts in various domains — trained in compositional modelling and in the usage of the GRAIL language, ie. the formalism used in GALEN — both to build the model and to validate it. Decentralization of modelling activities is mandatory, and the issues on coherence, uniformity and integrability of the various contributions are crucial. The cooperative development of a model implies frequent revisions and reconciliations towards a *common modelling style*, with explicit decisions that affect the previous work of each center. The process *must be iterative*, with different layers of agreements, from general to specific; the work on more specific items will refine the working agreements among the centers at the more generic layers. Moreover, it would be hard to integrate cooperative efforts without a *unique conceptual framework, ontologically based*.

Cooperative modelling should be therefore supported by a *methodology* to extract and represent knowledge in an uniform way, based on

- early discovery of potential sources for conflicts among modellers, by focusing on anticipated issues and early reconciliation;

- minimal interaction among cooperating experts (ie. maximal autonomy), preventing incoherence by adequate structured discussions based on precise intermediate documentation and by a consolidated set of rules and guidelines on a common modelling style.

We describe in this paper the methodology we worked out for the GALEN-IN-USE project; it was tested during 1996 in a cooperative effort by 4 "domain centers" in Europe (Italy — with 3 specialist teams —, Nederland, France, Sweden) interacting with a "GRAIL center" in Manchester, on more than 1000 phrases about surgical procedures. The final goal of the project is to demonstrate the feasibility of distributed modelling for a European nomenclature.

2. Working out a methodology for cooperative modelling

First in §2.1 we identify the kinds of skills of the various people involved in the analysis; then we outline in §2.2 the basic process of modelling an individual concept, from the expression in the original corpus to the canonical form in the GRAIL model. Finally, in §2.3 we describe the kind of activities to be perfomed in an iterative distributed process.

2.1. Define roles to assure effectiveness and quality

The first step was to identify the roles of the people that should interact; these roles correspond to skills that could be provided by one or more people; a person could have skills to perform different roles. We considered four different roles:
- the *specialists on the domain* that have to interpret the corpora and gradually produce a structured representation of the rubrics;
- the *experts on terminologies and classifications* that have to organize, revise and homogenize the efforts of the specialists;
- the *GRAIL modellers* that produced or will produce the formal model (e.g. GRAIL model);
- the *coordinator* in each center.

We defined their responsibilities in a set of inter-related activities, and an iterative process of development, with products that they have to produce and gradually refine.

2.2. The basic process on individual rubrics

The modelling process should bring developers from a set of terminological phrases selected from an existing corpus to a set of representations of the related concepts into the formal model of GALEN, according to the GRAIL formalism used in the project (fig.1).

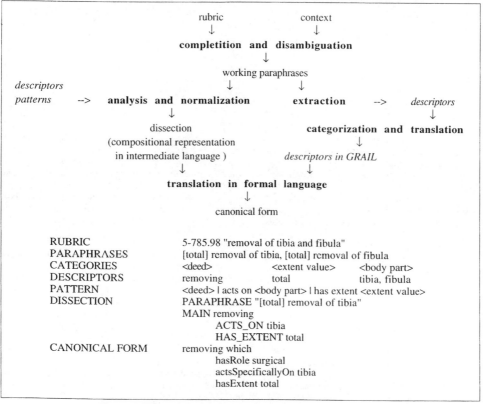

Figure 1. The modelling process and its application to an example
(items in italics are re-usable for other corpora)

2.3. Detailed description of the cooperative process

The basic process regarding an individual entry (Figure 1) implies three major activities :

- construction of unambiguous and explicit paraphrases that grasp hidden meanings and the context of the entry in the original corpus,
- their compositional representation in an intermediate language, and
- a semiautomatic translation into the GRAIL formalism.

In parallel, we extract and translate the atomic concepts needed in the compositional representation, ie. the building blocks (called "descriptors").

A preparatory phase of selection of sources — and of phrases within the sources — is also needed, with mutual awareness of the decisions among the cooperating centers.

In consequence, our methodology distinguishes five kinds of activities embedded in an iterative process; they can be schematized as in table 1.

Table 1. Description of activities in the iterative process of cooperative modelling

---

Activity 1. Prepare the subset of expressions to be analyzed

Each center specifies a corpus (one or more terminological systems) or collects a set of terminological phrases from patient files, textbooks, available paper forms or input layouts [Galeazzi 1994]. The domain specialist and the expert on terminological systems organize the corpus in "waves" (ie. they select a narrow subset of terminological phrases and harmonize them, by adding current phrases or removing too detailed or obsolete phrases). The results should be harmonized across centers.

Activity 2. Prepare working paraphrases

Each original terminological phrases in the wave should be checked for ambiguities, implicit information, errors, contextual information. From a rubric the expert can produce one or more "*paraphrases*", according to

- his/her interpretation of the meaning of the expression,
- the additional knowledge provided by the terminological system on that rubric, and
- the context of the rubric within the terminological system.

Paraphrases serve as reference for further modelling and do not replace rubrics in original sources. Each domain specialist should figure out — with the assistance of the expert — possible criteria to organize paraphrases of the current wave into medically meaningful clusters; each cluster suggests a concept ("*node label*" in the vocabulary of ISO TC46) that should be superordinate to all the elements of the cluster.

Activity 3. Extract candidate descriptors

Descriptors (activity 3) and dissections (activity 4) are strongly related. Within each working paraphrases, the domain specialist should separate the most general superordinate concept from differentiating characteristics that can be systematically expressed. Each superordinate concept is a candidate base concept (in our example, the descriptor "removing"). Each differentiating characteristic produces candidates for semantic links and associated concepts (in the example, the string "of tibia" produces the link "ACTS_ON" and the concept "tibia"). Descriptors belong to "*categories*" (eg. "removing" belongs to the category <deed>, tibia and fibula belong to <body part>). The domain specialist should systematize each descriptor under its own semantic category. The GRAIL expert should translate the set of descriptors using the GRAIL formalism.

Activity 4. Systematic production and harmonization of dissections

Starting from the paraphrase, the domain specialist uses (agreed) patterns and descriptors to dissect each paraphrase and to obtain an intermediate representation. The semi-formal representation in the intermediate language is called "*dissection*". A dissection is a semantic network made of a set of descriptors (eg. removing, tibia, fibula, total) related by means of semantic links (eg. ACTS_ON, HAS_EXTENT). Using the node labels (activity 2) domain specialists should verify that phrases within each cluster have similar dissections and harmonize the dissections in the whole wave. Local criteria for harmonization should be integrated into a common set of criteria across centers.

Activity 5. From dissections to canonical forms

The GRAIL expert translates the patterns into grammar-level statements in GRAIL; then, using the GRAIL descriptors already in the model (activity 3) he/she translates dissections into canonical forms. The feedback from this translation will assist not only in the discovering of errors and inconsistencies, but also in further harmonization among the representations of similar phrases (to increase the uniformity of style and to revise the common guidelines).

---

3. Discussion

The 'ideal' methodology should avoid as much re-modelling as possible by a preventive exercise (with timely reconciliations on problems), ie. it should:
- facilitate since the beginning interaction among teams working at different extensions;
- bridge between specialists and modellers.
- foster awareness and coherence in the modelling process.

To facilitate integration, the extensions produced by the individual teams have to use an explicit similar set of rules and the same "style", fully compatible with the ones already embedded in the model and compatible among them. These rules are partially enforced by the supporting software that is being developed by partners of the GALEN-IN-USE project, namely by the University of Nijmegen, the University of Manchester and CNR.

3.1. Requirements for a cooperative methodology

After our experience of direct GRAIL modelling in the first GALEN Project, it was clear that:
- the modelling effort requires a large amount of resources and different skills; therefore it had to be distributed among an adequate number of domain expert and terminological experts, and adequately coordinated;
- the GRAIL language has peculiar difficulties for "normal" physicians and cannot be used as the current formalism for distribute effort of analysis of expressions; therefore most of the experts should be enabled to focus on the issues of compositional modelling, independently from the additional difficulties of GRAIL modelling;
- the different subdomains are not homogeneous and the level of details that could be represented about each concept depends too much on the modelling style of the expert; therefore modelling activities in a field should be based on existing systematic corpora (in our case, mainly terminological systems on surgical procedures) and experts should use them to decide how many concepts they have to model, and how many details they have to represent about each concept;
- even if available corpora are systematic with respect to their needs, conceptual modelling requires a further systematization to obtain a set of phrase with homogeneous number of explicit details;
- issues and problems raised by the experimental work tend to increase to unmanageable levels, because discussions tend to diverge on too many subtopics, and the amount of resources allocated to discussions must be balanced with the amount of resources to populated the model; therefore interaction among experts should be focussed on really crucial issues, and experts have to be aware of which decisions can be taken locally and which ones are for a common debate and consensus.

Our methodology was designed in order to provide an answer to these requirements.

3.2. Separate semantic issues from GALEN-specific implementation

Our methodology is based on the idea of an "intermediate representation" of rubrics of terminological systems by descriptors, initially developed and refined by two of the Authors (EG, ARM) during the first GALEN project. This attitude is intended to:
- involve as much as possible of specialists in the first phases of analysis;
- separate "what has to be there" from "how to express it in GRAIL".

The goal is to separate what is related to *any compositional representation* (eg. according to the CEN approach [Rossi Mori, 1997]) from the peculiarities of the GRAIL formalism.

This attitude is motivated by cultural, organizational and practical reasons:
- decisions are taken in the most appropriate context;
- more domain specialists can be involved, not exposed to GRAIL;
- it allows to exchange experience and data with other "non-GALEN" initiatives;
- it allows to re-translate the intermediate representations according to different releases of the formalism and the model.

The intermediate representation is also more "tolerant" about initial contradictions and irregularities, and can be used in preliminary phases of structuring and refining a raw model.

4 . Conclusions

Advanced terminological systems are urgently needed. Conceptual modelling will be a bottleneck for the diffusion of clinical information systems in healthcare.

A methodology to assign responsibilities and tasks and to regulate interactions preserving coherence is a prerequisite to distribute modelling activities among cooperating centers.

Our methodology exploits 5 different constructs:

1. paraphrases   to decouple terminological systems with their context from the subsequent work on modelling;

2. descriptors   to detect issues of potential conflicts among centers;

                  to prepare the translation into the formal model and to provide an early feedback to experts and domain specialists;

3. patterns   to facilitate uniformity of style among centers and to prepare the grammar-level statements in the formal model;

4. dissections   to manage a semi-formal intermediate representation, as a bridge between specialists and GRAIL modellers;

5. node labels   to refine the previous analytical work by comparative views, thus facilitating comparison of potentially similar dissections and the extraction of patterns.

Our methodology was applied successfully to coordinate the modelling activities of three teams of surgeons in Rome with activities of other partners in the GALEN-IN-USE project.

Acknowledgements.
Work partially supported by contract HC1018 "GALEN-IN-USE" from European Union.

5 . References

Galeazzi 1994   Galeazzi E, Agnello P, Gangemi A (et al). What is a medical term ? Terms and phrases in controlled vocabularies and continuous discourses. In: Barahona P, Veloso M, Bryant J (eds): Proceedings of the 12th Congress of the European Federation for Medical Informatics, Lisbon, 1994, 234-9

Galeazzi 1996   Galeazzi E, Rossi Mori A. I servizi terminologici come elemento cruciale dei servizi informativi sanitari nell'era telematica. In "AIIM 96", Atti del IX Congresso Nazionale di Informatica Medica, Venezia ottobre 1996.

GALEN doc.   GALEN documentation, available from the main contractor AL Rector, Medical Informatics Group, Dept. Computer Science, Univ. Manchester, Manchester M13 9 PL, UK (e-mail galen@cs.ac.man.uk; URL=http://www.cs.man.ac.uk/mig/galen)

Nowlan 1994   Nowlan W, Rector A, Rush T, Solomon W. From Terminology to Terminology Services. 18th Annual Symposium on Computer Applications in Medical Care (SCAMC94). Washington DC, 1994: 150-4.

Rector 1994   Rector A. Compositional models of medical concepts: towards re-usable application-independent medical terminologies. In: Barahona P, Christensen JP eds. *Knowledge and Decision in Health Telematics.* Amsterdam: IOS Press, 1994; 109-14

Rector 1995   Rector A, Glowinski A, Nowlan W, Rossi-Mori A. Medical concept models and medical records: An approach based on GALEN and PEN&PAD. Journal of the American Medical Informatics Association 1995;2(1):19- 35.

Rossi Mori 1993   Rossi Mori A, Gangemi A, Galanti M. The coding cage. In: ReichertA, Sadan BA, Bengtsson S, Bryant J, Piccolo U eds. MIE 93 London: Freund Publishing House, 1993, pp 466-72

Rossi Mori 1995   Rossi Mori A. Coding systems and controlled vocabularies for hospital information systems. *Int J Biom Comp* 39 (1995) 93-8

Rossi Mori 1997   Rossi Mori A, Consorti F, Galeazzi E. Standards to support development of terminological services for healthcare telematics. to be presented at the Working Conference of IMIA WG6, Jacksonville, FL, January 19-22, 1997

Medical Informatics Europe '97
C. Pappas et al. (Eds.)
IOS Press, 1997

285

A Consultation System Integrating Chinese Medical Practice in Herbaltherapy, Acupuncture and Acupressure

Adina Raclariu[1], Simona Alecu[1], Maria Loghin[1], Lavinia Serbu[2]

[1] *Software ITC SA, 167 Calea Floreasca, 72321 Bucharest, Romania*
[2] *Institute for Postgraduate Studies in Medicine and Pharmacy, Bucharest, Romania*

Abstract The paper presents an informatic system offering the acupuncturist, herbalist and acupressurist a rich source of clinical information. It adapts the theory of Chinese Medicine to Western medical practice and is solidly based on the ancient Chinese classics.

The system provides an orientative diagnosis starting from the clinical picture of the patient consisting in syndrome differentiation. Based on the *Yin-Yang* and *5 Elements* theory the remedy associated with the energetic imbalance is determinated. Then the tastes, nature and tropism implied by the principle of treatment are used to prescribe the herbal treatment. The treatment variants through acupuncture and acupressure are also indicated. The system is also useful in teaching Chinese Medicine.

Introduction

Chinese medicine modalities play a larger role in the self-health care of citizens than previously understood. Despite the broad use of alternative medicine treatments, there is a paucity of data available to demonstrate convincingly whether these practices are efficacious, safe and beneficial, lead to positive clinical outcomes, improve the quality of life, reduce or eliminate adverse symptoms, prevent disease or enhance health. New findings in alternative and complementary medical research challenge conventional knowledge and reconnect us with the wisdom of our ancient heritage.

The central aim of our research is the design and implementation of a consultation system in Chinese Traditional Medicine. The main objectives pursued have been:

1. the choice of the quintessential trait of Chinese Medicine in diagnosis and therapy;
2. the use of the abundant resources of flora in the world;
3. the use of the information in the data bases for medical training.

Diagnosis assistance

Chinese diagnosis is intimately related to Pattern Identification as it provides the diagnostic tools necessary to identify the patterns. The correlation between outward signs and internal organs is summarized in the expression: "Inspect the exterior to examine the interior". The second fundamental principle of Chinese diagnosis is that "a part reflects the whole". Chinese pulse[1] or tongue[2] diagnosis are striking examples of this. Chinese diagnosis includes four methods traditionally described in four words: looking, smelling, asking and feeling. The symptoms are split in to 32 groups that include observation of elements such as: spirit, body, demeanor, head and face, eyes, nose, ears, mouth, teeth-gums, throat, limbs, skin, tongue, pulse, sweating, stools and urine, sleep, pain etc. Each group is assigned a weight. The main symptom groups are those referring to pulse and tongue, which for this reason are assigned the largest weights. The algorithm counts for each syndrome and each symptom group of the syndrome the proportion of symptoms found in the patient and uses these figures and the group weights to calculate the score of the syndrome.

The *diagnosis* algorithm allows the calculation of a score for each of the 170 syndromes among which the system seeks to differentiate. A list of syndromes is constructed in decreasing order of the scores thus calculated. The top of the list displays the most likely syndromes for the patient examined (Figure 1).

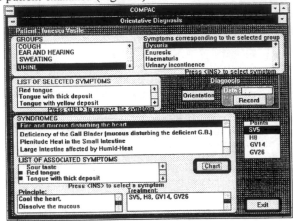

Figure 1 Diagnosis assistance

Determination of the energetic imbalance of the patient, used for syndrome differentiation, allows the indication of different variants of *treatment* based on: Herbaltherapy, Acupuncture and Acupressure.

Herbaltherapy

The Five Elements Law

Herbaltherapy is a vast subject in Chinese Medicine and it is based on the *5-Element model*.

Together with the theory of Yin-Yang, the theory of the 5 Elements constitutes the basis of Chinese medical theory. Chinese Medicine observes Nature and, with a combination of the inductive and deductive method, sets out to find patterns within it and, by extension, apply these in the interpretation of disease.

Each herb has a certain taste which is related to one of the Elements and other correlation and features of it can be established, as are illustrated in Figure 2. The five tastes are: sour for *Wood*, bitter for *Fire*, sweet for *Earth*, pungent for *Metal*, salty for *Water* [3]. Thus, if an organ is diseased one should avoid the taste related to the Element that controls that organ. Because the herbs have a more definite and somewhat less "neutral" effect than acupuncture the possibility of ill effect arising from a wrong treatment is greater. Thus it is essential to distinguish between the nature of the herbs, which can be: hot, cold, lukewarm, cool, neutral.

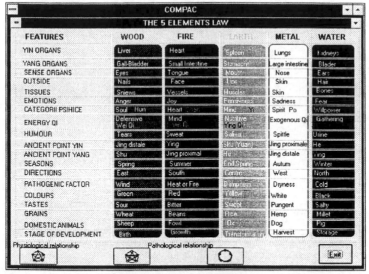

Figure 2 The 5 Elements Law

Beside the place of action of the herb, named also tropism and represented by the channels affected, taste and nature determine the herb which can be used for a syndrome [4].

Remedy determination

Based on the treatment principle, associated with the determined syndrome, a phytotherapeutical remedy is indicated, and also a subremedy in certain cases.

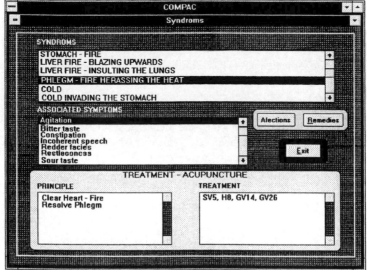

Figure 3 Integration of the three methods of treatment

Each remedy has associated tastes, natures and tropism. Tastes has a certain effect on the body: the *sour* taste generates fluids and Yin (it is astringent and can control perspiration and diarrhorea), the *bitter* taste clears Heat, sedates and hardens (it clears Damp-Heat and it subdues rebellious Qi), the *sweet* taste tonifies, balances and moderates (it is used to tonify deficiency and to stop pain), the *pungent* taste scatters (it is used to expel pathogenic factors), the *salty* taste flows downwards, softens hardness (it is used to treat constipation and swelling).

After the interpretation of the treatment principle for the syndrome (Figure 3) and of the features already discussed for remedies, the useful herbs are indicated [5].

The system includes the European medicinal plants (equivalent to Chinese plants), classified on the basis of traditional Chinese principles. The integration of herbaltherapy implies the correlation of medicinal herbs, used in treatment, with syndrome differentiation, based on taste, nature and tropism (Figure 4).

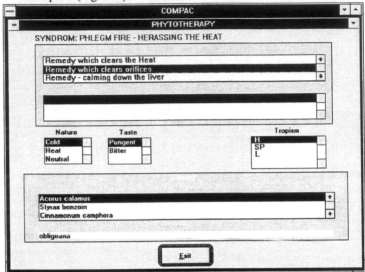

Figure 4 Herbaltherapy

Acupressure

Acupressure is a simple technique, which can be applied in self-therapy, following the same rules that were described thousands of years ago for acupuncture. Acupressure is similar to acupuncture, the only difference being that the fingertip is used instead of needles [6]. Based on the same syndrome differentiation, pushing the button "Affections", causes the system to display the allopathic affections, implied by the identified syndrome and information referring to the points indicated for the treatment, supplemented with further information that must be taken into account in the case of the given treatment.

Acupuncture

The establishment of the diagnosis is followed by the indication of the point formula and therapeutic principle [7].

The traditional Chinese chronoacupuncture methods Tzu Wu Liu Chu Liao Fa and Ling Kwei Ba Fa [8] can also be used in the establishment of the point formulae, allowing optimization depending on the opening times.

Based on one of the most important principles of acupuncture, that of considering the patient as a whole, the treatment can also be established using microsystems [9]:

- reflexology - the plantar reflexogen areas and the reflexogen areas of the upper and lower limbs, and the organs corresponding to them, are displayed;
- auricular therapy - the treatment of diseases by the stimulation with needles of points located on the ear.

Training

The system can also be used for *training*. It provides detailed information about: channels, points, "The 5 Elements Law" [10], syndromes associated symptoms and the recommended remedy, pulsology (following BOSSY and BORSARELLO), tongue examination, remedies and the associated plants .

Implementation

The system has been developed in FoxPro for WINDOWS and C++. The system is used by means of menus, being easily operable, and a powerful help facility is provided. The system has been installed and is being tested at the Institute for Postgraduate Studies in Medicine and Pharmacy and in other clinics in Romania. The performance has been assessed by analyzing how often the diagnosis module generated diagnoses identical to the opinion of the clinicians.

Conclusions

Non-drug therapy becomes more important with the accumulation of evidence of toxic and other side effects of drugs. In this context, herbaltherapy, acupuncture and acupressure begins to receive growing attention, since they have efficient and harmless results.
The system offers the advantage of providing a lot of information in a short time, contributing to the diagnosis and therapy in this domain. Also, the system can be used as a tool for medical training.

References

[1]. J.Borsarello, Pulsologie en medicine chinoise, Paris, 1981.

[2]. Y.Requena, Acupuncture et Psychologie - Pour une approche nouvelle de la psycho-somatique, Maloine, Paris, 1982

[3]. Z.Jinhuang, L.Ganzhong, Recent advances in Chinese herbal drugs - actions and uses, Science Press, Beijing, 1991.

[4]. Dr. G. Guillaume, Dr. Mach-Chien, Pharmacopee et Medicine Traditionelle Chinoise, Edition "Aubard", 1987.

[5]. Yves Requena, Acupuncture et Phytotherapie, Maloine Editeur, Paris, 1983.

[6]. S.Ivan, Presopunctura, Bucuresti, 1992

[7]. *** Essentials of Chinese Acupuncture. Foreign Languages Press, Beijing, 1980.

[8]. H.Lu, The time-honored Chinese techniques of acupuncture, Acad.Orient.Herit., Vancouver , 1978.

[9]. L.Tureanu, V.Tureanu, Microsisteme, timpi optimi si puncte extrameridian in acupunctura, Ed. All, Bucuresti, 1994.

[10]. Giovanni Maciocia, The Foundations of Chinese Medicine, Longman Singapore Publishers Ltd. , 1990.

Medical Informatics Europe '97
C. Pappas et al. (Eds.)
IOS Press, 1997

A study of Dermatoglyphics in Gonadal Dysgenesis: a computerised analysis applicable in under-developed countries

Professor Bernard Richards, Medical Informaticist, Manchester, England
Dr Silvia Mandasescu, Consultant Endocrinologist, Roman Hospital, Romania

Abstract. Dermatoglyphics, the study of finger-tip and palmar prints, can play an important role in suggesting or confirming the diagnosis in the case of certain congenital syndromes. The paper discusses the prints in the cases of two important syndromes viz Turner's and Klinefelter's, and shows how to differentiate between the two.

1. Introduction

Some work has been done in the past in using computers as an aid in Dermatoglyphics. One aspect that is new in this paper is that the computer has been used to house a database on young people which has enabled some interesting results to be obtained for two Syndromes, Turner's Syndrome (first reported in 1938) and Klinefelter's Syndrome (first reported in 1942), results which are very new. Previous work has been concerned with examining the Dermatoglyphics of patients with Klinefelter's Syndrome [1] and with Turner's Syndrome [2]. What is new in the work described below is that our cohort contains both these types of patients allowing cross-comparisons.

The earliest work on Dermatoglyphics was done by Purkinje[3] in 1823. It has been known for many years that the Dermal Ridges (the lines and ridges on the palms of the hand, and on the feet and on the fingers), begin to form between the thirteenth and nineteenth week of foetal gestation [4]. The study of the development of such patterns and their association with subsequent conditions in later life is termed "Dermatoglyphics".

The dermal ridge patterning thereby provides an indelible historical record that indicates the form of the early foetal hand (or foot) [5].

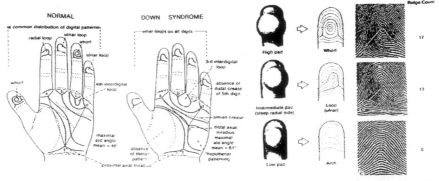

Figure 1. Palmar Prints, Normal, and DOWN   Figure 2. Foetal prints at 18 weeks

Mild to severe alterations in hand morphology occur in a variety of syndromes. Whilst not conclusive evidence in themselves, these patterns enhance the clinicians' ability to arrive at a specific overall diagnosis of a congenital syndrome [6].

There are two general categories of dermatoglyphic alterations, viz. an aberrant pattern, and an unusual frequency of ridges and/or a distribution of a particular pattern on the finger-tips. A good example of such abnormalities occurs in Down Syndrome, a Syndrome caused by an additional chromosome number 21., otherwise known as Trisomy 21 Syndrome. Figure 1 shows a normal palm and that of a Down Syndrome palm.

Figure 2 shows the development of foetal fingertip pads at 16 to 19 weeks and the resulting fingertip dermal ridge patterns. The "ridge count" is obtained as the number of ridges between the centre of a pattern and the more distant tri-radius. (The upper print has two such tri-radii: the count to the more distal one is 17).

The significant patterns are those identified as (I) Open areas; (ii) Arches; (iii) Loops, open towards the thumb being radial, those away from the thumb being ulner (See Fig 1); and (iv) whorls. There are six zones of patterning, viz the hypothenar (distal to the thumb, (see Figure) the Thenar (nearest the thumb), and the four interdigital areas. There are also four tri-radii situated at the base of the fingers (see Figure) identified by the letters a, b, c, d. Finally there is a major tri-radius located near the wrist, this is denoted by t (See Figure): there may be a secondary tri-radii nearer the fingers denoted by t^1, noticeably in the Down Syndrome (See Figure).

The other important parameter is the atd angle. Its value depends on the position of t and is normally about 48°.

Finally, the sum of the ridge counts on all ten fingers is denoted by TRC. (Total Ridge Counts).

2. The Genetic Significance of Dermatoglyphics

Researchers carried out by various experts e.g. Holt (1961) lead to the conclusion that one's dermatoglyphics are an essential part of one's constitution and are an important genetic characteristic. An identical configuration is never passed on from the parents but only a tendency to inherit some of the characteristics. These characteristics are influenced in part by the genes in the parents; each parent being homozygous (same) or heterozygous (different) in the various genes. However during foetal development, these dermatoglyphic structures can be modified. The most serious dermatoglyphogencsis occurs in the compartments of the thumb, next in order of seriousness come the irregular patterns in the third finger and the little finger (fourth finger), then the middle finger (2nd) and lastly the forefinger (1st).

Syndromes in which abnormal patterns are very characteristic include Down Syndrome, Turner's Syndrome (females) and Klinefelter's Syndrome (males). One might notice in passing that these syndromes are all characterised by missing or additional chromosomes, viz. Down Syndrome (an additional number 21 chromosome), Turner's Syndrome (XO, i.e. a missing Y chromosome) and Klinefelter's Syndrome (XXY, an additional, female, X chromosome)

3. The Methodology of this Study

Dermatoglyphic studies were carried out between 1985 and 1986 on subjects having Turner (six female cases) and Klinefelter (four male cases) Syndromes, in comparison with a control group of 100 unrelated individuals (namely 50 girls and 50 boys), those latter being between the ages of 12 and 14 years in good health and randomly selected.

A dermatoglyphic record was made for each patient including digital and palmar prints, diagnosis, and other clinical parameters of each patient.
The following dermatoglyphic characteristics were recorded.

1. The frequency of lacy form fields
2. The inter-digital prints
3. The terminations of the main lines (the palmar type)
4. The Thenar and Hyperthenar palmar prints
5. For digital prints, the total number of crests (TRC)
6. The number of digital crests (RC)
7. The A-D Index (ADI)
8. The number of palmar tri-radii
9. The position of the palmar t point (see Fig 1)
10. The size of the atd angle (see Fig 1)
11. The dat angle
12. The number of palmar crests Rcab, Rcbc, Rccd
13. The distance between the palmar tri-radii, ab, bc

For each palm, 30 items of data were recorded; hence each person had 60 items in total
These were recorded in the database. Of the above 13 characteristics, items 1 to 5 inclusive were allocated a code, whilst items 6 to 13 were accorded a numerical value.

4. Results

	Girls		Boys		Turners		Klinefelters	
	Left	Right	Left	Right	Left	Right	Left	Right
A								
T								
L^U	100%	66%	100%	67%	50%	50%	34%	50%
L^R								
W^d		17%			34%	34%	16%	16%
W^s				33%	16%	16%	34%	16%
W^c		17%					16%	16%
W								
Totals	100%	100%	100%	100%	100&	100%	100%	100%

Table 1: The distribution of print types for Finger 1 of each hand
(In the Table, all figures are percentages. The actual numbers involved are 50 girls, 50 boys, Turner Syndrome 6 cases, Klinefelter Syndrome 4 cases).

Many interesting results were obtained. Space prevents a full and demonstrative discussion of these. However two results can be shown here. Table 1 below shows the distribution of the digital prints for Finger 1. Similar results have been produced for the other fingers. This Table shows the significant differences between the two abnormalities and the prints of the normal cohort. The other figures are similar. (In the Table, A represents Arches; T. the tri-radius; Lo and LR Ulnar Loops and Radial Loops; Wd, W 5, wc are Whorls, double, singular, and circular; and W is a normal whorl). The absence of Ulnar Loops in the left hand of a patient clearly indicating an abnormality. The full set of results for all five fingers of both hands, when taken together, clearly provide evidence suggestive of an abnormality. Using "Palmar types" (results not shown here) will distinguish between Turners and Klinefelters.

5. Conclusion

The following important conclusions are to be noted.

1.   Diseases with genetic predispositions are accompanied by mutations in the papillary prints which remain unchanged during the person's life. Hence the study of dermatoglyphics will be a meaningful aid in congenital diagnosis. It does not replace other methods but helps to establish the diagnosis.

2.   Examination of a patient's hand and foot prints does not require special apparatus nor expensive reagents: paper and ink will suffice and these latter can be used outside the hospital, even on domicilliary visits. Hence as a diagnostic aid, these results are more economical, in monetary terms, then chromosomal analysis. This aspect is of great importance in the poorer countries.

3.   The main types of syndromes in which dermatoglyphics can play a part are:

(i)   the chromosomic syndromes, eg Down (Trisomy 21), Edwards Trisomy 18), Patau (Trisomy 13), Cri-du-Chat (deletion on Chromosome 5), Turner, and Klinefelter;

(ii)   the genetically determined syndromes, e.g. autosomal dominants (Huntingdon's Chorea) and sex-linked syndromes (Haemophilia);

(iii)   syndromes of undetermined aetiology, e.g. Vater Association

(iv)   teratological syndromes, e.g. Fetal Hydantoin Syndrome, Fetal Alcohol Syndrome

4. The results of our study are:

(a) The appearance of very complex prints, more complex than those we adopted as our "standard", and a significant variation from other groups in different regions of the country.

Our observations were, nevertheless, in accord with those found in other large centres of genetics, e.g. the Kennedy-Galton Centre in St Albans, UK.

(b) we would not claim that only one fingerprint is specific for gonadal   dysgenesis, but the totality of spread over all fingers is significant.

(c) The appearance of complex patterns and palmar-asymmetry is more frequent in abnormal cases: in normal cases the alpha-type predominates, whereas in, for instance the Turner Syndrome, several different types were encountered, viz. alpha type 1, beta, beta types 1, 2, and so on.

(d) The increase in the TRC number is very significant, especially in 45XO cases.

5. Our results are in accordance with those from the international literature [1, 2]

6. The statistical methodology used here can be applied to the determination of predictors for the other syndromes. It is only necessary to determine the parameters for the other syndromes (e.g. Trisomy 18, Edward's Syndrome, and also the XXXXY Syndrome) and to compare this with those of the normal population whose parameters are contained in this study.

7. The methodology described above can be very useful in establishing a rapid postnatal diagnosis for those conditions which will give rise to many medical and socio-economic problems in the patient, problems which will have an impact on the public-health programme of a nation.

6. References

1. Petremand-Hyvarinen, R. Morphologic and dermatoglyphic aspects of Klinefelter 47XXY syndrome. J. Genet Hum (Switzerland) 26, 1978 SUPP pl-38

2. Reed T et al. Dermatoglyphic differences 45X and other abnormalities of Turner's Syndrome. Hum Genet (Germany), 7th April 1977, 36 (1) pl3-23

3. Purkinj e J. E, " Commentatio de Examine Physiologico Organi Visus et Systematis Cutanei" . Breslau: Vratislaviae Typis Universitat, 1823

4. Popich, G A and Smith D. W.: The genesis and significance of digital and palmar hand creases: Preliminary report. J Pediatr., 77: 1917, 1970

5. Mulvihill, J and Smith D W.. Genesis of dermal ridge patterning. J Pediatr., 75 1969

6. Uchida, I.A. and Soltan, H.C. Evaluation of dermatoglyphics in medical genetics. Pediatr. Clin. North Am., 10: 409, 1963

Medical Informatics Europe '97
C. Pappas et al. (Eds.)
IOS Press, 1997

XBONE: A Hybrid Expert System for Supporting Diagnosis of Bone Diseases

I. Hatzilygeroudis[1, 2], P. J. Vassilakos[3], A. Tsakalidis[1, 2]
[1]University of Patras, School of Engineering, Dept of Computer Engin.
& Informatics, 26500 Patras, Hellas(Greece)
[2]Computer Technology Institute, P.O. Box 1122, 26110 Patras, Hellas
[3]Regional University Hospital of Patras, Dept of Nuclear Medicine,
Patras, Hellas(Greece)

Abstract. In this paper, XBONE, a hybrid medical expert system that supports diagnosis of bone diseases is presented. Diagnosis is based on various patient data and is performed in two stages. In the early stage, diagnosis is based on demographic and clinical data of the patient, whereas in the late stage it is mainly based on nuclear medicine image data. Knowledge is represented via an integrated formalism that combines production rules and the Adaline artificial neural unit. Each condition of a rule is assigned a number, called its significance factor, representing its significance in drawing the conclusion of the rule. This results in better representation, reduction of the knowledge base size and gives the system learning capabilities.

1. Introduction

Expert systems are increasingly used to support medical diagnoses [1, 2, 3]. Diagnosis of bone diseases is greatly facilitated by the use of nuclear medicine methods, such as scintigrams (or scans), and a number of relevant expert systems have been developed [4, 5], which are based on a single representation scheme. Expert systems technology is moving towards hybrid representations [6, 7]. A promising integration is that of a symbolic representation, e.g. rules, with a connectionist one, i.e. various artificial neural networks.

In this paper, we present a hybrid medical expert system, called XBONE, which uses a hybrid representation formalism integrating rules and the adaline artificial neural unit. In section 2 the medical knowledge involved is presented. In section 3 the architecture of the system is discussed. Section 4 deals with the hybrid knowledge representation formalism, and finally Section 5 concludes.

2. Medical Knowledge

2.1 Patient Data

Patient data can be distinguished in three types: demograhic, clinical and nuclear medicine image (NMI) data. *Demographic data* concerns information such as patient's age, sex etc. *Clinical data* is further distinguished in physical findings and laboratory results. *Physical findings* are those detected by a physical examination of the patient, like the existence and the kind of a pain, called clinical *symptoms* as well. *Laboratory results* are those detected via laboratory tests, e.g. blood tests. Finally, *NMI data* is that extracted from scintigrams that depict the concentration of an administered radio-pharmaceutical (99m Tc-MDP) on patient's osseous tissue. Patient data are related to *domain knowledge*.

2.2 Diagnostic knowledge

Diagnostic knowledge concerns the way a diagnosis is performed. It is distinguished in two types. The first type, *procedural diagnostic knowledge*, reflects the diagnostic procedure. Diagnosis of bone diseases is considered a two-fold procedure. An initial diagnosis, called the *early diagnosis*, is made based on the demographic and clinical data of the patient. This is then used either to specify the kind of the scan needed (simple or 3-phase) or to be compared with the *late diagnosis*, which is based on the NMI data.

The second type of diagnostic knowledge, *heuristic diagnostic knowledge*, concerns experience and represents the way an expert uses patient data to make diagnoses. We acquired heuristic knowledge from an expert and constructed a *diagnostic tree* based on criteria such as the sex and the age of the patient, the existence and the acuteness of symptoms (e.g. pain, fever) etc., as far as non NMI data is concerned. As to the NMI data, criteria are related to the recognition of the *characteristic pattern* of the radio-pharmaceutical concentration, which is based on qualitative features (such as the uniformity of the concentration) and quantitative features (such as the extent of the concentration). Each pattern gives an indication for one of the following bone disease categories: metastases, hyperplasia of spinal cord, traumas, orthopedic abnormalities, arthrites, metabolic diseases, spinal cord diseases, Paget disease, benign tumors and malignant tumors.

3. System Architecture

The architecture of the system is illustrated in Fig.1. It consists of six main modules. *Patients database* (PDB) contains the demographic data and the scintigrams of the patients. Scintigrams are acquired by a γ-camera and then automatically transferred to the system [8]. *Hybrid knowledge base* (HKB) contains the domain and the heuristic diagnostic knowledge, represented as (neu)rules. *Working database* (WDB) contains the case-specific data, that is the (initial) patient data, partial conclusions and answers given by the user, represented as facts. *Hybrid inference engine* (HIE) realizes the diagnostic procedure and uses the available knowledge in HKB to draw conclusions. *Explanation mechanism* (EM) creates explanations when asked to do so. *Training mechanism* (TM) is used for rule training. Finally, *user interface* (UI) performs a number of functions related to user interaction with the system.

4. Knowledge Representation in XBONE

4.1 The Hybrid Formalism

We introduce *neurules* alongside conventional rules. Each neurule is considered as an adaline unit (Fig.2a,b). The inputs C_i, $i=1,...,n$ of the unit are the conditions of the rule. Each condition C_i is assigned a number sf_i, called a *significance factor*, that represents the significance of the corresponding condition in drawing the conclusion.

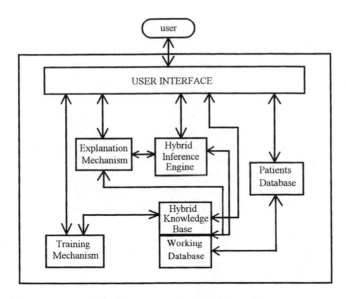

Fig.1 The Architecture of XBONE

Moreover, each rule itself is assigned a number sf_0, called the *bias factor*. Each input takes a value from the following set of discrete values: '1' if condition is *true*, '0' if it is *false* and '0.5' if its value is *unknown*. This gives the opportunity to easily distinguish between the falsity and the absence of a condition, in contrast to conventional rules. The output D, which represents the *conclusion* (decision) of the rule, is calculated as the weighted sum of the inputs filtered by a threshold function(see e.g. [9]):

$$D = f(\mathbf{a}), \quad \mathbf{a} = sf_0 + \sum_{i=1}^{n} sf_i \; C_i \tag{1}$$

where **a** is the *activation value* and $f(x)$ the *activation (threshold) function* (Fig.2c). Hence, the output can be one of '-1' and '1', representing failure and success of the rule respectively.

The general syntax of a rule is the following:
<rule> ::= [(<bias-factor>)] **if** <conditions> **then** <conclusions>
<conditions> ::= <condition> {, <condition>}
<conclusions> ::= <conclusion> {, <conclusion>}

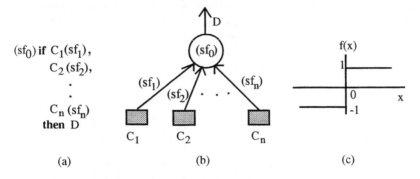

Fig.2 (a) A neurule (b) Corresponding adaline unit (c) Activation function

<condition> ::= <object> <l-operator> <value> [(<significance-factor>)]
<conclusion> ::= <object> <r-operator> <value>.
('[]' denotes optional occurrence, '{ }' denotes zero, one or more occurrences of the enclosed expression and '<>' denotes a nonterminal symbol.)

<object> acts as a variable and represents a concept in the domain, e.g. "sex", "pain" etc. <l-operator> can be a symbolic (e.g. is, isnot) or a numeric (e.g. <, =, >) operator, whereas <r-operator> can be only "is". <value> denotes a value of <object>, numeric or symbolic. Finally, <bias-factor> and <significance-factor> are real numbers. Significance factors and the bias factor are optional in a rule. Thus, neurules (with factors) and conventional rules (without factors) may coexist in the knowledge base. (The terminal symbol ",", in the case of a conventional rule denotes a conjunction).

The formalism also supports *variable declarations* that have the following syntax:

<variable-declaration> ::= <variable> : <multiplicity> : <value-domain>

and declare the types and the value domains of the variables.

<multiplicity> can be either "s" or "m" and denotes whether a variable is *single-valued* or *multi-valued* respectively. <value-domain> declares the possible values or the numeric type of a variable. Examples: "fever:s: (high, medium, low)", "symptom :m:(pain, fever)" and "age:s:integer".

Finally, the formalism supports *facts*. A fact has the same format as a conclusion of a rule. Facts represent either initial conditions or conclusions and are stored in WDB.

4.2 Hybrid Knowledge Base

HKB consists of the *domain knowledge base* (DKB) and the *hybrid rule base* (HRB). DKB contains domain knowledge, as variable declarations. HRB consists of two parts which contain knowledge concerning the early and the late diagnosis respectively. HRB may contain both conventional rules and neurules (Fig.3). Conventional rules are typically used to represent conclusions produced in a unique and exact way, in contrast to neurules, or conclusions that cannot be represented by a neurule (see Section 4.3). Thus, a neurule is actually a merger of more than one conventional rule. This greatly reduces the size of HRB.

4.3 Training neurules

The factors assigned to neurules are determined by TM. Each neurule is individually trained. To this end, a number of training patterns, called a *training set*, are supplied to TM for each rule. Training of the neurules takes place prior to the initial use of the system and every time the system is updated. The training sets are extracted from known (old) patient cases and/or the diagnostic tree. The standard least mean square (LMS) learning algorithm (see [9]) is used to determine the values of the factors.

However, there are cases where TM fails to find converging factors (case of non-separable functions, see [9]). This is an inherent weakness of the Adaline model. Then, conventional rules should be employed.

R1:	**R2:**
if sex **is** man ,	(-8) **if** pain **is** continuous (5) ,
age > 20 ,	patient_class **isnot** man_36_55 (2.5) ,
age < 36	fever **is** medium (2) ,
then patient_class **is** man_21_35	fever **is** high (2)
	then disease_type **is** inflammation

Fig.3 A conventional rule and a neurule

4.4 Inference Process

An inference process is performed in two stages, the *early diagnosis stage* and the *late diagnosis stage*. During the early diagnosis stage the first part of HRB is activated, the system asks questions about patient's clinical data and produces a first diagnosis. During the late diagnosis stage, the second part of HRB is activated. Activation of this part requires that a series of scintigrams of the patient be automatically loaded. Afterwards, the system asks questions about NMI data. Finally, it suggests a diagnosis that may or may not coincide with the first one. It is then up to the user-physician to decide on the final diagnosis. The inference mechanism is based on a backward chaining strategy.

5. Conclusions

In this paper, a hybrid medical expert system that supports diagnosis of bone diseases via scintigrams is presented. NMI data are extracted by the user-physician. Although there are systems using computer-based methods for NMI data extraction (e.g. [5]), image processing techniques are not very reliable and are not preferred (e.g. [4]). On the other hand, this makes participation of the user-physician more active.

Knowledge is represented via a formalism integrating rules and the adaline neural unit, to combine modularity and naturalness of rules with the representation and learning capabilities of neural units. This results in better representation, since one can easily represent imprecise relations, significantly reduces the size of the knowledge base, since each neurule is a merger of more than one conventional rule, and gives the system learning capabilities, since rules can be automatically updated.

A weak point of neurules is their inability to represent non-separable training patterns. To overcome this, a more complex (two layer) neural network is required. This, however, may make representation more complex, less comprehensible and modularity may be lost.

References

[1]   B.N. Prasad, S.M. Finkelstein and M.I. Hertz, An expert system for diagnosis and therapy in lung transplantation, *Computers in Biology and Medicine* 26(6) (1996) 477-488.
[2]   S.D. Likothanassis, P. Adamidis and C. Giogios, Use of neural networks in medical expert systems, *Medical Informatics* 20(4) (1995) 349-357.
[3]   M. Fathi-Torbaghan and D. Meyer, MEDUSA: a fuzzy expert system for medical diagnosis of acute abdominal pain, *Methods of Information in Medicine*, 33(5) (1994) 522-529.
[4]   S.V. Ellam and M.N. Maisen, A Knowledge-based System to Assist in the Diagnosis of Thyroid Disease from a Radioisotope Scan, in Pretschner D.P. and Urrutia B. (Eds), Knowledge-based systems to aid medical image analysis, vol.1, Commission of the European Community, 1990.
[5]   J.H.C. Reiber, G. Bloom, S.S. Gerbrands, E. Backer, H.J. van de Herik, A.E..M Reijs, I. van der Feltz and P. Fioretti, An Expert System Approach for the Objective Interpretation of Thallium-201 Scintigrams, in the same as [4].
[6]   C.A. Huges, E.E. Gose and D.L. Roseman, Overcoming deficiencies of the rule-based medical expert system, *Computer Methods and Programs in Biomedicine* 32(1) (1990) 63-71.
[7]   B. D. Leao, E. B. Reategui, A. Guazzelli and E.A. Mendonca, Hybrid systems: a promising solution for better decision support tools, *Proceedings of the 8th World Conference on Medical Informatics* (1995) 823-827.
[8]   I. Hatzilygeroudis, P.J. Vassilakos and A. Tsakalidis, An Intelligent Medical System for Diagnosis of Bone Diseases, *Proceedings of MPBE'94* (1994) 148-152.
[9]   S.I. Gallant, Neural Network Learning and Expert Systems, MIT Press, 1993.

Medical Informatics Europe '97
C. Pappas et al. (Eds.)
IOS Press, 1997

From Hospital Information System Components to the Medical Record and Clinical Guidelines & Protocols

Mário Veloso[a], Nuno Estevão[a], Pedro Ferreira[b], Rui Rodrigues[b], César Telmo Costa[a], Pedro Barahona[b,c]

[a] CENTIS / Hospital Egas Moniz, Rua da Junqueira 126, 1300 Lisboa, Portugal
[b] Faculdade de Ciências e Tecnologia / UNL, Quinta da Torre, 2825 Monte da Caparica, Portugal
[c] UNINOVA, Quinta da Torre, 2825 Monte da Caparica, Portugal

Abstract. This paper introduces an ongoing project towards the development of a new generation HIS, aiming at the integration of clinical and administrative information within a common framework. Its design incorporates explicit knowledge about domain objects and professional activities to be processed by the system together with related knowledge management services and act management services. The paper presents the conceptual model of the proposed HIS architecture, that supports a rich and fully integrated patient data model, enabling the implementation of a dynamic electronic patient record tightly coupled with computerised guideline knowledge bases.

1. Introduction

Clinical activities are the heart of a hospital life, not only because they correspond to its reason of existence (the provision of care to patients), but also because most hospital information processing is related to the patient, namely to the clinical activities patients incur. This explains the current emphasis on the patient and patient related (clinical) activities when developing information systems for healthcare organisations like hospitals [1, 2]. This new generation of Hospital Information Systems (HIS) is oriented towards medical activity, while integrating administrative functions of previous HIS generations.

Domain knowledge is a key element for the design and implementation of such systems if they are to provide intelligent support to the professional activities in the hospital [3]. This includes knowledge about "acts and linked data" (following the concepts defined in RICHE [4]), as well as knowledge about the organisation and actors. In addition, it ought to include knowledge about the strategies concerning professional activities, to enable a customised exploitation of information and knowledge by application programs. A formal representation of the concepts, semantic relationships and behaviours is crucial for such purpose, particularly when the integration of knowledge-based systems assisting the clinicians daily professional activities is also envisaged.

This paper introduces an ongoing project in CENTIS / Hospital Egas Moniz [5] towards the development of a new generation HIS aiming at the integration of clinical and administrative information within a common framework. A particular emphasis is put on the clinical information and knowledge related to the hospital professional activities with a special focus on the role of the electronic patient record. This is regarded as a basis for co-operative care planning including the use, in the daily practice, of clinical guidelines and protocols which have been shown to be effective in improving the healthcare process in terms of quality, efficiency and outcome. The rational for the implementation of clinical guidelines comes from real needs of professional bodies and health authorities, but also, as outlined in the Epistol study of the AIM programme [6], because guideline implementation might constitute a less demanding task concerning system design and implementation than developing expert systems or general-purpose decision support systems.

The explicit knowledge about domain objects and professional activities to be processed by the system together with related knowledge management services and act management services, represents a key element in the adopted approach, well illustrated by the conceptual model of the proposed architecture. This architecture supports a rich and fully integrated patient data model, thus enabling the implementation of a dynamic electronic patient record tightly coupled with computerised guideline knowledge bases.

The paper is organised as follows. In section 2, an overall description of the system is informally introduced. Section 3 shows in more detail the Electronic Patient Record, including a brief presentation of how protocol-based care is handled by the system. Finally, in section 4 a few relevant issues are discussed.

2. Description of the system

An object-oriented modelling approach has been used to build a conceptual model of the information system components. This knowledge representation model (figure 1) is implemented in various levels of abstraction from generic models of objects, to reference models describing the application domains, and finally to data models concerning the actual data regarding the patients through the instantiation, by the applications, of more general classes and their semantic links.

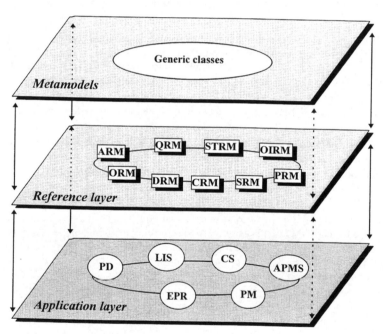

Figure 1 - Knowledge representation model

This approach aided us to cope with the complexity of HIS requirements and will enable results to conform to the emerging medical informatics standards (e.g, CEN TC251). Two types of results need to be considered: i/ conceptual results, consisting of an architecture and open interface specifications; ii/ software services, i.e. a kernel of common functions and data to be shared by the different applications which together will compose the HIS.

2.1 Meta-structure layer (metamodels)

This layer provides a description of the generic types of concepts and domain objects class models (in terms of generalisation/specialisation and composition) and their semantic relationships, using an object oriented approach. These metamodels aim at guiding the implementation of the reference models of the following system layer, and are also utilised by the application modules for validation and system access purposes.

2.2 Reference layer

This layer provides a detailed description of the domain objects of the hospital and professional activities (sub-classes of the above metamodels). Two types of services are available: i/ database management services for building up the reference models according to the defined metamodels and the needs/characteristics of the organisation; ii/ application services through which applications may access the reference models. A brief overview of the components of this layer follows:

- Concept Reference Model (CRM) - description of the actual structure and semantic relationships of the domain objects used by the system, including medical knowledge.
- Organisation Reference Model (ORM) - characterisation of the organisation (i.e. hospital) in terms of structure (generalisation/specialisation), composition, utilisation of resources, etc.
- Subject Reference Model (SRM)- description of structure and semantic relationships of the actual classes of objects composing the patient (subject of care) data model.
- Object Interface Reference Model (OIRM) - specification and (display) methods for every defined object in the system, in order to provide a coherent interface.
- Act Reference Model (ARM) - characterisation of the acts used in the organisation in terms of their attributes, classification (generalisation/specialisation), composition, composition rules, objectives, act result (types of generated data), etc.
- State Transition Reference Model (STRM) - acceptable state transitions of act classes.
- Data Reference Model (DRM) - characterisation of the data generated by the acts.
- Quality Reference Model (QRM)- classification of acts usage by means of quality indicators expressing a judgement about the utilisation of the acts in the organisation.
- Protocol Reference Model (PRM) - characterisation of the guidelines and protocols used in the organisation in terms of their attributes, classification, composition, composition rules, objectives, act result (types of generated data), etc.

This last component is being developed within the Prestige project [7] as a Generic Protocol and Guideline Model (GPGM). This generic model, which is being made available as a public domain resource, aims at the effective delivery of guideline-based care with basis on the modelling of knowledge services for clinical management.

2.3 Application layer

This layer comprises a set of run-time applications end-users will interact with, including:

- Act Processing Management System (APMS) - it manages all the events in relation with state transitions of actual acts. APMS is based on the assumption that all the events occurring in the organisation depend on the interaction between agents: typically, the *requester* (an organisation object, such as a department or actor) requests a *performer* (another organisation object) to perform some *act* with respect to a specific *patient*. The APMS keeps a record of all the actions and state transitions of an act during its life cycle.
- Legacy Information System (LIS) - it enables the exchange of information with legacy systems. User transparent services connect the EPR to legacy information systems (e.g the Hospital Patient Management System, SONHO, used in Hospital Egas Moniz) in order to access and/or update related tables).
- Patient Dossier (PD) - to store patient data together with generating acts.
- Communication Services (CS) - to exchange information on services shared between the organisation and the outside world (e.g. regional/national healthcare networks).

- Protocol Manager (PM) - to provide services supporting the selection and execution of protocols (also being implemented, as a generic technology, in the Prestige project).

3. The Electronic Patient Record (EPR) and protocol-based care

The implementation of the EPR is based on two major assumptions. Firstly, the patient clinical record must be envisaged as a repository of the patient related clinical interventions along his/her life, together with the data such interventions have produced. Clinical interventions follow the concept of "Acts" as defined in RICHE and used in several European projects [8, 9]. Secondly, the patient medical record must be regarded as a virtual record represented by all clinical activities performed within the hospital for a patient. The activity around a patient is thus represented by a succession of acts and generated data, the patient record being a view on these acts and data.

According to this, the EPR consists of an user interface together with an integrated engine enabling users to process patient related acts and linked data, which can be tailored in different clinical settings according to the user needs and preferences. The following is a short overview of the main characteristics of the proposed EPR:

- The user interface provides the means a) to enter new acts by selection of instances of the object classes specified in ARM for the given class of users, b) to perform some action on already created acts depending on the current state of the selected act and its allowed life cycle state transitions as defined in STRM or by composition rules specified in ARM (in the case of composite acts). The interface also provides the means to process the professional content of acts, that is data linked to the act according to the specified state transition. A specific interface object is dynamically evoked according to the generated type of data (i.e. OIRM service).
- The interface is managed by an integrated engine which handles validation procedures and patient database services, as well as generated events, through services provided by the reference models. The reference models provide declarative knowledge on domain objects allowing a dynamic adaptation of the interface to user requirements, as well as a proper management of available functions/actions different users can execute at any moment of the patient process of care. The run-time application layer components provide services for data storage (PD) and act life cycle management, in isolation (APMS) or integrated within a guideline/protocol (PM), as well as user transparent communication services (CS).

Protocol management deserves a few additional comments. Protocols model the process of care, specifying established and recommended best practice on a patient-specific basis. Protocols are thus composed of acts which ought to be performed in certain sequences taking into account some specified knowledge on the process of care, namely the clinical conditions where they are applied and the characteristics of the patient during the process of care. In our approach protocols are defined as a special kind of act, hence presented to the user by the interface as any other act. The main difference resides in that a specific manager, the Protocol Manager, handles the life cycle of selected protocols on the basis of patient clinical data (stored in the patient dossier) and specified protocol knowledge. Protocols will be specifically evoked by the user, as any other (composed) act. Generated output consists of messages either recommending acts to be performed, or warnings on the lack of protocol compliance, as well as indications on current protocol state.

4. Discussion

The new generation of HIS is oriented towards medical applications while integrating administrative functions of previous HIS generations. In the past, most care oriented applications have modelled medical information around a pre-defined medical record. However, in our opinion, such approach is not appropriate to cope with the complexity and diversity of the domain and of the process of care. Systems providing an intelligent support to the professional activities in the hospital require an extensive use of knowledge on hospital objects, on the medical domain they apply to, in the context patient care-plan management. The use of a knowledge-based approach to represent domain objects and their properties in knowledge bases, which can be exploited at run-time by application programs has already been successfully demonstrated [10].

The proposed architecture follows a similar approach allowing a sound representation of such knowledge and its consistent utilisation from different applications like the electronic patient record and knowledge based system. Furthermore, it enables the use of computerised clinical guidelines and protocols in the daily clinical practice, fully integrated with the electronic patient record, dynamically customised according to the user's practice. In addition, because representation of the medical knowledge is extensively modelled, from superficial to deep modelling, the future integration of some general purpose decision support system is also facilitated.

Finally, the proposed system architecture follows CEN TC251 recommendations [11] on that such healthcare system should be built "as an open federation of autonomous but interworking systems, capable of meeting the following objectives: i/ to provide optimised support to the specific needs of the individual centres and units ...; ii/ to ensure the overall integration of the organisation ...".

Acknowledgements

This work was partially supported by the Commission of the European Union under the TAP project PRESTIGE n° HC1040.

References
[1]   Hammond WE. *Hospital Information Systems: A Review in Perspective*. Yearbook of Medical Informatics. 1994: 95-101.
[2]   Blum BI. *The evolving role of hospital information systems*. In: Barahona P, Veloso M, Bryant J, (eds), Proceedings of the Twelfth International Congress of the European Federation for Medical Informatics. Lisbon, Portugal, 1994: 23-26.
[3]   Kanoui H, Joubert M, and Favard R. *Knowledge-based Model and Query language to Medical Databases in a Hospital Information System*. In: Barahona P, Veloso M, Bryant J, (eds.), Proceedings of the Twelfth International Congress of the European Federation for Medical Informatics. Lisbon, Portugal, 1994: 23-26.
[4]   Frandji B, Schot J, Joubert M, Soady I, Kilsdonk A. *The RICHE reference architecture*. Medical Informatics, 1994, 19: 1-11.
[5]   Veloso M, Costa C-T. *Integrated Hospital Information System: Conceptualisation and Implementation* (in Portuguese). Descartes Prize, Portuguese Institute of Informatics, 1994.
[6]   *Knowledge and Decision in Health Telematics*. In: Barahona P, Christensen J P (eds.), IOS Press, 1994.
[7]   Gordon C, Veloso M. *The PRESTIGE Project: Implementing Guidelines in Healthcare*. In: Brender J, Christensen J P, Scherrer J-R, McNair P (eds.), Proceedings of the Thirteen International Congress of the European Federation for Medical Informatics, IOS Press, 1996: 887-891.
[8]   Joubert M, Kanoui H. *The knowledge-based management of medical acts in NUCLEUS*. In: Andreassen S, Engelbrecht R, Wyatt J (Eds.), Proceedings AIME 93, IOS Press, 1993: 377-380.
[9]   Nicklin P and Frandji B. *Act Management and Clinical Guidelines*. In: C Gordon and JP Christensen (Eds.), Health Telematics for Clinical Guidelines and Protocols. IOS Press, 1995: 117-124.
[10]   Kanoui H, Joubert M, and Favard R. *A Knowledge-Based Modelling of Hospital Information System Components*. In: Barahona P, Stefanelli M, Wyatt (eds.), Proceedings of the fifth Conference on Artificial Intelligence in Medicine (AIME '95), Springer, 1995, 319: 330.
[11]   CEN TC251 Pre-Standard, Healthcare Information System Architecture, 1995.

Medical Informatics Europe '97
C. Pappas et al. (Eds.)
IOS Press, 1997

Clinical Protocol Development using Inter/IntraNet Technology: the FENARETE System

A. Errera[1], P. Merialdo[2], A. Orsano[1], G. Sindoni[2] and G. Rumolo[2]

[1]Università di Roma La Sapienza
Policlinico Umberto I: IV Clinica Chirurgica
Via del Policlinico, 5 00161 Roma

[2]Università di Roma Tre
Dipartimento di Informatica ed Automazione
Via della Vasca Navale, 84 00146 Roma

Abstract: In this work we present FENARETE, a software tool to design and distribute clinical protocols in an Inter/IntraNet framework. We consider a medical protocol as a clinical behaviour scheme, formally and clearly defined with sufficient details. Our work allows the knowledge content of any clinical protocol to be fully represented in a symbolic style. A computer based support tool that works as an interface between clinicians and the protocol knowledge base is regarded by the authors as a basic building block developing an integrated environment for medical protocols design and management. The FENARETE application has been developed in Java and it is available for any Internet-linked machine with a Java-compatible browser.

1 Introduction

Nowadays, the development of an Integrated Health Information Environment finds in the Inter/IntraNet technology [3, 13] an adequate answer to most of the internetworking problems. This technology can improve the quality and the cost-effectiveness of hospital activities. Contemporary medicine has to deal with an increase of prices, specialisation levels and information needs. The information technology (IT) is able to give a real support to formalise and to develop a large set of medical guidelines and clinical protocols [7, 8, 2, 9]. This objective fulfils many medical requirements such as: medical knowledge diffusion, medical practice training, health service cost-effectiveness evaluation and clinical activities monitoring. The adoption of standard guidelines for healthcare management improves the quality of patient treatment allowing the circulation of medical protocols independently from any particular hospital infrastructure. The physician who follows a standard clinical protocol, is provided with a support tool able to clarify and improve his action plane. Moreover, the protocol safeguards the clinician from mistakes or from excluding relevant hypothesis. The hospital is recognised as a heterogeneous environment where inter-communication represent a critical activity. However communication can be set up with other hospitals and healthcare centres. This two kinds of communication can be improved using standard technologies as the Inter/IntraNet one. From a technical perspective, the Java development environment [10] is a valid tool to build and to distribute software products that meet the above requirements.

In this work we present FENARETE, a software tool to design and distribute clinical protocols in an Inter/IntraNet framework. The presentation is organised as follows: in section two, we present our general framework for clinical protocol design; in section three, we describe the prototype tool that has been realised to support effective use of clinical protocols in our environment; in section four we discuss related proposal and future evolution of the FENARETE project.

2 Developing clinical protocols

The clinical protocol is a central element for the management of effective patient care processes. It allows to set up, to monitor and evaluate the clinical activities plane. Protocols can be considered real healthcare tools, only when they are adequately represented and when the adopted formalism enables computer based management. We consider medical protocol as *a*

clinical behaviour scheme, formally and clearly defined with sufficient details. Moreover, in a local organisation it has to be considered as a normative statement.
The protocol is a path through different interleaved physiological and pathological states. The clinician, during the decision-making activity, has to choose between different alternatives. The protocol representation has to give more attention to the decision activities then to the therapeutic and diagnostic ones. The opportunity to reuse a protocol, or its parts, in different organisations or moments can be a real improvement for the healthcare service. Moreover, the clear definition of medical protocols allow patient to know what is the care process in which he or she is involved. However healthcare management can quantify necessary resources and improve the service quality. A medical protocol is a symbolic description of a healthcare process. Besides it has to be represented using a finite set of symbols (i.e. graphic symbols) each one used to individuate a different basic activity type. Instead, a healthcare process is a medical knowledge fragment useful for the care of a specific disease. The medical protocol reorganise this knowledge giving it a format that is valid for an effective use. This help physicians to explore the continuos, often messy, information flow proposed by medical knowledge sources. Anyway each application of a medical protocol to a single pa-

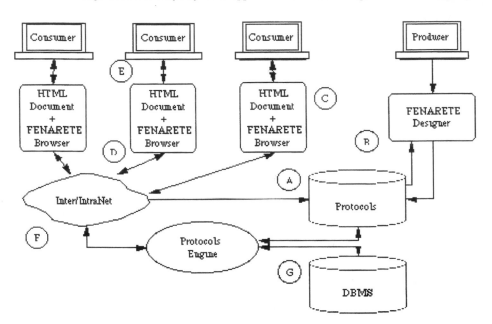

Figure 1: The FENARETE System Architecture

tient is a delicate task under the physician responsibility. The definition of a medical protocol representation formalism is composed by a syntactic and a semantic description. The first one characterise the way how the protocol appears to physicians while the latter define, in a formal and clear style, how it can be used. The formal semantics has the role of an instrument to investigate the expressive power and the algorithmic complexity of the protocol description language. Moreover, only the formal specification of the language semantics allows to compare our proposal with other already formalised.

3 Using FENARETE

Our work allows the knowledge content of any clinical protocol to be fully represented in a symbolic style. A protocol describes how to perform some tasks and describes each task with its atomic parts. We adopt a symbolic description where every activity type is represented by an appropriate icon. The main benefit of a symbolic and graphical description of medical protocols is to encapsulate and hide details until they become relevant. A computer based support tool that works as an interface between clinicians and the protocol knowledge base is regarded by the authors as a basic building block developing an integrated environment for medical protocols design and management. The interface can help doctors in defining and consulting medical protocols and in applying protocols in real cases. Two requirements are to be met by the system:

- the *network centric* paradigm (multimedia management in distributed systems);
- a friendly and intuitive user-system interaction.

Taking into account this requirements - and as the great diffusion of the World Wide Web has well-established a new paradigm that allows to easily create and manage distributed hyper-media - it seemed natural to choose WWW technologies to develop the system.

The FENARETE system[1] has been developed in Java and it's available for any Internet-linked machine with a Java-compatible browser. In this manner we have maximum protocol spread and we offer an instrument that is virtually accessible from everywhere.

Java permits to write programs (applets) that can be sent, by a server and that can be executed on the client. The language is an interpreted object oriented language and it is C++ like. One of the Java main peculiarities is to allow to write machine independent applets. Client safety

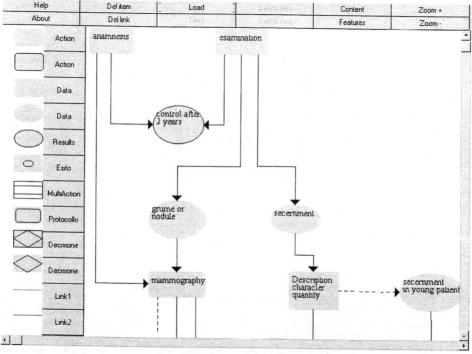

Figure 2: The FENARETE User Interface

is guaranteed from language restrictions, like the impossibility to write on the client itself.

The FENARETE system (fig. 1) is composed by two autonomous software tools: the proto-cols browser and the protocols designer. The designer tool allows to create new medical protocols, reusing and organising the already developed protocols. The browser tool is a Java-applet able to consult protocol from a remote client.

The FENARETE system offers graphic primitives that represent the above mentioned seman-tic hierarchies. All clinical activities are supported by a wide medical knowledge concerning general aspects (anatomy, pathology, physiology) and specific aspects joined to the single clinic cases faced by the single medical institutions (ambulatory, hospital, day hospital). The wide medical domain must be subdivided into little manageable fragments, which are derived by different institution and which concern different specialities. This problem has to be com-pared with that of diffusion and reuse of medical knowledge.

---

[1] URL:http:// poincare.inf.uniroma3.it/Medinfo/Fenearete

The main request in this specific domain is a representative formalism with an high expressive power that can catch temporal aspects, structural aspects inherent to single information related to a single patient and the related medical concept structure, the control of the single activities to carry on, and finally all the aspects linked to the concurrence of simultaneous activities that use shared resources. The formal definition of an iconographic and textual language that describes protocols, represents the most important goal of the project. This formalism answers, in a practical but scientifically rigorous fashion, to the set of requirements that come from the previous considerations.

The FENARETE user interface (fig. 2) is developed in the same way for both tools. It looks like a graphic editor but it allows to represent and manage all the knowledge useful to describe a clinical protocol. The user interacting with the system can browse inside the behaviour described by the protocol and he/she can record all the information useful to monitor the patient care process.

4 Conclusions and related work

The FENARETE system for medical guideline and protocol management has been presented. The network-centric paradigm allows to share the implicit medical knowledge through the incoming information highways. Java and WWW have been chosen as the reference technologies to develop the running prototype. The system is available at the URL:http:// poincare.inf.uniroma3.it/Medinfo/Fenearete. With respect to related works [8, 9], the authors of this paper tried to exploit those contribution to add sharing capabilities to protocol management systems through the Internet.

References

[1]   S. Andreassen, R. Engelbrecht, J. Wyatt *Artificial intelligence in medicine* AIME'93 conference on Artificial Intelligence in Medicine Europe, 3-6 October 1993, Munich

[2]   P. Barahona *Resource management constraints in guideline-based care* MIE'96

[3]   T. Berners-Lee, R. Cailliau, A. Luotonen, H. Nielsen, A. Secret *The World Wide Web* Comm. ACM 1994; 37(8): 76-82.

[4]   L. Brodie, J. Mylopulos Eds. *On Knowledge Base Management Systems* Springer-Verlag 1986

[5]   P. Barahona, R. Walton, Z. Ilic et al. *Deep medical knowledge to design clinical guidelines* In proceedings of the MIE 94

[6]   M. Cléret, P. Denier and P. Le Beux *Exploitation of a large knowledge data base: analysis and extraction of required data for construction of a computer assisted diagnosis system* In proceedings of the MIE 94 Conference 1994

[7]   B. De Carolis, F. Giovagnorio, V. Cavallo *An approach to multimedia guidelines in diagnostic radiology* In proc. of the CAR 96 Conference 1996

[8]   J.Fox, N. Johns, A. Rahmanzadeh, R. Thompson *PROforma: a method and language for specifying clinical guidelines and protocols* MIE 96

[9]   C. Gordon, I. Herbert, P. Johnson *Knowledge representation and clinical practice guidelines: the DI-LEMMA and PRESTIGE projects care* MIE 96

[10] J. Gosling, H. McGilton *The Java™ language environment: A white paper.* See: http://java.sun.com/whitePaper/java-whitepaper-1.html

[11] M. Helander *Handbook of Human-Computer Interaction* Amsterdam: North Holland 1988

[12] S. Herbert, C. Gordon, A. Jackson-Smale et al. *Protocols for clinical care* In proceedings of the MIE 94

[13] B. Johnsen, S. Vingtoft et al. *A common structure for the representation of data and diagnostic processes within clinical neurophysiology* In proceedings of the MIE 94

[14] H. J. Lowe, E. C. Lomax, S. E. Polonkey *The World Wide Web: a Review of an Emerging Internet-based Technology for the Distribution of Biomedical Information* JAMIA 1996; 3(1): 1-14.

[15] P.Lagouarde, R.Thompson, J-L Renaud-Salis, P. Ferguson, S Hajnal, P. Robles. *The PROMPT Electronic Health Care Record* MIE 96

[16] M. Rossol *Automatic analysis of the medical diagnosis: a basis for retrieval of pathological reports* In proceedings of the MIE 94

[17] H. Sitter, H Prünte, W. Lorenz *A new version of the program ALGO for clinical algorithms* MIE 96

[18] J.D. Ullman *Database and Knowledge Bases* Computer Science Press 1989

[19] Wahlster W and Kobsa A.: *User Models in Dialog Systems.* In User Models in Dialog Systems, Springer verlag, Berlin, 1989, 4-34.

Medical Informatics Europe '97
C. Pappas et al. (Eds.)
IOS Press, 1997

An Ontology-based Framework
for Guideline-driven Medical Practice

S. Quaglini, L. Dazzi[a], R. Saracco[a], M. Stefanelli, F. Locatelli[b]

Dpt. Computer Science and Systems - University of Pavia
[a] *Consorzio di Bioingegneria e Informatica Medica - Pavia, Italy*
[b] *Clinica Pediatrica - IRCCS Policlinico S. Matteo, Pavia, Italy*

Abstract

This paper describes a general framework for clinical practice guidelines development, dissemination and use. We propose an ontological description of the medical knowledge and of the organizational context, in order to produce clinical guidelines which, on one hand, can be widely shared between different institutions and, on the other, can be efficiently tailored to consider the peculiarities of each clinical context.

1. Introduction

The USA Institute of Medicine defined clinical practice Guidelines (GL) as "systematically developed statements to assist practitioner and patient decisions about appropriate health care for specific clinical circumstances" [1]. The importance of appropriate use of GLs to provide optimum patient management and to ensure high quality of care is widely recognized, yet, there is a significant gap between the development of a generic GL, i.e. a GL provided by a consensus conference, and its utilization into a real clinical context. Clinician acceptance and utilization of GLs is hindered by several factors, first of all, very often generic GLs do not consider peculiarities of each organizational context. That's why recent research efforts have been done to build *site-specific* GLs [2] starting from more general documents.

Our goal is to develop a framework of tools for GL-driven medical practice capable of dealing with the problem of site-specification, so that each institution could implement its own GLs, perfectly consistent with the intentions of the *official* generic GL, but which introduce different methods to satisfy the same goals. From a computational point of view, all our tools have been developed using Java and HTML languages, in order to create an environment in which knowledge sources (ontology libraries, GL servers, etc) can be easily shared and distributed.

As a test bench for the proposed methodology, we have chosen the generic GL for the management of Acute Myeloid Leukemia (AML) in children, developed in 1992 by the AIEOP (Italian Association of Pediatric Haematology and Oncology). In the following, this GL will be referred as "AML-GL".

2. The Framework Architecture

The framework which is under development is based on a computable and highly structured GL formal representation and on an ontological representation of the clinical knowledge and of the organizational context. The overall functionalities implemented by this framework are shown in Fig. 1. To support the clinical expert at specifying the GL according to the formal specification, we have developed a tool called Generic Guideline Editor (GGE). In practice, the GGE should be used by clinical experts and knowledge engineers to encapsulate a traditional GL into a formal representation meant to be capable of capturing the knowledge contained in the text in a form which can be

interpreted by a computer. There are two other tools which can be invoked by the GGE:
(1) *a Validating Tool*, capable of verifying the logical correctness of the represented

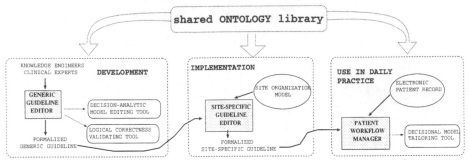

Fig. 1 The framework architecture for the GL development, implementation and dissemination

GL; and (2) *a Decision-Analytic Model Editing Tool* to face those situations in which the GL itself highlights a choice that must be based on a proper management of uncertainty and patient's preferences (the description of these tools can be found in [3]).

The Site-Specific GL Editor exploits the organization model to tailor the GL for a context-specific implementation, and allows the quantification of those parameters which have been left unbound in the generic version of the GL (a typical example is the maximum cost which each institution allows for a certain task). Moreover, the computerized GL is integrated with the electronic patient record, if the scheme of the latter is based on the same ontology. This integration improves compliance to GL's prescriptions, as shown in [4] and provides inputs to a Patient Workflow Management System [5]. From our point of view, such a system would imply an agent-based architecture for the whole Hospital Information System (HIS) [6]. An ontological description of all the entities managed by the various tools underlies the whole system. This means that we plan to develop an ontology server capable of facilitating the GL definition and use at the various levels described in fig. 1.

3. The Formalized Generic Guideline

The formal representation is based on a modular, top down structuring of the health care process. Each module is nested in a more general module, which represents the context for its proper use, or, in other words, each module can be decomposed into a certain number of sequential or parallel subtasks. Tasks which cannot be further decomposed in subtasks are called atomic tasks. Each task in the GL (atomic or not) is described by a Task Frame, which stores all the attributes specifying that task. Three main attribute categories may be distinguished: attributes to describe the task (description, type, intention), to allow the management of the task in an agent-based system (skills, location, time and economic constraints), and to allocate the task within the whole GL (activation condition, termination condition, subtasks, next task).

By means of the GGE all the tasks composing the AML-GL are specified, and a computational representation (Lisp structures) is produced. An inference engine interpreting the knowledge embedded in these structures can be implemented, leading to patient-specific advices. Of course, this implies the use of a database storing temporal information, i.e. patient data with associated time-stamps, of an inference engine carrying out temporal reasoning, and of a tool showing the results of a database query through dynamically created HTML pages.

3.1 Site specification

The GGE has been designed to support, first of all, the development of a *generic* GL, that is the GL as it is provided by national or international health care organizations. A site-specific GL editor should be used by health care professionals in a specific environment, i.e. a hospital, to tailor the generic GL according to organization constraints. Modifications needed to make a generic GL site-specific can be very different in entity: it could be just a change in the time schedule of controls and drug delivery, but it could also be necessary to alter a recommendation dramatically, for example because the required resources are not available at the site. The process of GL site-specification requires three basic components: 1) a generic GL, annotated so that criteria and intentions leading each recommendation are made explicit; 2) an organizational model of the clinical context, in which roles, resources, policies and preferences must be explicit; and 3) a set of rules specifying the legal modifications. These three components are the input of a tool capable of developing site-specific GLs in a semi-automatic way. The following paragraph is focused on point 2).

3.1.1 The organizational model

Let us describe what we mean by "organizational model by means of an example, i.e. the problem of accountability of a professional for tasks of a certain kind. The assignment of roles and responsibilities during the patient's workflow management is something which is strictly dependent on the clinical context we are referring to: the hierarchical position required to become accountable for tasks of a certain kind may vary from site to site, while the professional skills required to perform the same task do not change. If a generic GL could be developed so as to specify just the professional skills required for a certain task, the agent who will physically perform this task could be decided when the GL is accepted inside a certain context, taking into account the organizational model. We propose an ontological description of the health care unit organization, linked to Databases storing details for each relevant entity and entity-relationship. The ontology was developed using Ontolingua, and its computational implementation is obtained by means of a translating tool towards a KEE-like frame-based environment. Through a proper analysis of the frames' structure and of the hierarchical links between them, it is possible to derive the relational scheme of a database, which stores the information describing each clinical unit.

3.1.2 An example

Let us consider a fragment of our organizational ontology (see top of Fig. 3), i.e. the part describing the concept of physical resource: the bottom half of Fig. 3 shows the mapping of the ontological subclass "machinery" to the corresponding database tables. In this way, the database derived from the ontology would store the minimum set of data required to achieve the kind of cooperation between different organizational contexts stated by the shared ontology paradigm. To show how this description of the clinical unit could affect the process of GLs' site-specification, let us consider a case in which the AML-GL specifies the intention to be achieved, but leaves the choice of the clinical action to be performed to the target institution: in such a situation, the organization ontology could guide this choice taking into account resources, utilities, preferences and policies. The AML-GL gives a certain number of precise indications, but when it comes to the conditioning regimen before autologous BMT, there is no unique prescription available. The intention of this intervention is to provide an immunosuppressive therapy to the patient, in order to facilitate the marrow engraftment. However, the choice between Total Body Irradiation and Busulfan (TBI-BU), or Cyclophosphamide and

Busulfan (CY-BU) is left to the hospital. By now, there are no controlled clinical trials showing with statistical evidence that TBI-BU provides better results than CY-BU, even if some local studies seem to give this indication, that's why this choice is left open by the GL. These two immunosuppressive therapies are very different: to perform a TBI, complex and expensive devices are required (particle accelerators), while the CY-BU treatment can be performed almost everywhere and is less expensive (order of 1000 ECU versus 100 ECU). If irradiation facilities are available on the site, usually TBI is chosen, but, otherwise, several factors must be considered: for example the hospital needs to have agreements with other equipped institutions. And even if these agreements exist, the cost of the irradiation, the geographical distance of the hosting site, the waiting list are factors which can influence the hospital policy. All these aspects can be modelled by the organization ontology. When the AML-GL is implemented into a particular context, committees of medical experts and administrators tranform this generic GL into a site-specific one.

3.1.3 Running a site-specification for the test-bed guideline

We considered here three different health care institutions: Policlinico San Matteo in Pavia, Ospedali Riuniti in Bergamo and Ospedale di Cagliari. Their characteristics were described as instances of the ontological class "health care unit", and stored in database tables. The Hospital in Bergamo has its own Irradiation Unit, Pavia and Cagliari do not, but there is a convention for TBI interventions between Pavia and Bergamo, and another one between Pavia and Varese (another medical centre capable of providing TBI). Some rules have been implemented, to describe the process of choice between the two immunosuppressive therapies, and these rules are triggered by the content of the various database tables. Some examples are listed below: [1]

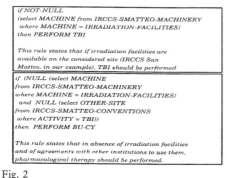

Fig. 2

Results can be inferred straight forwardly applying the above mentioned rules to the ontologies describing the 3 different clinical sites.

4. Conclusion

We propose a formalism for specifying clinical practice GLs, so as to make them sharable by human and software agents acting in a distributed health care environment, and reusable by different institutions, with different organization peculiarities. As a matter of fact, GLs are most effective when they are customized for the institution that will use them. Unfortunately, this customization makes it difficult to share GLs between different institutions and to maintain them in face of organizational changes.

We believe our formalism will help solving some of these problems, by providing on one hand logically correct computer-formalized GLs, and, on the other, tools to guide

---

[1]for sake of simplicity, the SQL sintax is not fully complied in these rules description

the process of site-specification, where it is needed.

```
(in-package "ONTOLINGUA-USER")
(define-theory economic-concepts (socio-concepts))
(in-theory 'economic-concepts)                                              a)
(define-class RESOURCE (?r)
   "Resources: physical and human,they have a cost."
   :def   (and (individual ?r)(can-have-one ?r resource.cost))
   :axiom-def  (subclass-partition resource
                                   (setof human-resource physical-resource)))

(define-class PHYSICAL-RESOURCE (?phres)
   "A physical resource is some equipment or machine (e.g. TAC machinery) or
   consumer good."
   :def (and (resource ?phres)(not (person ?phres)))
   :axiom-def  (subclass-partition physical-resource
                                   (setof consumer-good timed-physical-resource)))

(define-class CONSUMER-GOOD (?cg)
   "Class of consumer goods."
   :def (and  (physical-resource ?cg)(can-have-one ?cg storage-cost)
             (has-one ?cg consumer-good.cost)))

(define-class TIMED-PHYSICAL-RESOURCE (?tps)
   "Physical resource with use time."
   :def (physical-resource ?tps)
   :axiom-def (subclass-partition timed-physical-resource(setof machinery room)))

(define-class MACHINERY (?mach)
   "The machinery is a physical-resource,has a purchase-cost, a purchase-date,
   a purchase-mode, an amortization-period, a residual-value, it uses some
   consumer-good, has an unitary-cost and performs An action."
   :def  (and (timed-physical-resource ?mach)
              (has-one ?mach machinery.purchase-cost)
              (has-value-of-type ?mach machinery.purchase-date calendar-date)
              (has-value-of-type ?mach machinery.purchase-mode purchase-mode)
              (has-value-of-type ?mach machinery.amortization-period duration)
              (has-one ?mach machinery.residual-value)
              (has-some ?mach machinery.consumer-goods)
              (has-one ?mach machinery.unitary-cost)
              (has-some ?mach machinery.action)))
```

b)

IRCCS_SMATTEO_MACHINERY

MACH-ID	MACHINE	PURCH_COST	PURCH_DATE	PURCH_MODE	AMORT_PER	RESID_VALUE	UNIT_COST
RX1	RX DEVICE	100.000	01/01/92	LEASING	5	80	50
RX2	RX DEVICE	180.000	01/01/92	LEASING	5	80	50

IRCCS_SMATTEO_MACHINERY.CONSUMER_GOODS

MACH-ID	CONSUMER_GOOD
RX1	FILM
RX2	FILM

IRCCS_S_MATTEO_ACTION.MACHINERY

ACTION	MACH-ID
RX-LEG	RX1
RX-TORAX	RX1

Fig. 3 a) A fragment of the organizational ontology and b) some of the tables derived from the ontology

Acknowledgments The authors thank Dr. Douglas Fridsma, from the Section on Medical Informatics, Stanford University School of Medicine, for helpful discussion on guideline representation.

References

[1]. Institute of Medicine (MJ Field and KN Lohr Eds.). Guidelines for Clinical Practice. From Development to Use. National Academy Press, Washington D.C., 1992.

[2]. Fridsma DB, Gennari JH, Musen MA. Making Generic Guidelines Site-Specific. Proceedings of the 1996 AMIA Annual Fall Symposium (JJ Cimino, Ed.), 597-601, 1996.

[3]. Quaglini S, Saracco R, Stefanelli M, Fassino C. Supporting Tools for Guidelines Development and Dissemination. Accepted for presentation to AIME97 Conference.

[4]. Lobach DF, Hammond WE. Development and Evaluation of a Computer-assisted Management Protocol (CAMP): Improved Compliance with Care Guidelines for Diabetes Mellitus. Proceedings of the Symposium on Computer Applications in Medical Care, 18: 787-791, 1994.

[5]. Yousfi F, Beuscart R, Geib JM. PLACO: a Cooperative Architecture for Managing Workflow in Critical Care Units. Proceedings of the Symposium on Computer Applications in Medical Care, 19: 454-458, 1995.

[6]. Falasconi S, Lanzola G and Stefanelli M. Using ontologies in multi-agent systems, accepted for presentation at the KAW'96 Workshop, Banff, Canada, November 9-14, 1996.

Medical Informatics Europe '97
C. Pappas et al. (Eds.)
IOS Press, 1997

Telematics for Clinical Guidelines: A Conceptual Modelling Approach

Colin Gordon[1], Ian Herbert[2], Peter Johnson[3], Peter Nicklin[2], David Pitty[1], Philip Reeves[1]

1. Royal Brompton Hospital, London
2. NHS Information Management Centre, Birmingham
3. Sowerby Unit for Primary Care Informatics, University of Newcastle

Abstract. *PRESTIGE* is a project for applying telematics to assist the dissemination and application of clinical practice guidelines and protocols. Previous publications have described *PRESTIGE*'s technical approach, including the use of a generic model for representing the knowledge content of clinical guidelines. This approach offers the possibility of 'plug-and-play' electronic distribution of clinical guidelines produced by multiple authoring bodies for use on multiple healthcare clinical management software platforms. A recent joint workshop held with the Section on Medical Informatics, Stanford University School of Medicine compared the European consensus approach developed in *PRESTIGE* with a parallel series of projects for computer-assisted protocol-based healthcare undertaken at Stanford and other American centres over the past, which confirmed the convergence and complementarity of our approaches, and holds out prospects of world-wide standardization in healthcare protocol knowledge representation. This paper summarises *PRESTIGE* conceptual model set which is the design of the project's approach.

1. Background: elements of the models

1.1 Knowledge

Guideline applications are *knowledge-based* applications. Guidelines are modules of clinical knowledge and the function of telematics guideline applications are to assist the availability, accessibility and appropriate use of that knowledge where it is relevant in clinical practice. *PRESTIGE*'s approach, derived from the DILEMMA project and other earlier work in clinical knowledge-bases systems, uses an explicit, declarative representation format in knowledge bases which facilitates the adaptation, flexible use and maintenance of clinical knowledge. This approach to knowledge representation requires an explicit knowledge model defining common and standard formats for computerised representation and use of items of knowledge. The *PRESTIGE* models incorporate and refine the *DILEMMA Generic Protocol Model* which offers a common electronic format for representing all clinical guidelines across specialities, user sites and application software platforms.

Clinical guidelines contain knowledge about medical concepts such as diagnoses, therapies and symptoms. They also contain knowledge about how to perform specific healthcare acts and activities such as monitoring consultations and treatment planning. Therefore a model of clinical guideline knowledge needs to call on a *model of healthcare activities and processes*. In DILEMMA this need was addressed by use of the UK National Health Service's *Common Basic Specification* (CBS: now retitled the NHS Healthcare Model), a model describing all forms of business performed by a health service.

1.2 Types of protocol entities

The *PRESTIGE* Protocol Model, which forms part of the *PRESTIGE* Conceptual Model, provides rules defining the knowledge statement constructs which may or must be present in a *PRESTIGE* protocol knowledgebase. As an Object model, it defines the kinds of entities (objects) which may appear in the protocol, with their permitted relations and attributes. Several main types of these objects can be identified.

- As protocols are knowledge, they will involve the use of general *concepts* (concepts of activities, acts and case-specific phenomena such as diagnoses and symptoms);
- protocols will have a structure consisting of the overall protocol and its component parts (which are all *individual, named instances* of the concept 'protocol version');
- protocols will include *expressions*, built out of concepts, instance names and syntax operations ('and', 'or', 'at least...'...) as prescribed in the BNF grammar rules for an expression type (cf. above), which can be used in several roles within the protocol:
  * conditions governing the appropriate use of a protocol or its parts (such as when a specific act should be performed). A condition is a (sometimes complex) specification of a (simple or composite) 'phenomenon' which can be shown to be true or false in the current context of an individual healthcare case. A phenomenon may consist of
  * individual patient attributes, symptoms and diagnoses (subject characteristics),
  * facts about things done (recorded acts and their attributes and states),
  * facts pertaining to a context of care ('patient already in the care of a chiropodist'; 'local availability of open access echocardiography'),
  * 'method' expressions to define the specific attributes of an act to be performed (e.g. a drug dosage),
  * 'templates' which define a set of data items which are to be collected.

1.3 How parts of the Conceptual Model are interlinked?

Several of the same types of object occur (either as uses of concepts or as named instances of a concept) in the other Conceptual Models, so that the different segments of the models are interlinked. Clinical concepts are used in the patient record to describe individual (instance) patient characteristics; act concepts are used to record things done; 'protocol use' instance objects will reference the individual (instance) protocol version, defined in the knowledge base, which is being used in an individual patient case. Patient records will identify specific agents as observing data or performing acts; an enterprise database will identify the agent type (concept) to which an individual agent belongs, and the roles and accountabilities which it can take on; a protocol knowledgebase may identify the agent types needed to execute a part of a protocol, or as recipients of a referral action specified in a protocol. The use of clinical terms used to express all concepts mentioned here will be constrained, in each application site, by a common terminology/semantics model.

For example: if a protocol is to specify the activity in which it is providing support to a clinician, the term it uses must exist in the application site terminology/semantics model, and must be classified in that model as a subtype of the concept 'activity'.

2. Patient Data

To implement telematics support for clinical guidelines, we need not only knowledge bases and knowledge models, but a mature electronic patient record. Clinical guidelines define patient-specific recommendations where the option selected is a function of the patient's medical condition and other factors. A useful computerised aid will be able to detect which options are relevant for an individual patient by directly interrogating the patient record. (Patient-specific prompts have been shown in randomised controlled trials to enhance the effectiveness of guideline implementation). Moreover a record should be capable of keeping track of how a guideline is used over time, since later options are also determined by earlier choices made. An important part of the *PRESTIGE* models is therefore the Electronic Patient Record [EPR] model specification which defines what facts and data a *PRESTIGE* application EPR must be able to represent.

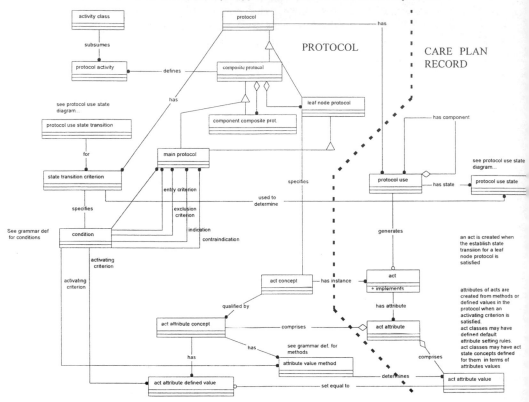

Figure 1. Protocol and care plan record: syntax and semantics of the protocol model

3.   The Healthcare Enterprise

As part of the planning and designing *PRESTIGE* applications, we analyse and document the existing clinical business process which a guideline is intended to assist, and which form the context where it will be used. This activity uses a methodology for business process re-engineering developed during the 3rd Framework AIM project SHINE. This approach identifies the organizations, professionals, data items and transactions involved in the cooperative delivery of healthcare by health services to patients. The models produced also allow a definition of how guidelines and associated technology will be inserted into modified versions of these processes (and, in some cases, how use of the guideline is intended to modify an existing process).

This type of analysis is not directly dealt with in the *PRESTIGE* conceptual model set since the models produced do not have to be expressed in a formalised notation and, although a vital step for application requirements definition, are not an immediate basis for software design. The project conceptual model set does, however, need to provide a formal representation of some healthcare organizational and administrative concepts which need to be explicitly addressed within software design. These include concepts about the healthcare *enterprise* (healthcare professionals, service units and services provided; types of resources required in providing specific services), together with administrative, demographic and *identification* data about individual patients. (Identification data about patients do not often play a significant role in clinical guideline themselves, but a consistent overall model of such information is nevertheless important in guideline applications, because cooperative healthcare professionals involved in applying a shared guideline (e.g. hospital staff and GP) may use different means to identify the same patient.)

Enterprise information enters in guideline applications in two ways. Often clinical guidelines need to be tailored to fit the specific constraints and circumstances of the local healthcare enterprise (such as the availability of specific skills and services): the local version of a guideline knowledgebase may then need to be extended or modified to refer explicitly to some local resource criterion; in applying a guideline, it may be necessary also to test such criteria by querying the current availability of local resources or services in an enterprise database. For both these services, a standard vocabulary and syntax must be provided for each enterprise to maintain its own such database and express enterprise constraints or criteria in its locally adapted guidelines.

4.   Clinical concepts and terms

PRESTIGE provides a set of generic models for guidelines, patient records and enterprise information which are independent of language and clinical domain. Within the language and clinical context of a given application site, it remains essential that a common and consistent clinical language is used in representing the site's clinical guideline knowledge, patient data and enterprise information. Without this common vocabulary, the telematics application will be unable to make proper combined use of these information sources in order to assist clinical professionals using a guideline. Standard clinical coding systems such as ICD, ICPC, SNOMED and (in the UK) Read Codes are currently able to meet part of this requirement, but are insufficient to express the knowledge or data entities used in typical clinical guidelines. The 3rd Framework project GALEN developed a compositional and generative approach to modelling medical concepts which provides a consistent means to create clinical termsets of any required scope and complexity ('acute chest pain with sudden onset precipitated by cold and exercise'). [6] In *PRESTIGE*, this model (the GRAIL Model) will be utilised to create supplements to standard codesets in current use (ICD, Read, ICPC) for each specific guideline application. GRAIL is not itself a part of the *PRESTIGE* Conceptual Model, but a harmonization process is being undertaken to ensure that the system of concepts used within GRAIL to model clinical concepts is consistent with (or mappable to) the assumptions and vocabulary of the Conceptual Model.

Note that this Model will not be a simple list of permitted terms. It will be a dictionary and (simplified) grammar for constructing noun phrases including legal qualifier phrases, together with a built-in classification of terms and term components which can be used to constrain the legal uses of a term within a knowledgebase or a patient record (and to guide the selection and browsing of terms by a patient record user interface or a knowledge authoring tool).

5.   Discussion

The models of the Protocol and the Patient also comprise specifications of the dynamic behaviour of various objects in the model. For example we describe formally how the dynamics of a *protocol use* object in the EPR [see figure] will involve creating objects to monitor the conditions specified in the protocol to govern its stages of execution, and creating *act* objects where specific protocol recommendations are being generated. This dynamics modelling effectively provides the semantics of the protocol model: it specifies the operational meaning of a guideline in terms of inferences performed on the basis of a protocol and a patient record, and its consequences in terms of recommended additions to a Care Plan within the EPR.

Different parts of the model will be used to constrain the final implementation of various components of the *PRESTIGE* technology:

* Both the Protocol Model and Terminology/Semantics Model will constrain the Guideline Authoring and Dissemination Tool (GAUDI) which is used to create and edit protocol knowledgebases.
* The EPR model will determine an API interface specification for all *PRESTIGE* application EPR implementations, to ensure that they deliver the care plan recording capabilities necessary for guideline applications.
* The Protocol Model (including dynamics) and EPR model will jointly directly determine the engineering implementation of the Protocol and Act Manager which performs the inferencing functions necessary to support protocol use.

See [3] and [4] for discussions of the requirements addressed by these model sets and the development methodologies for their utilisation in specific healthcare applications. The EON and INTErMED projects at the Section on Medical Informatics, Stanford University School of Medicine and associated American centres are pursuing similar objectives to *PRESTIGE* and have adopted a generic protocol modelling approach partly influenced by studying the results of the DILEMMA project which preceded *PRESTIGE*. [5] Comparisons conducted by SMI and *PRESTIGE* at a recent joint workshop indicates that the models and their operational semantics are broadly convergent; a full cross-mapping to demonstrate their formal equivalence is planned.

References

[1] C Gordon and JP Christensen (Eds.), Health Telematics for Clinical Guidelines and Protocols. IOS Press, 1995.

[2] C Gordon and M Veloso, The *PRESTIGE* Project: Implementing Guidelines in Healthcare. Medical Informatics Europe '96, IOS Press 1996, 887-891.

[3] C Gordon, SI Herbert, P Johnson, Knowledge Representation and Clinical Practice Guidelines: the DILEMMA and *PRESTIGE* projects. Medical Informatics Europe '96, IOS Press 1996, 511-515.

[4] C Gordon, P Johnson, C Waite, M Veloso. Algorithm and care pathway: clinical guidelines and healthcare processes. Proceeding of AIME97, Grenoble 1997.

[5] M A Musen, S W Tu, A K Das, Y Shahar, A Component-Based Approach to Automation of Protocol-Directed Therapy. JAMIA, forthcoming.

[6] A L Rector, J E Rogers, P Pole. The GALEN High Level Ontology. MIE 96, 174-178.

Medical Informatics Europe '97
C. Pappas et al. (Eds.)
IOS Press, 1997

Informatic support for processing the data regarding the environment factors possibly involved in the etiopathogenesis of insulin-dependent diabetes mellitus ETIODIAB

Simona Alecu[1], Viorel Dadarlat[1], Emilia Stanciu[1],
Constantin Ionescu-Tirgoviste[2], Ana Maria Konerth[2]

[1] *Software ITC, Bucharest, Romania*
[2] *"N.Paulescu" Institute of Nutrition and Metabolic Diseases, Bucharest*

Abstract. Diabetes represents a heterogeneous group of disturbances, which can have a different aetiology, but have in common glucidic, lipidic and proteinic metabolic disturbances. Insulin-dependent diabetes appears in genetically susceptible persons, as an autoimmune disease activated by environment factors. Epidemiological studies performed in different countries, notice the increasing of diabetes cases in the last decades.
Therefore the informatic system **EtioDiab** (from Etiopathological diabetes) has been developed. The purpose of this system is to assist the medical research regarding the environment factors involved in the etiopathogenesis of insulin-dependent diabetes. The system offers the possibility of calculation of many statistic indicators, of graphic representation of the recorded data, of verification of the statistical hypotheses.

1. Introduction

The **ETIODIAB** system has been designed to assist the medical research regarding the environment factors possibly involved in the etiopathogenesis of insulin-dependent diabetes mellitus [1]. The principal factors involved in the insulin-dependent diabetes we study are: alimentation mode, infections, vaccines, etc.

The system provides facilities for recording the information considered in the **EURODIAB ACE** - substudy 2 [2] and for complex processing of this information.

For system testing two control groups will be considered: one of diabetic persons, the other of non-diabetic persons. In the first stage the diabetic group will include 100 persons and the non-diabetic group 300 persons.

ETIODIAB allows the registration of a large amount of information (over 400 data items), like:

- identification data (date of birth, sex, date of first insulin injection etc.);
- family history (date of birth, insulin dependent diabetes presence, age at onset etc. for the parents and brothers/sisters of the child) (figure 1);

- birth characteristics (gestational age, birth weight, caesarean section etc.);
- problems in the neonatal period (severe infections, respiratory diseases etc.);
- mothers pregnancy history (pre-eclampsia, gestational diabetes, auto-immune diseases, infectious diseases etc.);
- medication during pregnancy (antibiotic, analgesic, antihypertensive etc. at any time and on trimesters);
- diseases in the child after the perinatal period (common contagious diseases, chronic diseases, allergic diseases, other severe diseases/illness requiring hospitalisation);
- growth patterns;
- vaccinations (tuberculosis, polio, tetanus etc.);
- early nutrition (length of exclusive breast feeding, age at first introducing formula etc.);
- hospital recording data (birth details of the child, child's diseases in the neonatal period, medication to child in the neonatal period, mother's diseases during pregnancy, regular medication during pregnancy).

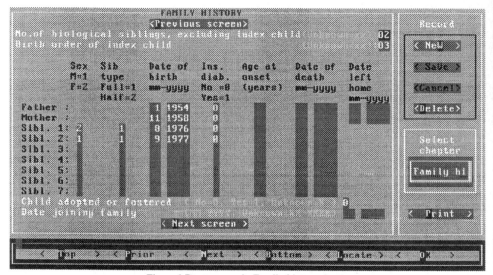

Figure 1 Person record - Family history chapter

2. Statistic processing and graphic representation

The **ETIODIAB** system allows the processing of a lot of recorded information in short time with accuracy. A flexible mechanism has been implemented for dynamic selection of the analysed set (figure 2), which can be:

- a group of records
- all records.

The selection criterion can be:

- simple (Example: sex=male)
- complex (Example: sex=male AND age<5 AND antipolio vaccination).

The specification of the selection criterion is easy, the system offering lists of adequate options. The parameters for the specified type of processing can also be selected from the lists offered by the system (figure 3).

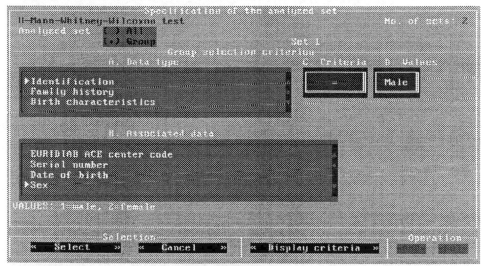

Figure 2 "Set selection" screen

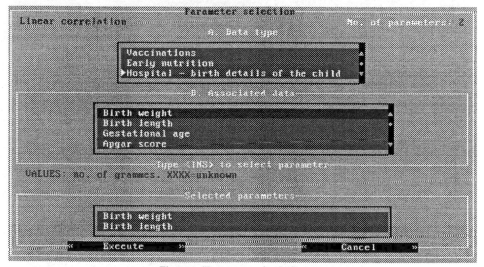

Figure 3 "Parameter selection" screen

The system offers the possibility of calculation of many statistic indicators, of graphic representation of the recorded data (figure 4), of verification of the statistical hypotheses. The tests implemented are: t-Student, χ^2, U-Mann-Whitney-Wilcoxon, Fisher-Snedecor, Shapiro-Wilk, iteration test [3] [4] [5]. Methods such as: dispersional analysis, correlation, regression have also been implemented.

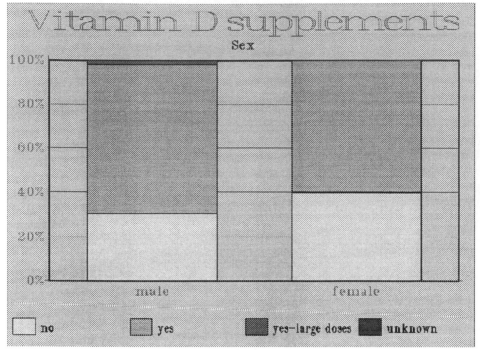

Figure 4 Graphic representation

ETIODIAB offers a friendly interface for recording the data and also allows their validation (for each type of the data verifies if the value is between the accepted ones, for the calendaristic dates is verified the correlation between them, between the recorded ages etc.).

3. System structure

The system components are:
- databases that contain information about investigated persons, selection parameters for testing, etc.
- programs that implement the functions provided by the system.

The main functions offered by the **EtioDiab** system are (figure 5):
- person records;
- statistic processing;
- graphic representation;
- system administration.

The system has been developed on IBM compatible personal computers under the FoxPro 2.5 environment and offers the user a modern, friendly interface.

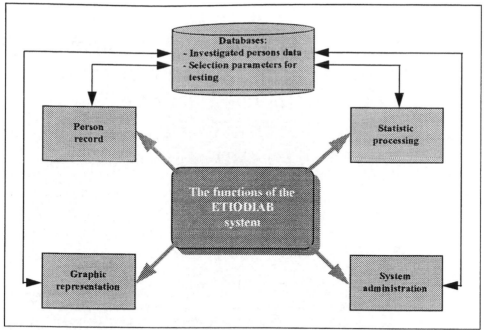

Figure 5 System structure

4. Conclusion

The system will be installed in the first stage in all diabetic centres involved in this study and then in all diabetic centres in the country.

The use of **EtioDiab** in medical research will allow:
- easy management of information
- high-quality processing of the recorded information
- information exchanges between all diabetic centres in our country.

References

[1] Genetic and environmental risk factors for type 1 diabetes (IDDM) including a discussion on the autoimune basis. Freund Publishing House, England, 1992.

[2] EURODIAB ACE - Substudy 2: Environmental determinants of IDDM in childhood. Protocol, 1993.

[3] Geoffrey J. Bourke. Interpretation and Uses of Medical Statistics. Blackwell Scientific Publication Oxford and Edinburgh.

[4] Ilie P. Vasilescu. Informatized statistics for sciences about men. Vol. 1 and 2, Military Publishing House, Bucharest, 1991 and 1992.

[5] Ioan Constantinescu, Dan Golumbovici, Constantin Militaru. Processing of the experimental data using computers. Technical Publishing House, Bucharest, 1980.

Medical Informatics Europe '97
C. Pappas et al. (Eds.)
IOS Press, 1997

A Hypertext Information System
for Standard Operating Procedures
in Haematological Intensive Care

A. Horsch[1], R. Sokol[1], D. Heneka[2], G. Lasic[2]

[1]Institute of Medical Statistics and Epidemiology, Technical University of Munich, Germany

[2]Department of Haematology and Oncology, Technical University of Munich, Germany

Abstract. In times of cost reduction efforts the role of standard operating procedures for both medical and nursing procedures gets increasing importance. Such
standards are necessary if the quality of patient care shall not suffer but even improve. While some sophisticated approaches are coming up with generation of clinical processes from formal protocol models in connection with documentation systems the clinical practice actually looks quite different: Paper-based „operating
standards" are used in day-to-day work, if any. In this paper a simple and powerful
WWW-based hypertext information system for easy provision and maintenance of
nursing standards is presented.

1. Introduction

Quality management is getting more and
more important on the background of ex-
ploding costs in health care. One basics for
the implementation of quality management
are Standard Operating Procedures (SOP)
for the all clinical processes. In order to
achieve wide range quality improvement
such SOPs have to be established in collaboration between a couple of expert
centres of the respective domain. For
nursing there are no fixed standards up to
now in Germany. Some kind of guideline

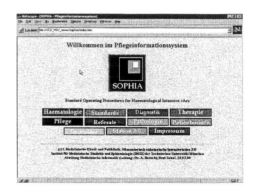

Fig. 1: SOPHIA homepage

exists in the form of classical text books like [1]. But the implementation of quality assurance lies in the responsibility of each individual hospital, clinic or department.

An important preparing step for the establishment of a widely recognised standard is the
communication of existing standards between expert centres and from the expert centres to
non-experts. A paper-based documentation of standards is in our opinion inadequate for this
purpose (and not only for this purpose). In order to support communication as well as updating of the standards a web-based computerised information system for nursing standards
in haemato-oncological intensive care has been implemented at the I. Medical Clinic of the
University Hospital Klinikum rechts der Isar of the TU Munich.

2. Related work

In [2] a formalised generic protocol model is supposed to provide protocol-based decision support for clinical care. The semantics of the model is defined in terms of a protocol knowledge base subsumed by a protocol model, and active care plan records deduced from the knowledge base. The authors suggest the usage of such a system as a „standard" or as a „less imperative guideline" that may also include „sets of alternative actions upon which the clinician is invited to exercise his or her judgement and to make a selection". In our opinion, guidelines as a preparation for standards can be implemented in a much more natural and intuitive way by a hypertext information system.

There are from our observation only few approaches to support nursing quality assurance. One of them is subsumed in the very formal general protocol-based approach of [2] to decision support in clinical care. Most approaches concentrate on nursing planning and documentation [3,4,5,6]. They have been triggered by new German laws aiming at cost reduction in health care. But as far as we know, nowhere such a system is in routine operation [7]. Despite this finding, due to our own experience and to that of colleagues the acceptance of computer systems by the nursing personnel is highly encouraging.

3. Objectives and requirements

The SOPs in the intensive care unit 3/0 are used as paper documents in several standing records. The whole collection has about 1000 pages and is organised quite similar to a book with chapters, sections and subsections. Its articles are printed MS-WORD documents.

The objective of the study were 1) to implement a part of the nursing guidelines as a Web-based information system and 2) to evaluate the new system in comparison with the conventional paper-based system.

The objectives of the evaluation were to investigate, whether 1) the new structure of the information, its presentation layout and its extent meet the users needs, 2) the new system brings, in comparison with the paper-based system a benefit with respect to speed of information retrieval.

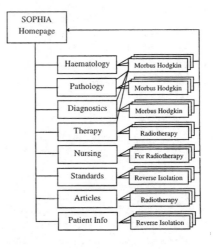

Fig. 2: Main structure of SOPHIA

The system had to be designed to meet the following requirements:

R1) *Fast access:* In practical use the access is very time-critical. A question rising during daily care must be answered immediately, i. e. without any delay. There is very few time. The information must be presented in a form suited for 'reception at one glance'.

R2) *Adequately detailed information:* As to the comprehensiveness of the information, different levels are required. An experienced user should not be burdened with too many well-known details. On the other hand, the system must also cover the needs of colleagues who are new in the department or are inexperienced.

R3) *Easy content update and maintenance:* One of the most serious obstacles of the paper-based procedure collection is the limited amount of updates that can be made on the sheets. In our experience many of the instructions become more and more unreadable due to the many hand-written corrections. Therefore the content of the system must be simply to update and maintain by non-professionals.

4. The application

To get a system with fast access to the needed content (requirement R1) the information has been structured in different chapters containing sections (figure 2). Sections contain the information or are once more divided into sub-sections. There is no further sub-division of the content. The access to any information requires at maximum 3 mouse clicks. The choice of chapter topics reflects the different views of users consulting the system in different situations and with different expertise. Together with additional cross-links between (sub-) sections and chapters a very quick access is guaranteed. On any page there is a button for direct return to the SOPHIA homepage (figure 1) with the chapter buttons.

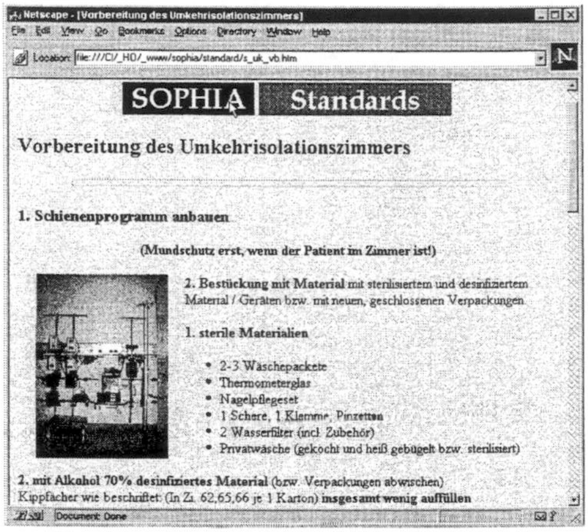

Fig. 3: Content page in chapter *Standards*

The chapters offer information with different completeness of explanations (requirement R2). The chapter *Standards* contains the SOPs for well-defined sub-tasks explained step-by-step for use in time-critical routine. There is no superfluous word in these texts (see example in figure 3). In the chapter *Nursing* one finds overall instructions for what procedures are required or recommended in the course of a certain therapy, for example radiotherapy (decision-support). This is also short but complete information for nursing routine as general background to the application of related SOPs. The chapters *Pathology*, *Diagnostics* and *Therapy* give background information about the disease and the medical procedures in relatively short form. Deep information for learning during quiet phases in day-to-day work are offered in the chapter *Articles* (Button *Referate* in the German homepage). The chapter *Patient-Info* contains information material for the patients and their relatives to inform in simple words about the disease and the treatment and nursing of the patient. An example for such a patient information is shown in figure 4.

In order to provide easy facilities for update and maintenance (requirement R3) the system SOPHIA has been implemented as a Web-based information system. That means, that the text has been broken down into thematically closed (sub-)sections. Each section is formulated as a HTML document (content page). The access to these content pages is provided by index pages (chapter pages; section pages referring to sub-sections). These pages are easy to update and maintain using a simple text editor or, more comfortable, a HTML editor.

Up to now SOPHIA is installed locally on a PC. Netscape Navigator 2.01 (Netscape Communications Corporation, Mountain View CA, USA) has been used as browser in the pilot project.

5. Evaluation

From April 1 to June 15 of 1996 the prototype has been evaluated. At this time it comprised a representative selection from different chapters with a volume of about 7% (73 machine written DIN A4 pages) of the complete paper-based SOP collection having a total volume of about 1000 written pages. The evaluation was done by a questionnaire. 15 of the 17 questionnaires distributed to the users in the haematological intensive care unit were filled in by 7 nurses, 2 doctors and 4 students of the unit and 2 guests from other departments. Here the questions and summarised answers:

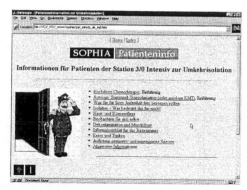

Fig. 4: Patient info about reverse isolation

Question 1: Is the information adequately structured in order to fasten access in comparison the paper-based SOP collection?

All users have found the information structured better than before („clearly arranged", „practicable", „easy to understand"). Retrieval has become easier. There are several paths on which an information can be reached depending on the user's view. Some users missed an index. Most users wish an online help facility. The layout and readability of the information was found to be not as good as on written paper, but acceptable. The majority of user sessions had a duration of 5-10 minutes.

Question 2: Is the depth and quality of information sufficient with respect to questions about general and special nursing and medical problems?

As expected, the different groups of professionals judged differently about the information offer. The main critics are that the information is not as comprehensive as it could be or needs to be. The partial incompleteness of the paper-based sources and missing related information that has not yet been incorporated in the system are probably the reasons for this. Some users missed a separate chapter *Hygiene*.

Question 3: What are the reasons for use of the system and how successful are they felt?

The system was most frequently used to get answers to time-critical questions on nursing procedures (chapters *Standards* and *Nursing*). On the next place in the ranking are general medical questions. Due to the partial incompleteness of the content only about half of the uses were felt to be a full success.

6. Discussion

The pilot project has proven that a WWW-based information system like SOPHIA is adequate to provide a high quality information service for an intensive care unit. Following a clear and simple hypertext structure the access to SOPs can be speeded up. The information can easily be updated and maintained. This supports the use of nursing standards. Furthermore, the standards can be communicated electronically with partners from other expert centres. When provided in the Internet, a broad and continued discussion about the standards of different institutions becomes possible. This can promote the evolutionary establishment of de facto standards.

Up to now, the system SOPHIA is installed on a local PC. It contains just a small part of the information needed. Step by step, the system is being completed by leading personnel of the intensive care unit. It is planned to bring the system into the Internet when it contains enough information. In parallel to the content import the system is continuously improved with regard to access comfort and user friendliness.

7. Acknowledgement

We with to thank Prof. Rastetter, chief of the Department of Haematology, and Prof. Neiß, director of the Institute of Medical Statisitics and Epidemiology, for supporting the pilot project SOPHIA. We thank our colleagues at the intensive care unit, their students and guests for testing our prototype and filling in the questionnaire.

References

[1] Juchli J: Pflege. Praxis und Theorie der Gesundheits- und Krankenpflege. 7., neubearb. Aufl., Georg Thieme Verlag, Stuttgart, New York, 1994

[2] Herbert SI, Gordon CJ, Jackson-Smale A, Salis JLR: Protocols for Clinical Care, MIE'94, 30-35

[3] Bott OJ, Penger OS, Terstappen A, Pretschner DP: Zur Spezifikation der Anforderungen an ein rechnergestütztes Pflegeinformationssystem für psychiatrische Kliniken, GMDS'95, 360-365

[4] Schrader U, Balint R, Marx R: CareBase - Eine Informationsdatenbank für den Pflegeprozeß, GMDS'95, 351-354

[5] Hütter-Semkat H, Eichstädter R, Herr S, Schrader U: Informationsverarbeitung aus pflegerischer Sicht. In: Haas, Köhler, Kuhn, Petrzyk, Prokosch (Hrsg.): Praxis der Informationsverarbeitung im Krankenhaus, ecomed Verlag, Landsberg, 1996, pp. 15-19

[6] Opitz E: Informationsverarbeitung im Pflegebereich - Checklisten und Marktlage. In: Haas, Köhler, Kuhn, Petrzyk, Prokosch (Hrsg.): Praxis der Informationsverarbeitung im Krankenhaus, ecomed Verlag, Landsberg, 1996, pp. 123-130

[7] Schulz B, Karll A: EDV in der Krankenpflege. Ergebnisse einer Erhebung in Hessischen Krankenhäusern, GMDS'95, 355-359

Corresponding author

Dr. Alexander Horsch
Institut für Medizinische Statistik und Epidemiologie
TU München, Ismaninger Str. 22, D-81675 München
Tel +49-89-4140-4330, Fax +49-89-4974
Email alexander.horsch@imse.med.tu-muenchen.de

Medical Informatics Europe '97
C. Pappas et al. (Eds.)
IOS Press, 1997

The Place of SGML and HTML in Building Electronic Patient Records

David Pitty, Colin Gordon, Philip Reeves, Andrew Capey, Pedro Vieyra, Tony Rickards
Healthcare Informatics Team, Royal Brompton Hospital NHS Trust, London, UK

Abstract. The authors are concerned that, although popular, SGML (Standard Generalized Markup Language) is only one approach to capturing, storing, viewing and exchanging healthcare information and does not provide a suitable paradigm for solving most of the problems associated with paper based patient record systems. Although a discussion of the relative merits of SGML, HTML (HyperText Markup Language) may be interesting, we feel such a discussion is avoiding the real issues associated with the most appropriate way to model, represent, and store electronic patient information in order to solve healthcare problems, and therefore the medical informatics community should firstly concern itself with these issues. The paper substantiates this viewpoint and concludes with some suggestions of how progress can be made.

1. Overview of SGML and HTML

SGML is a standard for creating and storing documents and document archives in a platform independent way. Facilities for managing and searching documents can be provided as long as the documents are all members of a class of documents which share the same Document Type Definition (DTD). The DTD consists of a set of tags that define the type of data elements from which documents are composed. For example, if we were building a Discharge Summary DTD the tags we would use might include <PATIENT NAME>, <PROBLEM>, <DIAGNOSIS>, <PRESCRIPTION>, <REFERRAL DATE>, etc. By searching on a tag such as <PATIENT NAME> all the associated discharge summaries for a particular patient can be retrieved. HTML is one instance of an SGML DTD which is used by the authors of Web pages as a document interchange and display standard. So the tags in the HTML DTD are, for example, <TITLE>, <CENTRE> etc. Web browsers such as Netscape understand the HTML DTD and can therefore read the tags and display the information in the appropriate form for the type of workstation being used. For further information see [1] and [2].

2. What is an Electronic Patient Record?

The term 'electronic patient record' has many different interpretations ranging from a set of unstructured scanned documents that can be indexed and browsed, to a structure for representing healthcare concepts in a form that supports routine clinical practice, audit, healthcare administration, research, decision support, and so on. Development of an electronic patient record is no different from developing any other information technology based solution to a problem, except perhaps that the multi-disciplinary healthcare environment is particularly complex. Using a rational approach to problem solving we should first identify problems to be addressed and then evaluate appropriate solutions, taking measurements at each stage so that success of the implementation can be judged.

Following the argument that technology can be employed to solve problems, the authors agree that the term 'electronic patient record' should be used to describe a mechanism for storing patient data that facilitates solving recognised healthcare problems. A strategy that solves many problems is therefore preferable to a strategy that solves few, within the constraints of cost effectiveness.

3. Problems and requirements

So, what are the existing problems with information management in healthcare? The following list of known problems and requirements is categorised by the different players involved. The list is not exhaustive but is broad enough to illustrate the technical arguments that follow.

Clinicians

C1   There is often poor availability of clinical information relating to the patient, such as medical history, current treatments, allergies, test results etc.

C2   Healthcare professionals (HCPs) rarely have access to management plans of other HCPs.

C3   Results are rarely accompanied by an explanation of how they should be interpreted.

C4   Information is usually represented in the format used by the originator, rather than what is useful to the recipient.

C5   Information relating to 'best practice' according to evidence or consensus is not available.

C6   HCPs do not have access to on-line reference data, particularly in a context sensitive form.

Administrators

A1   Tests are often duplicated at several sites and patient histories are taken at each stage in the healthcare process which results in wasted resources.

A2   Lack of dissemination of 'best practice' also means that the most appropriate or efficient diagnostic tests or treatments are not always used.

A3   Good quality audit information to improve efficiency and outcome is not available.

A4   The healthcare process itself is poorly defined and so co-ordination of activities is difficult, leading to repeated administrative activities such as recording names and addresses.

Researchers

R1   It is very time consuming and expensive to perform research using paper medical records.

R2   Epidemiology and other studies can only be performed against coding schemes which do not always have the relevant level of detail.

R3   There is little consistency in the treatment of patients with the same condition which makes outcome analysis difficult.

Patients

P1   There is little information available to patients about the healthcare they are likely to receive.

P2   There are considerable delays in obtaining appointments at clinics.

P3   They are asked the same questions by many different HCPs.

P4   HCPs seem unaware of what treatments, procedures etc. have been carried out at other sites.

Other Requirements and Problems

O1   Warnings for drug contraindications and similar dangers.

O2   Reminders or prompts for performing particular tests or making particular observations.

O3   Notifications of result availability etc.

O4   Support for user friendly data entry.

O5   Validation of data entry (such as patient identifiers).

O6   Important information held in the paper notes can easily be overlooked.

O7   Co-operative care and real-time resource management cannot be provided with paper records.

4.   Potential solutions

As with the many varied interpretations of what an electronic patient record is and what is should do, there are at least as many potential solutions. For example, if a formalised approach to administering healthcare was implemented, then use of telephones and fax machines would solve problems such as C1, C2, C3, A1, R3, P3, and P4, with contributions also being made to solutions for C4, C5, and A2. However, an opportunity to re-engineer healthcare in this way is unlikely to arise.

Information technology can be used to support process changes, particularly in the areas of distribution and exchange of information, for example exchanging EDIFACT messages, exchanging SGML or HTML documents, and exchanging scanned documents. These approaches tend to help solve the same problems as use of telephone and fax in terms of exchanging information, but are perhaps more likely to succeed as the process engineering required to enforce their use is not so great - that is, the Consultant is not forced to talk to the GP but the GP gets to share the relevant information anyway. This is not an ideal way to introduce better communication between HCPs, and it is likely that use of information technology in this way will forfeit solutions to requirements C2, C3, C5, R3 and A2 which rely on co-operation between clinicians.

Although these approaches allow data to be viewed in many places at once and support exchange of documents between HCPs, neither of them solve the remaining problems identified as they do not allow data to be structured and searched in a meaningful and efficient way. By duplicating the document format of the paper records the weaknesses are also duplicated which makes research, decision support, context sensitive reference searching, medical audit, etc., difficult and inefficient to perform, and impossible to perform if standard DTDs are not used.

5. SGML and HTML as a solution

5.1 Data capture and storage

SGML could provide a standard way of describing healthcare documents and their structure but only if a common set of DTDs is used. This standardisation problem is the same as attempting to produce a standard for ECG reports, test results, referral letters, care plans, prescription forms, etc. This is a difficult task that is suited more to the professional bodies than to the medical informatics community. The use of SGML also restricts data entry mechanisms to forms where the information to be collected must be configured in advance, and the order in which data is collected is dictated by the forms. This is undesirable, particularly in General Practice where a broad spectrum of observations and symptoms may be elicited in a short consultation. In addition, SGML does not provide the facilities to capture semantic or temporal relationships between data items and thus the record can only support simple inefficient searches and cannot offer interpretation along with the data.

Consistency of data captured is also a problem without adequate facilities to refer to previously captured information or reference information. As an example, it would be difficult and inefficient to check that data entered in a field is consistent with an established vocabulary such as Read or ICD10.

Consider an example which demonstrates the inelegance of an SGML based EPR. A patient undergoes a diagnostic angiogram followed by surgery. After the angiogram a report is written by the cardiologist using a DTD for an angiogram, and the surgeon writes an operation note using a DTD for a surgical intervention. From the data in these two documents many others are created, such as audit reports, discharge summaries, invoices etc., but each of these documents, or 'views' of the data, will need to be defined a stored separately because SGML does not support concurrent structures across multiple document types, and a different set of these documents will be required for each site according to their local preferences. The important relationship between the documents (i.e. they are all derivatives of the angiogram report and operation note) will be lost.

5.2 Data retrieval

The basic requirement for retrieval of electronic patient information is that any subset of one or more patient's records can be retrieved and displayed in a form that is appropriate for the user. For example, the needs of a General Practitioner and a surgeon are quite different but both information views should be derived from the same data. SGML only allows data to be displayed in the format it was entered. Medical equipment manufacturers may use HTML as a way of providing industry standard open access to their data, and they may even define their own 'proprietary' SGML DTDs in order to describe their data sets, but without standardised SGML DTDs across the manufacturers the information will serve no other purpose than being displayed because it cannot be interpreted.

Figure 1 shows a typical SGML-based architecture where a number of different SGML based servers holding a variety of clinical and administrative information can all be accessed by a low cost workstation using HTML, but its functionality is limited to viewing information because there is no semantic relationship between the data from the various sources. Even if standardised tags are used across the various DTDs the querying and searching mechanisms that can be applied to SGML documents are inadequate as they do not work across documents that are derived from different DTDs. In addition, the viewer is limited to retrieving documents in the form specified by the originator. The use of low cost technology described in [3] does not therefore meet requirements.

6. Alternative solutions

In order to solve the additional problems identified in section 4 an alternative approach is required that provides more than just a document based mechanism for storing healthcare data. It is necessary to model data sets, data structures, and semantic and temporal relationships between data items without worrying about the documents that hold these data items. Figure 2 illustrates this approach. The electronic patient record may be distributed across sites, such as General Practices and hospitals, but each record is compliant with the models. Unification and integration of data sets is thus provided in the structure of the electronic patient record itself rather than at the workstation.

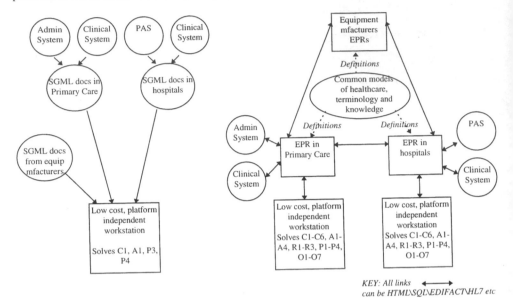

Figure 1 - Typical SGML based architecture

Figure 2 -Typical architecture using common models for EPR design

Note that links between systems can be of any suitable type, whether that be HTML, SQL, EDIFACT, etc. There are already high level object oriented conceptual models that can be applied to this scenario that also allow new technology such as Common Object Request Broker Architectures (CORBA) to be exploited. By using a well engineered model for the electronic patient record it is possible to present documents and views of data in any user-required format from the same data set without additional definitions. Generic viewing tools can utilise this freedom, user interfaces can be tailored to the type of user, and information can be provided in a form that the user is familiar with. In addition, healthcare organisations can tailor reports and documents to their own preferences.

This technology supports the use of guidelines in routine clinical care which has the benefit of improving quality, efficiency and outcome of the healthcare process. It can also provide context sensitive reference information, alerts for potential problems, generation of reminders, ensure consistency in interpretation of data, and provide good quality audit and research information. Data entry systems and data retrieval systems can be provided by any appropriate mechanism according to the requirements and cost constraints of each particular organisation. This could include HTML based browsers, Visual Basic front ends, 4GLs, Visual C++ systems, etc. In addition, references to the various data sources can be of any convenient form such as URLs or other pointers.

Looking at other work in this area, the proceedings of Medical Informatics Europe '96 returned three papers covering similar work [4][5][6]. Paper [6], and on further investigation paper [4], both explicitly separate the patient record from the HTML based view of patient information. The remaining paper is unashamedly based on emulating the paper records and presents a fair argument to support this view. However, there are countless papers in the same proceedings that approach the issues of distributed healthcare environments, open standards, information interchange, electronic patient records, interoperability, advanced user interfaces and so on with little mention of SGML although this does not of course prove conclusively that the approach is wrong.

7. Conclusions

SGML is based around the concept of documents. As such there is no separation of functions for capture and display from those of storage and representation. We know that each user group requires views of the data suited to the tasks they must perform which are not always document based. Benson proposes that the failure of information technology in healthcare is due to modern databases not being up to the job and that the SGML document based approach may be better [3]. The more realistic answer is that the problem is inherently difficult, in which case SGML will restrict our ability to solve the problem rather than enhance it. We know that many computer systems have failed in healthcare (and many other domains) because of the poor quality of user interfaces. Again, the SGML \ HTML solution does not solve this problem, instead it restricts our ability to solve the problem. We know that introducing computer systems into routine clinical care is a more difficult task than building software solutions so we need to use every software engineering tool available to build high quality user friendly systems, and this means technology such as visual programming environments, re-usable designs, re-usable code modules, careful requirements work, user customisable interfaces, pen based and voice based technology and so on. Building forms in SGML simply will not do.

SGML is concerned only with syntax and is therefore unable to capture temporal and semantic relationships between the data items in a record, particularly between documents derived from different DTDs. SGML is therefore not suited to providing different views of the same data for different types of user, it is not suited to providing dynamic views of data that can be constructed by the user at run time, and it is not able to provide anything but the most simplistic searches based on sequential parsing of the SGML documents.

These functions can only be achieved by storing information in a format that is independent of the way it is entered or viewed. Such a representation must also be able to support the correct semantic and temporal relationships between data items. Section 6 describes such an approach using a common electronic patient record model based on an object oriented model of healthcare, plus associated models of terminology and knowledge.

In the absence of a meta-model for defining DTDs, healthcare organisations and manufacturers will doubtless create their own DTDs. These documents will not be interchangeable and cannot be searched as a whole. Defining a meta-model for DTDs will help but the task is immense. Using a top-down model of healthcare is the only practical way to manage such complexity. Such a model is the same as that required to build electronic patient records in the architecture described in section 6.

On the plus side, SGML and HTML offer benefits for the exchange of healthcare information from departmental systems and the electronic patient record, or between electronic patient records, but this is only one approach. Section 6 proposes a solution that utilises the benefits of SGML and the benefits of using core models for representing patient data as well as accommodating other exchange formats such as EDIFACT and DICOM. The key point is that SGML DTDs and the electronic patient record must be derived from the same models. If so, the two approaches are complimentary.

SGML and HTML are popular technologies at the present time and have advantages in wide availability and acceptability, but this should not be seen as a reason for utilising inappropriate technology to solve a problem. In the words of Fred Brooks "there is no silver bullet" [7].

8. References

[1] A Gentle Introduction to SGML: TEI Guidelines for Electronic Text Encoding and Interchange, http://etext.virginia.edu/tei-tocs1.html.
[2] Colby M, Jackson D, Special Edition Using SGML, Que Corporation, 1996.
[3] Benson T, SGML and EPR Application of the Standard Generalized Markup Language (SGML) in Electronic Patient Records Version 1, 6th August 1996, for the NHS Executive's EPR Project Board.
[4] Karlsson D, Ekdahl C, Shahsavar N, Gill H, Forsum U, Wigertz O, A WWW-based Decision-Support System using Medical Logic Modules and Hypertext, Proceedings of Medical Informatics Europe '96, IOS Press, 1996.
[5] Bouaud J, Seroussi B, Zweigenbaum P, An Experiment towards a Document-Centered Hypertextual Computerised Patient Record, Proceedings of Medical Informatics Europe '96, IOS Press, 1996.
[6] Laforest F, Frenot S, Flory A, A New Approach for Hypermedia Medical Records Management, Proceedings of Medical Informatics Europe '96, IOS Press, 1996.
[7] Brooks F, The Mythical Man-Month, Addison-Wesley, 1975.

Medical Informatics Europe '97
C. Pappas et al. (Eds.)
IOS Press, 1997

Design and functional specification of the Synapses Federated Healthcare Record Server

Petter Hurlen[1] and Knut Skifjeld[1]
on behalf of the Synapses Consortium[2]

[1] Siemens Nixdorf Informasjonssystemer, Oslo, Norway
[2] St. James's Hospital/FDVH, Dublin , Ireland

Abstract. Synapses is a project funded under the EU Health Telematics Framework IV Programme. Synapses sets out to solve problems of sharing data between autonomous information systems, by providing generic and open means to combine healthcare records or dossiers consistently, simply, comprehensibly and securely, whether the data passes within a single healthcare institution or between institutions. This paper presents the specification of the Synapses server, the kernel concept of Synapses. It describes the basis in the European prestandard for Electronic Healthcare Record Architecture, the interfaces to the Synapses server and different integration mechanisms for systems providing information to the server. The specification will be verified at a number of validation sites, and the final result will be in the public domain.

1. Introduction

The delivery of healthcare is undergoing a change from having a single carer relationship to one where the patient is managed by several health professionals at the same time - shared care. A major impediment to progress towards shared care and cost-containment is the inability to share information across systems and between carers automatically. Today, patient information may be found in paper records, electronic healthcare records and other independent information systems, each with its own technical culture and view of the healthcare domain. There is general agreement that no single vendor will be able to meet all the information processing needs of an individual hospital, let alone of the whole healthcare sector [1, 2]. Thus, there is a need to define mechanisms for sharing data between different systems.

Synapses (HC 1046) is a three year project, starting in 1996, funded under the Health Telematics Programme of the European Commission. It sets out to solve problems of sharing data between autonomous information systems, by providing generic and open means to combine healthcare records or dossiers consistently, simply, comprehensibly and securely, whether the data passes within a single healthcare institution or between institutions. By facilitating data sharing, Synapses can provide potentially immediate access by the carer to all relevant healthcare information wherever and in whatever format it is stored.

Some developments do address problems related to sharing data, but most are not in the public domain or do only focus on specific types of the healthcare information. Synapses uses the healthcare record as basis for its approach to data sharing, and the result will be placed in public domain. The kernel of Synapses is the specification of the Synapses server supplying a set of services which support access to distributed components of healthcare records.

The background for Synapses has previously been described [3]. The Initial phase of Synapses focused on drawing together and building on the extensive work and results in the field of Telematics IT and Telecommunications and in CEN TC/251 [4, 5]. User requirements were collected and analysed [6, 7], and the consequences for the Synapses server described in the first draft Synapses Object Model and Object Dictionary specification [8, 9]. This paper focuses on the second step of the Synapses project, the Synapses integration mechanisms and the Synapses server services. This is described in the Synapses server specification [10].

The Synapses specifications will be implemented and validated in a wide variety of clinical domains with different patterns of usage - within hospitals, among primary carers in a local area, across carers for chronic illness; a total of 11 sites in 10 countries will be involved in the validation process. The experience from the validation will be reflected in the final version of the Synapses specifications.

2. Basic Synapses Concepts

The kernel concept of Synapses is that of a *Synapses server* supporting access to distributed components of *federated healthcare records* (FHCR). Record components may be requested by *Synapses clients*. A Synapses *feeder system* is a system that supplies record components to the Synapses server on a routine basis or on request.

Synapses takes an object-oriented view of the FHCR. All record components are regarded as *objects*. The base (super) class definitions for the objects are found in the *Synapses foundation classes* (object model). These class definitions are shared among all the participants of the Synapses consortium. The derived (sub) class definitions for a specific set of records are found in *Synapses class dictionaries* (object dictionaries) and *Synapses record structure dictionaries*. The class definition for each object (component) of a federated healthcare record can thus be found in a class dictionary. The class dictionary may vary between validation sites, but a maximum degree of consistency is attempted. The record structure dictionaries defines relationships between classes of record components, that is, legal structures hierarchies that can be found in records.

A request for data from a federated healthcare record would thus be a request for an object (component) of the record. The object would return the data it comprises, if necessary after retrieving them from a feeder system. An object may comprise its own data or the methods for retrieving the data, possibly from 'synapses' feeder systems. If a record does not comprise the appropriate object to provide the requested data, for instance comprising the necessary method to retrieve data from a feeder system, it must be created according to the class definition in the class dictionary.

3. ENV 12265

Synapses uses the European prestandard ENV 12265 *Electronic healthcare record architecture* [11] as basis for its definition of electronic healthcare records and record components. According to this prestandard, a record is both a virtual concept and a real entity with defined boundaries.

The record's information *content* can be divided in separate units. Each unit is called a *Record item*. It is recommended that the record information is divided into medically meaningful units, and that record items represent what the user or the developer of the record system regards as the smallest meaningful units of information. This could, e.g., correspond to data items in data base systems and paragraphs or sentences in text based systems.

It is generally agreed that parts of the record information can only be interpreted correctly in its full context. The context may be the result of other tests, other medical considerations, comments, plans, etc. The context must thus be preserved as part of the record, and be presented when a Record item is requested or exchanged when a record item is exchanged. The constructs used to represent the context is called the record's *structure*. It provides aggregation mechanisms for the record information and the context for this information. The ENV 12265 establishes a set of concepts to describe this structure.

A *Record Item Complex* (RIC) is the basic construct used to represent a record's structure. Two types of RICs have been defined. The *Original record item complex* (Original RIC) provides the primary context for Record items and RICs. A Record item must have one, and only one, Original RIC as its primary context. Original RICs must also have one, and only one, Original RIC as its primary context. In this way, a data structure composed of Original RICs constitutes a tree structure. The *View Record Item Complex* (View RIC) provides additional context for Record items and RICs. Two sub-types have been defined. The *View RIC 1* represents selection criteria for Record items, supporting the selection of Record items independent to the record structure in the cases where this can be done in a controlled manner. This may, e.g., be used to present record items of the same type selected from different parts of the record. The *View RIC 2* represents a reference or hyper link to another RIC. This can be used to describe that information that has its primary information context in one part of the record should be presented also in the context of another part, e.g., that the medication section in the medical chart also should be presented as the medication section in the nursing chart. The View RIC 2 construct extends the data structure into a directed graph.

Record Items and RICs are called *Record components*. Record components are composed of *attributes*, representing the properties of the record components. A number of attributes are defined in ENV 12265. In addition to the component's position in the record data structure, attributes may cover log information, organisational context, medical responsibility, etc. Attributes of a record component may either be represented explicitly, or implicitly derived from other components.

4. Proposed interpretation of, and extension to, ENV 12265

The ENV 12265 is a generic and open standard. It is intended as a base standard for consecutive standardisation work. In order to be implemented, some limitations and extensions needs to be defined.

The most important extension proposed in Synapses is the definition of a construct to describe the minimum set of information to be provided to the end users upon request. It is called *ComRIC*, and can be seen as a derived class of an Original RIC of the ENV 12265. The construct enables the user to define the minimum necessary information context for the information they record to be correctly interpreted, and has its basis in healthcare professional as well as legal and ethical requirements. It is intended to be a generic concept covering the 'Transaction' concept of the GEHR architecture [12] as well as the 'Document' concept of the DocuLive architecture [13]. The exact definition of a ComRIC class, that is, the minimum set of information that can be provided, will be defined by the users at each validation site and represented in the local Synapses class dictionary.

As a supplement, two additional derived classes of Original RICs have been defined. They are called FolderRIC and DataRIC. A *DataRIC* represents a smaller aggregation of Record Items, and is always a part of a ComRIC. If a Record Item or DataRIC is requested, the enclosing ComRIC is returned, to ensure that the sufficient information context for correct interpretation is provided. ComRICs are enclosed in *FolderRICs*. A FolderRIC is always regarded as part of another folder RIC, except for the Federated Healthcare Record, which in itself also is a FolderRIC. If a FolderRIC is requested, a list of its content is returned.

Another proposed extension to the ENV 12265, is the ability to cluster Record Items independently of their information context represented by the Original RIC. This is facilitated through introducing an additional attribute for the Record Items. Additional attributes are allowed by the ENV. Through this mechanism, information structure and record structure can be described independently and separately.

The ENV 12265 only indicates a set of attributes, and aside from requiring that they should have a name and a value, does not describe how they should be implemented. In Synapses, some attributes are represented as *simple attributes*, composed of only a name and a value. Record ID and log information are examples of attributes represented in this way. Other are represented by derived classes of Record items, as *compound attributes*. Comments, signatures and access rights are example of attributes represented in this way. Using a Record item to represent an attribute enables the recording of, not only what its value is, but also who recorded it, when it was recorded, etc.

5. Interfaces to the Synapses server

Synapses clients, server and feeder systems communicates through *interfaces*. Security aspects of a Synapses server is not a part of the Synapses project. However, some hooks are provided to enable such functions to be added at a later stage, and are referred in the following. Five interfaces to the Synapses server have been defined:

- *Synapses interface retrieval interface*
  This interface gives information about the interfaces implemented in a specific system. A system does not have to have all interfaces implemented to be Synapses compliant.
- *Information retrieval interface*
  This interface is used for information retrieval. It identifies records using custom search criteria, checks access rights and retrieves information. According to the principles described above, only ComRICs and FolderRICs can be requested and provided. This interface can also be used for retrieving the class definition for a given RIC.
- *RIC creation interface*
  This interface is used to create (instanciate) ComRICs and FolderRICs, including records, according to the class definition of the class dictionary.
- *Record item entry interface ("data input")*
  This interface supports Record Item entries from clients and feeder systems into the record structure composed of RICs.
- *Class definition interface*
  The class definition interface is used to create and modify the class dictionary in a Synapses compliant system. The Synapses foundation classes will be common to all Synapses installations. The Synapses class dictionary contains the object class definitions for the record components (Record items and RICs), and are derived from the Synapses foundation classes. New derived classes are defined and existing definitions are modified through the class definition interface. Inheritance is supported. Default values are included and can be modified.
- *Class definition interface*
  This interface is also used to define the relationship between record components.

Interfaces to basic system services and interfaces comprising functions that exclusively are related to security aspects are not defined at this stage, other than as hooks for further work. Later projects may define the basic requirements for such interfaces.

6. Synapses feeder systems integration models

As mentioned, the kernel concept of Synapses is that of a Synapses server supporting access to distributed components of electronic healthcare records. A record component of type ComRIC (or FolderRIC) may be requested by a Synapses Client through the Synapses information retrieval interface. A ComRIC may comprise a set of record components (Record Items and DataRICs) and/ or methods for retrieving record components. When a ComRIC is requested, the ComRIC's methods for retrieving record components from feeder systems may be invoked before returning the ComRIC and its components to the Synapses clients.

The most clean and powerful result is achieved when feeder systems are build from native Synapses components. In such cases, the subset of the federated healthcare record information that is stored in the feeder system will be represented as record components, and the feeder system itself will behave as a Synapses server. The same mechanisms are then used for Fetching and updating information residing within the feeder system as for record components stored in the Synapses server.

In some cases, feeder systems can be encapsulated to behave as Synapses compliant systems. If encapsulation is done outside of the Synapses server, the feeder system will appear to the Synapses server as a feeder system composed of native Synapses components. Such feeder systems will typically only provide a limited set of record component classes.

Encapsulation can also be made inside the Synapses server. In such situations, one or more object classes are defined in the Synapses server comprising non-standard methods for retrieving data from the feeder system.

The most typical integration model in the near future will probably be message based. The feeder systems publishes the information, and the Synapses server subscribes to it. The Synapses server must then comprise methods for incorporating the received data in the record structure.

7. Conclusions

While Synapses is an ambitious project, the Consortium is confident that by building on existing results and avoiding "re-invention of the wheel" it can succeed. Validation is being carried out on an extensive scale in many countries and in a variety of clinical settings. Different parts of the specification will be verified in different sites, according to the local clinical and technological setting.

It is our belief that the most reliable approach to healthcare information sharing, a prerequisite for shared care, is the sharing of records in whole or in part. Through the Synapses project, we hope to facilitate a development in this direction. The benefits of Synapses are potentially very far-reaching. For patients, immediate access by the carer to all the relevant healthcare information, ensure that the patient receives the appropriate treatment as quickly as possible avoiding unnecessary duplication of examinations, tests and other procedures, and errors due to missing information. For the end-users, Synapses will make more data immediately available to professionals and carers involved with a patient, and widen the catchment for researchers, teachers, administrators, and providers of resources and finance. From the point of view of industry, Synapses will increase the impact of any product or service that uses medical records, but widening the range of data available to them, and making the data compatible and comprehensible. Moreover, it will help industry to expand their potential market by facilitating synapsing between their systems and other systems elsewhere in Europe.

References

1 van de Welde, van der Werff A, Kilsdonk A, Damen W, Hubert M, *Towards a European framework reference model and architecture for the development of open hospital information systems*, Procs. MEDINFO 92, 188-193.

2 Bleich HL, Slack WV, *Design of a hospital information system: a comparison between interfaced and integrated systems*, Procs. MEDINFO 92, 174- 177.

3 Grimson J et al, *Synapses - Federated healthcare record server,* Procs. of MIE 96, Copenhagen 1996, J Brender et al (Eds), IOS Press, 695-699.

4 Toussaint P, Kalshoven M (Eds), *Impulses to Synapses*, The Synapses Project, 1996, Deliverable USER 1.2, AIM Office, DG XIII, Brussels

5 Toussaint P et al, *Supporting Shared Care for Diabetic patients*, Procs. of Toward an electronic health record Europe '96, London 1996, CAEHR, 117-121

6 Kalra D (Ed), *Synapses User requirements and functional specification (part A)*, The Synapses Project, 1996, Deliverable USER 1.1.1a, AIM Office, DG XIII, Brussels

7 Grimson W et al (Eds), *Synapses functional specification*, The Synapses Project, 1996, Deliverable USER 1.1.1b, AIM Office, DG XIII, Brussels

8 Kalra D (Ed), *Synapses object model and object dictionary*, The Synapses Project, 1996, Deliverable USER 1.3.1, AIM Office, DG XIII, Brussels

9 Kalra D, Lloyd D, *Synapses Object Model and Object Dictionary*, Procs. of Toward an electronic health record Europe '96, London 1996, CAEHR, 78-87

10 Hurlen P, Skifjeld K (Eds), *Design and functional specification of the federated healthcare record server and interfaces*, The Synapses Project, 1996, Deliverable SPEC 2.1.1, AIM Office, DG XIII, Brussels

11 Electronic healthcare record architecture, European prestandard ENV 12265, CEN 1996.

12 Ingram D, *GEHR: The Good European Health Record*, In *Health in the New Communications* Age, MF Laires, MJ Ladeira and JP Christensen (Eds), IOS Press, 1995, 66-74.

13 Skifjeld K et al, *From idea to product - Experiences from the development of DocuLive Electronic Patient Record system*, accepted for publication in British Journal of Healthcare Computing, March 1997.

Medical Informatics Europe '97
C. Pappas et al. (Eds.)
IOS Press, 1997

A computerized record hash coding and linkage procedure to warrant epidemiological follow-up data security

Catherine QUANTIN , Hocine BOUZELAT   and Liliane DUSSERRE
Department of Medical Informatics (Pr. L. DUSSERRE), Teaching Hospital of Dijon France
e-mail :cquantin@u-bourgogne.fr

Abstract : A computerized record hash coding and linkage procedure is proposed to allow the chaining of medical information within the framework of epidemiological follow-up. Before their extraction, files are rendered anonymous using a one-way hash coding based on the SHA function, in order to respect the legislation on data privacy and security. To avoid dictionary attacks, two keys have been added to SHA coding. Once rendered anonymous, the linkage of patient information can be accomplished by the means of a statistical model, taking into account several identification variables.

1. Introduction

To carry out epidemiological studies, many medical data users wish to be able to link nominal files.

However, in France, the linkage of nominal files within the framework of medical research is submitted, to law n° 78-17 of January 6th 1978, completed by law n° 94-548 of July 1st 1994 relative to nominal data processing. Moreover, before October 1998, all European countries will have to integrate the demands of the European directive of October 24th 1995, which is very close to the French legislation. Concerning the linkage of nominal files, the position of the French data protection commission (Commission Nationale de l'Information et des Libertés: CNIL), according to the legislation, is to render each file anonymous in an irreversible way before its export, so that returning to the nominal information becomes impossible.

As a consequence, in order to respect the legislation concerning medical file linkage, the application of an irreversible cryptology method to each nominal file before linkage would be necessary. However, implementation of cryptology methods in France is submitted to law n° 90-1170 of December 29th 1990 concerning telecommunication regulation completed by law n° 96-659 of July 26th 1996. These laws specify the condition of application of cryptology methods and, in particular, the type of encryption systems which have to be declared to the French Department for Information System Security (Service Central de la Sécurité des Systèmes d'Information : SCSSI)

This paper describes a recently implemented protocol, declared to CNIL and SCSSI, whose purpose is to render files anonymous in view of their extraction using the Standard Hash Algorithm (SHA). Once rendered anonymous, these files will be exportable so as to be merged, using a linkage statistical method, in the framework of epidemiological studies.

2. Methods

The protocol is composed of two steps. The first step concerns the irreversible transformation of identification data. The second step is devoted to file linkage using a statistical method in order to reduce the consequence of typing errors upon the linkage

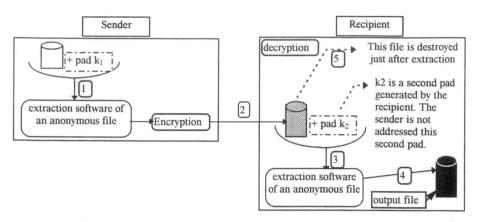

figure 1: Anonymous transmission of medical file

2.1 Anonymity of information

The principle is to ensure an irreversible transformation of variables which allow the identification of an individual (last name, first name, date of birth, sex). The aim is to obtain a strictly anonymous code, but always the same one for a given individual in order to link all information concerning the same patient. In fact, we cannot use encryption, in the literal meaning of this term, since encryption is by definition a reversible[1] process that allows the deciphering of the message by its legitimate recipient [2]. That's why we apply here a one way hash method, which is usually used for digital signature [3]and is strictly irreversible.

In agreement with SCSSI, we have chosen the Standard Hash Algorithm (SHA)[3] which, according to the American Federal Register, must be used every time a secure hash algorithm is required for federal applications.

Although mathematically irreversible, the hash computation does not completely warrant the information security. Thus, the algorithm could be used for a confrontation between hashed identities and the code to be deciphered.

To prevent this dictionary attack[4], two pads[1], have been introduced before the SHA application[5]. The first pad, k_1, is used by all senders of information and the second one k_2 is applied by the recipient, which anonymously ensures the file linkage. Nominal information is therefore hashed twice, consecutively with these two keys.

The aim of pad k_1 (resp. k_2) is to prevent a recipient (resp. sender) dictionary attack. As a consequence, the person in charge of the pad management should be kept outside the study and should not be given the hashed files.

However, the linkage of information related to a given patient requires the use of the same algorithm and the same pad k_1 by all senders. The security of the information hashed only once must then be ensured while it is transmitted to the recipient in order to avoid a dictionary attack by another sender. In particular, a network transmission should be secured by using a reversible encryption method, RSA for example[6].

2.2. File linkage

The aim of file linkage[7, 8] is to gather all information coming from different sources and concerning the same patient. Two types of linkage errors are of concern : erroneous links of notifications from two distinct patients, also called homonym errors, and failure to link multiple notifications on the same patient, also called synonym errors [9].

To reduce the impact of typing errors, a spelling treatment [10] has been introduced in the anonymity process, before the hash coding. The

---

[1] A pad is a large random file

principle is to transform the spelling of names according to phonetic rules.

Moreover, the linkage takes into account several identification variables such as, for example, first and last names, date of birth, gender and zip code. However, some variables provide more information and more reliability than others. As a consequence, Jaro[7, 8] proposed to associate a weight to each variable according to the reliability of the information provided by this variable. The weight given to date of birth is then higher than that given to gender, as two identical dates of birth are more discriminant than two identical genders. The more reliable a variable, the greater the weight will be, as the weight is computed from the logarithm of the ratio between the sensitivity and one minus the specificity of the studied variable (likelihood ratio). A composite weight is obtained by summing the weight of each variable.

The aim of the linking of two files F_1 and F_2 is to classify each pair of records obtained from crossing $F_1 x F_2$ as belonging to one of two sets: the set of matched record pairs M, and the set of unmatched record pairs U. From a statistical point of view, this problem is equivalent to the analysis of a finite mixture of two sets M and U, in proportions p and (1-p). The belonging of a pair to M (resp. U) is supposed to follow a binomial distribution characterized by the parameter m (resp. u). The m (resp. U) probability can be defined as the probability of agreement of the two records of the pair, for the considered variable, knowing that the two records (resp. U) correspond to the same individual.

The estimation of the parameters (m, u, p) is obtained through the maximization of the data likelihood. After having ordered the 2^n possible configurations of agreement and disagreement of pairs of records composed of n variables by the composite weight, one can compute the cumulative distribution functions of these configurations, conditionally to belonging to the sets M and U. Two threshold values can then be computed from which three sets of possible decisions are determined as follows: the pair is a match ; no determination is made ; the pair is not a match.

3. Performance assessment of the protocol

The performance of the computerized record hash coding and linkage procedure has been assessed by comparing record linkage based on exclusive use of the computerized linkage procedure with manual linkage considered to be the gold standard.

The computerized hash coding and linkage procedure was applied to two files. The first one corresponds to 305 colon cancer patients diagnosed in 1994 and recorded by the anatomopathological laboratory of the Dijon public teaching hospital The second gathers 264 458 patients hospitalized in the Dijon public teaching hospital in 1994.

The results of the application of these two files have been compared to those manually obtained by the Burgundy Registry of Digestive Cancers, this manual case resolution being considered as a gold standard procedure.

266 pairs of records were classified as a match by the computerized linkage procedure. All of these patients were actually hospitalized in the Dijon public teaching hospital, according to the manual results of the Registry.

However, among the 80 659 424 remaining records classified as not a match, two of them should have been considered as a match, according to the gold standard. In terms of patients, this means that 2 out of 39 patients were erroneously considered by the computerized procedure as if they were not hospitalized.

In fact, the computerized linkage procedure was not systematically applied to each pair, given that the total number of pairs was too great. The investigation was restricted to pairs (1 847)which have a good chance of being a match, using a blocking method. The blocking strategy[11] reference consists in the partitioning of the two files on one or more variables. For example, if both files were sorted by year of birth, the pairs to be compared would only be drawn from these records where the year of birth agrees. The rest of the pairs will automatically be classified as unmatched. It could be shown that the failure of matching, observed for two pairs in our application, was actually due to the use of the blocking method.

Finally, the estimations of the sensitivity and of the specificity of the computerized linkage procedure were respectively 99 % and 100 %.

4. Conclusion

The computerized record hash coding and linkage procedure proposed in this paper allow the linkage of medical information that has been rendered anonymous. The anonymity process is based on a one way SHA coding, preceded by a spelling treatment to reduce the impact of typing errors among the linkage. The security is reinforced by the use of two pads. The first pad is shared by the senders of information and the second one by the recipient only so that even the recipient could not manage a dictionary attack.

Once rendered anonymous, the linkage of patient information can then be accomplished while respecting the confidentiality of medical data. The linkage is realized by the means of a statistical model, taking into account several identification variables, and thus limiting the consequences of typing errors among non discriminating variables.

In the framework of Digestive Cancer Studies, the computerised record hash coding and linkage procedure have shown satisfying performances (sensitivity of 99 % and specificity of 100 %).

5. Acknowledgement

This research has been sponsored by the Burgundy Regional Council.

6. References

[1] -Beckett B. Introduction aux méthodes de cryptologie, Masson, 1990.

[2] -Brassard G. Modern Cryptology. Lecture Notes in Computer Science, 1993.

[3] -Schneier B. Applied Cryptography, Protocols, Algorithms, and Source Code in C. John Wiley & Sons, Inc., 1994.

[4] -Meux E. Encrypting personal identifiers. Health Services Research, 1994; 29(2): 247-56.

[5] -Bouzelat H., Quantin C., Dusserre L., Extraction and Anonymity Protocol of Medical File, Journal of American Medical Informatics Association, Washington, 1996 ; 26-30.

[6] -Rivest RL, Shamir A, Adleman L. A Method for obtaining Digital Signatures and Public-Key Cryptosystems, *CACM*, 1978; 2: 120.

[7] -Jaro M.A., Advances in Record-Linkage Methodology as Applied to Matching the 1985 Census of Tampa, Florida, Journal of the American Statistical Association, 1989.

[8] -Jaro M.A., Probabilistic-Linkage of large public health data files, Statistics in Medicine, 1995 ; 14 : 491-498.

[9] -Brenner H., Schmidtmann I., Determinants of Homonym and Synonym Rates of Record Linkage in Disease Registration, Methods of Information in Medicine, 1994, 35 : 19-24.

[10] -Dusserre L., Quantin C., Bouzelat H., A one way public-key cryptosystem for the linkage of nominal files in epidemiological studies. MEDINFO' 95, R.A. Greenes, H.E. Peterson, D.J. Protti (editors), Elsevier Science Publishers (North-Holland), 1995; 661-665.

[11] -Kelly R.P., Blocking considerations for record linkage under conditions of uncertainly. In Proceedings of the Social Statistics Section American Statistical Association, 1984, 602-605.

Medical Informatics Europe '97
C. Pappas et al. (Eds.)
IOS Press, 1997

SMART: a System Supporting Medical Activities in Real-Time

Domenico M. PISANELLI[1], Fabrizio CONSORTI[2], Paolo MERIALDO[2-3]

1. Consiglio Nazionale delle Ricerche - ITBM, V.Marx 15, I-00137 Roma
2. IV Clinica Chirurgica, Policlinico"Umberto I", V.Policlinico, I-00185 Roma
3. Università di Roma 3, Dip.Informatica e Automazione, I-00146 Roma

Abstract. This paper describes the system SMART whose goal is real-time assistance to physicians who execute diagnostic or therapeutic protocols in a clinical context. SMART is able to retrieve a protocol from its knowledge base and to monitor its execution step by step for a single patient. Different protocols for different patients can be followed at the same time in a health care structure. The prototype realized supports the execution of protocols for evaluating surgical risks. It has been implemented according to the specifications given by the 4th Surgical Clinic of "Policlinico Umberto I" and reflects the activities actually performed in that hospital. However, the protocol model defined is general-purpose and we envisage an easy application to other contexts and therefore to the informatization of other protocols.

1. Introduction

Guidelines for clinical practice are being introduced in an extensive way in more and more different fields of medicine [1]. They have the goal of indicating the most appropriate decisional and procedural behavior optimizing health outcomes, costs, and clinical decisions. Guidelines can be expressed in a textual way as recommendations or in a more formal and rigid way as protocols or flow diagrams. In different contexts they can be a either loose indication for a preferred set of choices or they can be considered a normative set of rules.

Although their diffusion is increasing, there are still concerns that guidelines could harm patient care, mainly because of their low flexibility. Tools helping in selecting the proper guideline for a specific patient and monitoring its execution step by step are highly needed. They could relieve the clinicians from the management of the guideline itself, letting them free to concentrate more on clinical decisions.

Several efforts have been devoted in the last few years in realizing computerized tools for guidelines management (see for example [2,3]). Formal representation models and methodologies have been investigated [4,5]. An essential role for telematics is expected, especially for World-Wide Web based tools [6-8].

In this paper we focus on the computerized support to clinical activities in the context of protocol-based care. By protocol we do not mean a mere list of actions, but a structured, flexible, and coherent descriptions of activities aimed at solving specific problems [9]. We present the system SMART (Supporting Medical Activities in Real-Time) whose aim is real-time assistance to physicians who execute diagnostic or therapeutic protocols in a clinical context. In the next paragraph we sketch out the architecture and the functionalities of SMART, the third paragraph reports its application at the University Hospital of Rome for supporting the evaluation of surgical risks. In conclusion we emphasize the added value that such a system can offer in a clinical environment.

2. Architecture and functionality of the system

We defined a simple graphic formalism for modeling the activities aimed at the execution of a protocol carried out in a clinical environment. Such a formalism is described in detail in [10]. It is possible to represent activities running in parallel, mutually exclusive activities, cycles and optional activities. SMART stores protocols represented according to this formalism. The system is able to retrieve a protocol from its knowledge base and to monitor its execution step by step for a single patient. It works like an automatic reminder system, showing the activity or the set of activities to be executed. Different protocols for different patients can be followed at the same time in a clinical structure.

Unlike other reminder systems, it keeps track of the status of an activity (e.g. started, suspended, executed, reported). This feature can be exploited at ward level for making queries like: "for all the patients show the activities planned but not yet executed". This facility is useful when a large number of patients is being cared simultaneously in a ward.

The system runs in a PC environment on a Windows™ platform and has been implemented using the Microsoft Access™ relational data base and the Access-Basic™ programming language. The modular architecture of SMART is shown in figure 1.

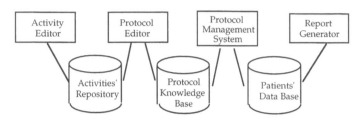

Figure 1
The architecture of SMART.

The Activity Editor captures the information describing medical activities related to the various protocols (e.g. agent, environment, resources needed). Such information is subsequently stored in the Activities' Repository in form of relational data.

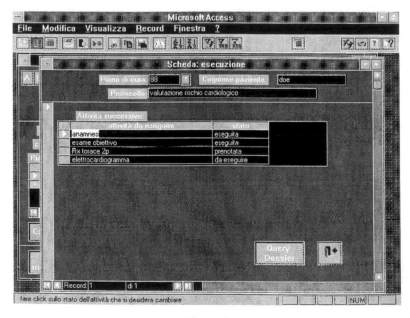

Figure 2
The system shows a list of activities to be executed
for a patient, in the context of the chosen protocol.

The Protocol Editor allows the user to pick up activities from their repository and to build up a graph which represents the protocol according to the formalism defined. The nodes of this graph are either activities or control symbols accounting for parallelization, cycles and conditional execution. The graph is stored in relational format in the Protocol Knowledge Base. Activities may be decomposed in sub-activities and such a refinement may be applied recursively.

The activity and the protocol editors are not employed directly in the patient management, but for defining the protocols which will be executed. Therefore their use is limited to the customization phase. On the contrary, the other modules of SMART support the process of care in real-time, and all the physicians performing care are enabled to interact with them.

The Protocol Management System allows the physician to match a protocol with a patient in the context of care provision. The physician reads the activity which has to be performed and updates the system when it is completed. Figure 2 shows a list of activities to be done as presented by the system. This module writes and updates the Patients' Database with data reporting the status of a patient with respect to the execution of his/her protocol. The physician can also insert comments and reports on a patient.

The completion of an activity is not always an immediate task, rather it goes through several steps which SMART is able to keep track of. We singled out those states relevant to be reported for each activity. The system allows to update the state of each activity and to retrieve the situation from the patient's point of view or from the ward's point of view.

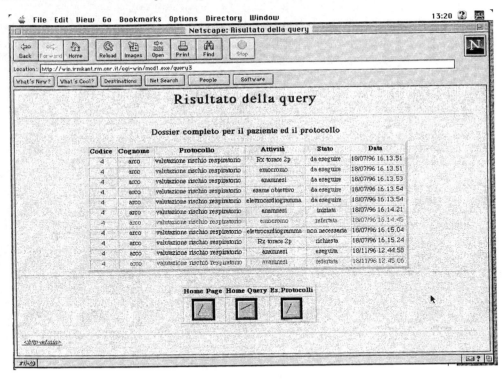

Figure 3
The Patients' Database queried by a HTML client via the Internet.

The Report Generator queries the patients' database for getting information such as: "Which protocol is the patient following?", "Is it completed?", "What must be done now?". It is able to generate a report with different levels of detail. For example it is possible to check – for each activity performed – when the single activity states occured (e.g. when a skull radiography was scheduled, executed and reported). The report generator is also useful in managed care, since it allows to keep track of activities executed and respective costs. From the quality point of view, the reports are able to show whether the process of care followed the optimal path.

We also implemented a common-gateway interface (CGI) which allows users to access the patients' database by means of the Internet using a HTML client (figure 3). Being the network an unsafe environment, this feature is still experimental (for a demo version, see the URL: http://win.irmkant.rm.cnr.it/smart.htm).

3. A case study: the evaluation of surgical risk

The 4th Surgical Clinic of "Policlinico Umberto I" (the Hospital of the first University of Rome) has developed a set of clinical guidelines for pre-operative and post-operative management of patients undergoing the most frequent types of surgery.

Many different data are collected in order to reach a decision, the investigation being carried on several domains. It includes the assessment of cardiac conditions and lung conditions as well as estimating the probability of haemorragy. Some routinary activities are always performed in order to check if the patient would risk too much in a possible operation (e.g. anamnesis, ECG). Should the situation be unclear, a deeper level is explored, i.e. further analyses and diagnostic images are made.

A special attention has been devoted to guidelines for the evaluation and reduction of risks related to surgery and a first attempt was made to integrate those guidelines with the clinical information system running at the department [11]. However, as soon as the number and the complexity of the adopted guidelines increased, it became evident the need for a more effective modelling of protocols and a more powerful management system for the protocol-related activities.

The system SMART has been conceived to answer such needs. The 4th Surgical Clinic is currently testing SMART for managing the protocol of surgical risk evaluation. The protocol actually followed in that clinical context has been modeled according to the graphic formalism defined. The formalism resulted adequate to represent the complex protocols used in everyday practice.

A fragment of the protocol is reported in figure 4: activities are represented by rectangles, control nodes by circles ("+in" and "+out" stands for "begin parallelization" and "end parallelization" of activities in the case not all of them have to be executed, whereas "-in" and "-out" stands for "begin parallelization" and "end parallelization" of mutually exclusive activities).

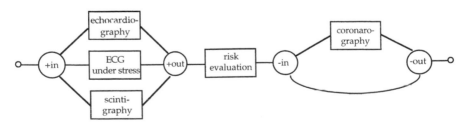

Figure 4
A fragment of the protocol of surgical risk evaluation.

After having successfully tested the expressive power of the graphic formalism, the case study involved the real-time management of patients. SMART was thus employed for monitoring the execution of the protocol of surgical risk evaluation.

As already pointed out, many patients and many protocols may run in parallel. Managing a single protocol for a single patient may be trivial, but tracing the numerous activities performed on many patients, as well as supporting their parallel execution is the real added value of this system.

4. Conclusion

It has been proved that adherence to plans may reduce cost of care up to 25% [12]. The optimization of patient management must consider two essential aspects of care provision: the interaction and co-operation of a clinical department with the diagnostic services (request of appointments, preparation of patients for the exam, scheduling, negotiation...) and the execution of different parallel activities pertaining to different protocols for the same patient.

For example, the treatment of a patient candidate to major rectal surgery who presents chronic respiratory failure, hypertension, and myocardial ischemic damages implies the execution of three different protocols. They could be optimised to run in parallel, requiring the interaction with a number of different services (respiratory physiopathology, cardiology, department of imaging).

The full potentialities of SMART can be exploited in such an environment where different protocols are executed in parallel on several patients. In this context the system is able to retrieve the updated situation of every patient, as well as to give an overall report on the ward. Keeping track of the parallel activities performed, it avoids unnecessary duplication of tasks, but it also prevents possible omissions.

The case study has confirmed the flexibility of the graphic formalism for representing protocols. An extension of the protocol knowledge base is foreseen in order to satisfy the requirements of our experimental site. A visual interface for entering and updating protocol will replace the present editor. Currently the system is as a stand-alone application, but the migration to a client-server architecture is foreseen. Other extension regards a tight integration with other information systems (e.g. computerized patient records, scheduling and resource allocation systems) in a context of interaction and co-operation of a clinical department with the diagnostic services.

References

[1]   Grimshaw JM, Russell IT. Effect of Clinical Guidelines on Medical Practice: a Systematic Review of Rigorous Evaluations. *Lancet,* 1993; 342: 1317-1322.
[2]   Vissers MC, Hasman A, van der Linden CJ. Protocol Processing System (ProtoVIEW) to Support Residents at the Emergency Ward.*Proceedings of 12th International Congress of European Federation of Medical Informatics,* 1994; 138-143.
[3]   Ertle AR, Campbell EM, Hersh WR. Automated Application of Clinical Practice Guidelines for Asthma Management. *Proceedings of the 1996 AMIA Fall Symposium,* 1996; 552-556.
[4]   Starren J, Xie G. Comparison of Three Knowledge Representation Formalisms for Encoding the NCEP Cholesterol Guidelines.*Proceedings of 18th SCAMC,* 1994; 792-796.
[5]   Tu SW, Mark MS, Musen MA. The EON Model of Intervention Protocols and Guidelines. *Proceedings of the 1996 AMIA Fall Symposium,* 1996; 587-591.
[6]   Barnes M, Barnett GO. An Architecture for a Distributed Guideline Server.*Proceedings of 19th SCAMC,* 1995; 233-237.
[7]   Cimino JJ, Socratous SA. Automated Guidelines Implemented via the World Wide Web.*Proceedings of 19th SCAMC,* 1995; 941.
[8]   Long WJ, Fraser H, Naimi S. Web Interface for the Hearth Disease Program. *Proceedings of the 1996 AMIA Fall Symposium,* 1996; 762-766.
[9]   Grifoni P, Lalle C, Luzi D, Pisanelli DM, Ricci FL, Serbanati LD, Modeling the Management of Protocols as the Kernel of a Healthcare Information System. *Proceedings of MEDINFO 95,* 1995; 502-505.
[10]   Pisanelli DM, Consorti F. Support to the Management of Clinical Activities in the Context of Protocol-Based Care. Proceedings of the *ACM Symposium on Applied Computing,* 1997.
[11]   Consorti F, Assenza M, Ferri F, Gargiulo A, Lombardi A, Martinis G, Di Paola M. MSR: A Decision Support System for the Decision Strategy of Surgeon. *Proceedings of 11th International Congress of European Federation of Medical Informatics,* 1993; 90-94.
[12]   Clayton PD, Hripcsak G. Decision support in healthcare. *Int. J. of Bio-Medical Computing,* 1995; 39: 59-66.

Medical Informatics Europe '97
C. Pappas et al. (Eds.)
IOS Press, 1997

A JAVA-Based Multimedia Tool for Clinical Practice Guidelines

Victor Maojo, Carlos Herrero, Francisco Valenzuela, Jose Crespo, *Pablo Lazaro,
**Alejandro Pazos
Medical Informatics Group, School of Computer Science
Universidad Politecnica de Madrid. Boadilla del Monte 28660 Madrid, Spain
*Health Services Research Unit. Instituto Carlos III. 28029 Madrid, Spain
** Department of Computer Science, Universidad de La Coruña, Spain

Abstract. We have developed a specific language for the representation of Clinical Practice Guidelines (CPGs) and Windows C++ and platform independent JAVA applications for multimedia presentation and edition of electronically stored CPGs. This approach facilitates translation of guidelines and protocols from paper to computer-based flowchart representations. Users can navigate through the algorithm with a friendly user interface and access related multimedia information within the context of each clinical problem. CPGs can be stored in a computer server and distributed over the World Wide Web, facilitating dissemination, local adaptation, and use as a reference element in medical care. We have chosen the Agency for Health Care and Policy Research's heart failure guideline to demonstrate the capabilities of our tool.
Keywords : Practice Guidelines. JAVA. Multimedia. World Wide Web

1. Introduction

Clinical Practice Guidelines (CPGs) are "systematically developed statements to assist practitioners and patient decisions about appropriate health care for specific clinical circumstances"[1]. Whereas paper-based CPGs are easy to read and can be rapidly browsed, they have different problems that restrict and difficult their use. These problems include: (1) checking consistencies; (2) cost of dissemination; (3) local adaptation to variable clinical environments and circumstances; (4) difficult evaluation of their impact in medical care; (5) update and introduction of new medical knowledge; and (6) lack of feedback to developers.

Various researchers have proposed that computer-based guidelines can solve those problems, facilitating their use in medical care. For instance, Greenes and his collaborators at the Decision Systems Group, Brigham and Women's Hospital, have been working in different computer programs to make extensive use of guidelines in medical care. This work has evolved from an preliminary tool[2] to a current system, GEODE, embedded in a whole clinical workstation[3]. The InterMed project is another example, carried out by a different medical informatics labs from Harvard, Stanford, Columbia, and Utah[4].

In the next sections we will describe a computer tool that we developed to facilitate translation of CPGs from paper documents to electronic format.

2. Methods

We have created an original specification language to represent graphically CPGs as flowcharts, linked to multimedia information, to facilitate distribution over the network and display them in computer screens at remote sites. Users can retrieve those guidelines by means of any WWW client. We have also developed tools that facilitates guideline edition and user interaction.

Once the guideline is retrieved by hypertext links from any WWW browser, users can automatically display CPGs in a flowchart format using software programs that we have created. We used an object-oriented methodology in the development process, with two different language implementations, based on C++ and JAVA. Multimedia information such as text, graphics, images, video, and sound can be linked to any part of the algorithm. AHCPR's of heart failure guideline[5] was considered as a benchmark to test performance and capabilities of the program.

3. Results

3.1. A Specification Language for Clinical Practice Guidelines

Our tool represents CPGs in a flowchart format, using an original Specification Language for CPGs. This is a simple data format to create ASCII text documents that represent clinical algorithms. Another approach using commercial databases has also been implemented. Functionalities of this latter version are the same as the ones explained below.

We use tags to represent the different elements of the CPG in a similar way as they are used in HTML (HyperText Markup Language). A description of this language has been reported elsewhere[6].

It is important the order of appearance of the language elements. There are elements which are optional and others that can appear many times. In some cases, elements are represented with only one leading tag and some tags appear within others, as it is shown in the following example:

<TITLE>Heart Failure: Evaluation and care of patients with left ventricular systolic dysfunction </TITLE>

<ACTION_BOX>

    <NODEID> 2

    <BOXTITLE>Initial Evaluation   </BOXTITLE>

    <DATA>...</DATA>

<NEXT> 3

</ACTION_BOX>

We have considered several different parts in the algorithm structure:

1. *Title* and *General Information* of the CPG. This part includes the description of the specific clinical problem of the CPG, their intended users, authors (name, degree and institutional affiliation), publication date, review dates, and the method used to elaborate the CPG.

2. The *Flowchart* contains the description of steps to follow in each clinical problem. All the nodes include the information that will appear in the diagram, specific information in dialog boxes, and can be linked to related multimedia resources. The description of dependencies among nodes determines the structure of the flowchart.

There are 4 kinds of nodes: Action, Clinical State, Decision and Council. The first three kinds of nodes were described in a proposal for clinical algorithm standards reported by a Committee created by the Society for Medical Decision Making (MDM) [7].

We have introduced some minor modifications to such proposal. For instance, splitting in more than two branches, and council nodes[5] , which are the fourth type of nodes in our language. These alternatives are included to accommodate our tool to different clinical algorithms proposed in CPGs published by different organizations.

3. *Glossary* is used to explain terms that appear in any part of the guideline document, to write down bibliographic references, and facilitate other kind of explanations, such as term definitions.

The description of a CPG in our specification language may be implemented in any hardware platform since it is ASCII text, with specific tags for special characters, —e.g., in Spanish. This is the same method used in HTML to describe platform independent ASCII files.

Our group has developed an ASCII text editor for Windows with an MDI interface for the specification language, with different aids. The most important function of this editor is to check the syntactic correction of the CPG document and its conformance to the specification language. Since the specification language is very simple it is also possible to use any ASCII text editor in any platform to directly edit those CPGs. We use these source files with our windows display tool, and we can generate target files in HTML with calls to our JAVA applets.

3.2. Edition and Visualization Tools for CPGs

There are several disadvantages in representing graphically clinical algorithms in paper format. When CPGs´ complexity is not trivial it is difficult to follow the algorithm, and sometimes it is impossible to avoid overlapping of arcs.

Using computer representations, users have a wide variety of browsing, abstracting and zooming techniques to navigate through the algorithm[2]. Display functions allow users to browse different paths in the clinical algorithm, expanding nodes forward or contracting paths backwards with a mouse click, or access descriptive text, tables, images, drawings, video and sound, taking advantage of computer multimedia capabilities. Other functions allow visualization of the graph, change of fonts, zoom of the whole graph or of a single branch, and search and edition of text strings.

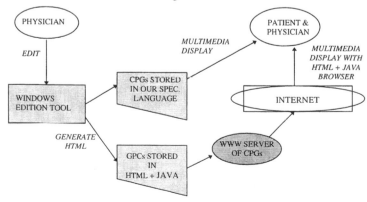

Figure 1: System for CPGs display and edition

Once users have edited a CPG, it is stored in an ASCII file according to the specification language. Either when users open an existing CPG or save a modified one, syntactic correction of the CPG is checked. Thus, unconnected CPGs or paths with no end are avoided.

4. Discussion

Our system allows guideline developers and organizations to create WWW servers where CPGs and protocols can be easily stored. Translation of CPGs to our specification language permits their storage as ASCII text files with independence of the platform and facilitates their distribution over the WWW. We have also implemented a database format to store guidelines, facilitating acceptance from different users that can be reluctant to use our specification language.

An important reason for local adaptation is variability in medical practice. For instance, a specific test or recommendation cannot be carried out at some medical centers. With this need in mind, we introduced functionalities for graphical edition in our tool. Thus, users can modify nodes, arcs, contents, and multimedia links to ensure that the guideline can be adapted to their specific clinical environments and circumstances.

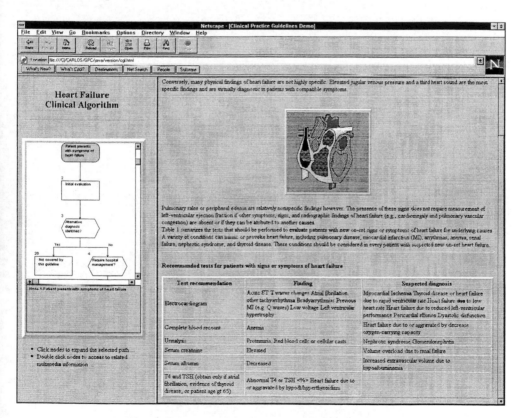

Figure 2: Java Visualization Tool for the Heart Failure CPG.
(note : Frame formats can be adapted to different monitors´ size and users´ preferences)

5. Conclusions and future directions

The computer tool that we have described in this article is part of a project that we are carrying out to address some of the problems related to practice guidelines —as explained above. For instance, we have created with other faculty members of our school a logic-algebraic method to check consistencies in CPGs represented by set of rules, and we collaborate with a Spanish medical center to evaluate physicians' attitude to computer-based guidelines.

We are currently working to integrate CPGs into medical information systems. Future incorporation of inference and knowledge representation modules, to access patient data to determine the transition logic between the states of the flowchart, will increase our tool's capability as a decision support system.

A JAVA version of the display tool has been completed (see figure 2). It is currently under evaluation and can be accessed over the net on request. All functions are easily available using a WWW browser with JAVA compliance, facilitating platform-independent access and display of multimedia information of any CPG.

Acknowledgments

This research was funded by the Fondo de Investigación Sanitaria (FIS), Ministry of Health, Spain (FIS 1952/95). Carlos Herrero is supported by a FIS grant (FIS 96/4016). We want to thank Ricardo Ruiz and Andres Lopez, two undergraduate students of our group, who collaborated in some parts of this research. Computer resources were donated by Hewlett-Packard through its HISE (Health Information Systems Engineering) 1996 Initiative.

6. References

1. Field M, Lohr K. (eds.). Guidelines for Clinical Practice. National Academy Press, Washington, D.C. 1992.

2. Abendroth TW, Greenes RA, Joyce EA. Investigations in the use of clinical algorithms to organize medical knowledge. SCAMC 1988; 12:90-95.

3. Liem EB, Obeid JS, Shareck EP, Shato L, Greenes RA. Representation of clinical practice guidelines through an interactive World-Wide-Web interface. SCAMC 1995; 19:223-227.

4. Oliver DE, Barnes MR, Barnett GO, Chueh HE, Cimino JJ, Clayton PD, Detmer WM, Gennari JH, Greenes RA, Stanley MH, Musen MA, Pattison-Gordon E, Shortliffe EH, Socratous SA, Tu SW. InterMed: An Internet-Based Medical Collaboratory. AMIA Fall Symposium 1995; 19:1023.

5. Konstam M, Dracup K, Baker D. et al. Heart failure: management of patients with left-ventricular systolic dysfunction. Quick reference guide for clinicians No. 11. , AHCPR Publication No. 94-0613. Rockville, MD: Agency for Health Policy and Research, Public Health Scrvice, U.S. Department of Health and Human Services. June, 1994.

6. Herrero C, Maojo V, Sanandrés JA, López A, Crespo J, Lázaro P. A Specification Language for Clinical Practice Guidelines. 18th IEEE Conference in Medicine and Biology. Amsterdam, 1996.

7. Society for Medical Decision Making Committee of Standardization of Clinical Algorithms. Proposal for Clinical Algorithm Standards. Medical Decision Making. 1992; 12(2): 149-154.

Medical Informatics Europe '97
C. Pappas et al. (Eds.)
IOS Press, 1997

Decision Support System for Designing Chemotherapeutic Regimens

D.Henderson, J.McCall and J.Boyle

School of Computer and Mathematical Sciences,
The Robert Gordon University, Aberdeen, Scotland, AB25 1HG

1.   Introduction

Over the last 40 years or so, more than 30 anti-cancer agents have been discovered and are now in widespread clinical use. For many of these agents it has proven impossible, using empirical clinical evaluation, to define an optimum administration schedule for many drugs and tumour types. Variation in tumour response and oncologists' preference to administer most drugs in combination, rather than as a single agent, make clinical evaluation complex. Furthermore, with the continued development of new anti-cancer agents, it is increasingly impractical to explore thoroughly treatment possibilities empirically. The costs, both human and financial, of running sufficient drug trials would be prohibitive. This problem among others is highlighted by [Cassidy and McLeod (1995)] when discussing a logical approach to drug trials.

Therefore in order to determine optimum administration schedules, it seems reasonable to develop a system which will allow oncologists to predict the influence of new cancer treatments on tumour growth before committing to clinical trials. There are few such systems currently available, however recent advances in both mathematical modelling and information technology suggest that their construction is now practical.

The authors are developing a system of inter-linked tools which will form the basis of an "Oncologists Workbench". The Workbench will allow oncologists to interactively define and experiment with simulated drug treatments and evaluate their likely outcome. In Section 2 we discuss the background to our work. The tools which constitute the Workbench are described in Section 3 and we conclude with a discussion in Section 4.

2.   Background

The authors have been investigating tumour growth and the response to chemotherapy under various scenarios. This research has lead to the translation of theoretical models of tumour growth and response into a form which is of use to practising clinical oncologists. The model in its current form [Usher and Henderson (1996)] displays the behaviour shown in the models of Goldie and Coldman (1979), Birkhead and Gregory (1984), and Martin et al (1992) and concurs quantitatively with what is observed clinically.

A considerable amount of theoretical work has been done on the optimisation of chemotherapy in particular by Swan (1990) and by Martin and Teo (1994). A major difficulty in this area is the translation of theoretical results into practical guidelines because suggested theoretical regimens can prove clinically unacceptable. Investigative work is currently under way into using heuristic search techniques to improve empirically determined treatments within clinically acceptable bounds [McCall and Petrovski 1996].

Most computational systems developed to date focus on the storage of drug trial data, though there are some which support clinical decision making (e.g. PRO*forma* [Fox et al (1996)]). There also exist cancer information databanks (e.g. PDQ), and there are new initiatives developing common standards for the interchange of clinical information (e.g. MACRO).

However, practising oncologists wishing to investigate the influence of new cancer treatment schedules on tumour growth without having to explicitly consider any underlying mathematical model(s), currently have no objective tools available.

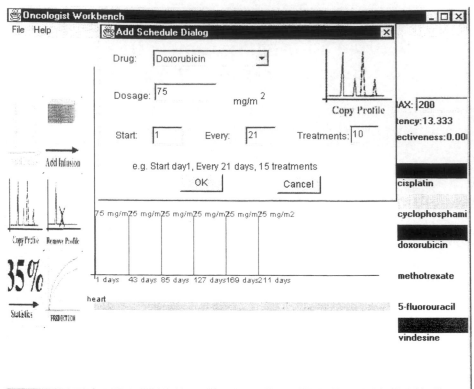

Figure 1: The regimen editor allows for the interactive design of treatment schedules. On the right is a palette of possible drugs, in the centre is the main design area, and on the right are controls for the editor. The controls allow the oncologist to edit the treatment (by removing or adding information), as well as a utility which allows for the quick specification of profiles (shown in the *add schedule dialog* box). There are also methods which send the treatment off to remote mathematical models.

3. Results and Methods

A prototype Workbench has been developed which consists of 3 main components; these are the regimen editor, the simulation engine and the interactive tumour response graph. The prototype is available as both a stand alone application and within the WWW [Boyle et al 1996]. Each of the Workbench components is described below.

The Regimen Editor

The regimen editor allows oncologists to graphically define a multi-drug treatment regimen using up to seven drugs. Currently, two different delivery strategies are permitted (a bolus or an infusion). Oncologists build up the required chemotherapeutic regimen by dynamically selecting the required drug, the method of delivery, and the time of administration. This process can then

be repeated so that schedules with multiple boluses and infusions can be constructed if required (see Figure 1).

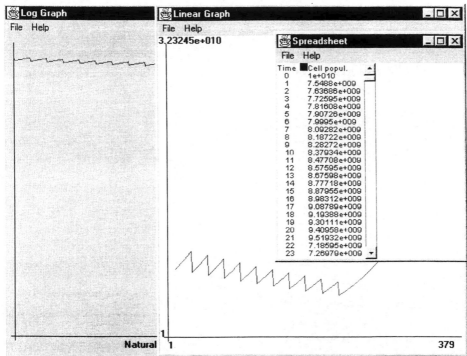

Figure 2: The mathematical model uses the information from a treatment regimen to predict how the tumour size (the number of cells) changes over time. We have provided a number of different views on these results, to enable the oncologist to examine the results. A log graph view, a tabular view and a standard graph view have been provided. As we have designed the system using a model/view mechanism any number of these views can be created and used in combination (so that a selection in one view is shown in all the other views).

The regimen editor contains three elements which relate to toxicity, and advise oncologists of possible problems. The first two are the maximum tolerated dose at any point in time and the maximum cumulative dose which can be administered. If either of these two constraints are exceeded , a warning is given to the user. Since oncologists have a variety of methods at their disposal for overcoming certain toxic side effects (e.g. bone marrow suppression can be overcome by a bone marrow transplant) these two values can be changed, thus allowing higher doses or a higher cumulative quantity of drug to be given. The third element is a mechanism which indicates visually to the user the additive side effects which are induced by the administration of each drug. There are bars along the horizontal (time) axis of the graph which darken as the cumulative toxic effect of the regimen approaches the maximum tolerable dose for a specific time interval.

The Simulation Engine
Different mathematical models may be utilised within this component of the oncologists workbench which describe tumour growth and response to chemotherapy. Two examples will be described here. Firstly the Gompertz growth model incorporating a cell kill term representing the administration of a chemotherapeutic drug can be seen below:

$$\frac{dN}{dt} = -\lambda N \ln\left(\frac{N}{\theta}\right) - \rho NC(t)$$

where   l and q are the tumour growth parameters

              r is the dose response parameter

and   C(t) is the concentration of the chemotherapeutic drug.

The second example is the Competition model (Usher and Henderson (1996)). The tumour consists of two subpopulations (drug sensitive and drug resistant cells) and there are mechanisms in operation for cells migrating between the subpopulations. The required differential equations governing the behaviour of the drug sensitive and drug resistant cell subpopulations are given below:-

$$\frac{dN_1}{dt} = \begin{cases} \left\{\lambda_1^* N_1\right\} & + \left\{\beta\gamma_2\mu\right\} - \left\{\psi\gamma_1 N_1\right\} - \left\{\rho N_1 C(t)\right\} & , N \le N_C \\[2em] \left\{\left(\lambda_1^* + \frac{\lambda_1}{\alpha_1}\left[1 - \left(\frac{N}{N_C}\right)^{\alpha_1}\right]\right)N_1\right\} & + \left\{\beta\gamma_2\mu\right\} - \left\{\psi\gamma_1 N_1\right\} - \left\{\rho N_1 C(t)\right\} & , N \ge N_C \end{cases}$$

$$\frac{d\mu}{dt} = \begin{cases} \left\{\lambda_2^*\mu\right\} & + \left\{\psi\gamma_1 N_1\right\} - \left\{\beta\gamma_2\mu\right\} & , & N \le N_C \\[2em] \left\{\left(\lambda_2^* + \frac{\lambda_2}{\alpha_2}\left[1 - \left(\frac{N}{N_C}\right)^{\alpha_2}\right]\right)\mu\right\} & + \left\{\psi\gamma_1 N_1\right\} - \left\{\beta\gamma_2\mu\right\} & , & N \ge N_C \end{cases}$$

where N_1 and m denote the number of cells in the drug sensitive and drug resistant subpopulations, respectively, at time t.

           $N = N_1 + m$ denotes the total tumour cell population

           N_C represents the size of the total tumour cell population at the transition point corresponding to the two phase growth of the "Generalised-Ex" model [Usher (1994)].

           l_1^*, l_1, a_1, are the growth parameters associated with the drug sensitive cells.

           l_2^*, l_2, a_2 are the growth parameters associated with the drug resistant cells.

           y is the migration rate of drug sensitive cells becoming drug resistant.

           b is the migration rate of drug resistant cells becoming drug sensitive.

           g_1, g_2 are the respective proportions of proliferating drug sensitive and drug resistant cells.

           r is the dose response parameter.

The information provided by the oncologists when designing novel chemotherapeutic regimens within the regimen editor is passed to the simulation engine. The information stored about each drug is retrieved, and the implemented mathematical models are utilised to predict the tumour response to treatment. The simulation results are then passed to the interactive tumour response graph where oncologists can view the tumour response, either graphically or in tabular form. The oncologists therefore never have to explicitly consider the mathematical models which are being employed. Only an understanding of the biological mechanisms incorporated in the models is required in order for the results to be correctly interpreted.

The Interactive Tumour Response Graph

The interactive tumour response graph allows for the representation and analysis of tumour response to treatment. The output produced provides oncologists with the ability to browse tumour size throughout treatment in both graphical and tabular form (see Figure 2). This tool therefore allows for easy comparison between the results for different chemotherapeutic regimens. Since the results can be viewed in tabular form it is straightforward to compute statistics which are of interest, for example, anticipated response rates for a specific treatment or the fractional reduction of the average tumour.

4.   Discussion

Clinical oncologists currently utilise empirical clinical evaluation for evaluating the effect of novel chemotherapeutic regimens upon tumour growth. This method is expensive and time consuming and as a result, is unlikely to ever produce the optimum dose and schedule for even a single agent. In order to try and address this problem the Oncologists Workbench has been developed which allows treatment schedules to be graphically constructed, and returns a predicted tumour response.

The Workbench could therefore:-
*   expedite clinical drug trials
*   lead to more cost effective experimentation
*   suggest optimal treatment regimens within the bounds of clinical acceptability

5.   References

BIRKHEAD B.G and GREGORY W.M, 1984. A mathematical model of the effects of drug resistance in cancer chemotherapy. Mathematical Biosciences, 72, pp.59-69.
BOYLE J, HENDERSON D, McCALL J, McLEOD H, and USHER J, 1996. Exploring Novel Chemotherapy Treatments using the WWW. Proceedings of MEDNET96.
CASSIDY J and McLEOD H, 1995. Is it possible to design a logical development plan for an anti-cancer drug ? Pharmaceutical Medicine, 9, pp.95-103.
FOX J, JOHNS N, RAHMANZADEH A and THOMSON R. PROforma: a method and language for specifying clinical guidelines and protocols. MIE 1996.
GOLDIE J.H and COLDMAN A.J, 1979. A mathematical model for relating the drug sensitivity of tumours to their spontaneous mutation rate. Cancer Treatment Reports, 63, pp.1727-33.
MARTIN R.B, FISHER M.E, MINCHIN R.F and TEO K.L, 1992. Optimal control of tumor size used to maximise survival time when cells are resistant to chemotherapy. Mathematical Biosciences, 110, pp.201-219.
MARTIN R and TEO K.L, 1994. Optimal control of drug administration in cancer chemotherapy. World Scientific.
McCALL J.A.W and PETROVSKI A, 1996. Searching for optimal strategies in cancer chemotherapy. Presented to the Seventh IMA Conference on Mathematics Applied in Medicine and Biology. Oxford, 1996.
SWAN G.W, 1990. Role of optimal control theory in cancer chemotherapy. Mathematical Biosciences, 101, pp 237-284.
USHER J.R, 1994. Some mathematical models for cancer chemotherapy. Computers Math Applic, 28 (9), pp73-80.
USHER J.R and HENDERSON D, 1996. A competition model for cancer chemotherapy in the presence of drug resistance. Presented at the 7th IMA Conference on Mathematics Applied in Medicine and Biology, Oxford, 1996.

Medical Informatics Europe '97
C. Pappas et al. (Eds.)
IOS Press, 1997

Implementation Problems of Decision Support System for Nosocomial Infection

Miran REMS[(1)], Marko Bohanec[(2)], Božo Urh[(3)], Zdenka Kramar[(1)],
[(1)] *General Hospital Jesenice, Surgery Unit, Jesenice, Slovenia*
[(2)] *Jožef Stefan Institute, Jamova 39, Ljubljana, Slovenia*
[(3)] *INFONET - Engineering of Medical Informatics, Kranj, Slovenia*

Abstract. Decision support system for nosocomial infection therapy Ptah can reduce antibiotic misuse with data about bacteria resistance and antibiotic ineffectiveness. Resistance vectors in time series show epidemiological problems with resistant bacterias, named house-bacteria. Most important implementation factors are integrated hospital information system and doctors, nurses and managers interested in problems of nosocomial infection.

1. Introduction

Nosocomial infection is every microbial disease that develops during an admission to hospital and is a consequence of treatment, procedures of treatment or work of hospital staff[1]. About 5–10% of patients admitted to hospital develop a nosocomial infection, and 3% of them die of consequences [6]. Particularly acute are infections that occur at critically ill patients in intensive care units. The therapy must be appropriate and timely, since the patients whose immune system is strongly deficient are affected. Studies of nosocomial infections mainly stress the need of permanent control of procedures and therapy at intubated patients and patients with central vein catheters [7–10].

Because of its importance, specially for critically ill patients, constant surveillance of nosocomial infection is vital. First step in surveillance is the control of infection rates of procedures. By controlling infection rates we can specially assess nursing part of procedures (for example cleaning of entrance port of vein catheters or right procedure of tracheal aspiration, desinfection). Infection rate control has also economic impact. Using single use materials (gloves, aspirating catheters..), which are expensive, but obligatory, price for nursing of critically ill patient is rising. Only such accurate procedure can preserve critically ill patient of possible nosocomial infection, which is much more costly in economic point of view. Surveillance has importance as a quality control measure, as well [7,8].

A clinical manifestation of disease depends on at least three factors: (1) the patient's resistance, (2) bacterial aggressiveness and resistance to antibiotics, and (3) environment in which the patient is treated. All the three factors behave biologically and vary fast. Therefore, the therapy itself should be fast and predefined [11]. A proper treatment requires:

- permanent microbiologic supervision,
- monitoring bacterial resistance,
- permanent control of diagnostic and therapeutic procedures.

The nfluential part of the environment is a doctor with his knowledge of antimicrobal therapy, biology of bacteria, antibiotics and environment as such. The Doctor is probably the most influential factor for the outcome of disease. He can also influence the bacterial resistance. With antibiotic therapy the patient is doing well, but with improper use of antibiotic the bacteria can also do well despite of antibiotics.

Particularly dangerous initiators of nosocomial infections are aggressive bacteria that are developed and transmitted within the hospital, reaching a high level of resistance to antibiotics. Such bacteria have to be identified as soon as possible, and their further progress must be stopped by appropriate procedures. All these characteristics call for a computer support in this area.

In order to detect such bacteria, called house-bacteria, strict protocols for all proccdures must be considered.

2. Decision support systems

Variety of bacterial and environmental biology promote decision support systems (DSSs) for therapy of nosocomial infections. Proper therapy in case of established nosocomial infection is very important, specially with critically ill patient.

There are data which support the opinion that DSSs could increase the antibiotic resistance. The study with over 160 000 patients show that antibiotic costs were halved with stable antimicrobal resistance patterns, with decreased mortality[10]. Result was reached with DSS for antibiotic management and not with limited physician access to certain antibiotics.

- DSS and surveillance programmes are appropriate in hospitals with integrated information systems [7,10,11]. In General Hospital Jesenice integrated hospital information system called *InfoMed* has been used since 1992. Surveillance of infection rates is a part of this system from 1994[12,13]. Subsequent analyses have shown that the collected data provide a valuable insight into the past events and activities, which can substantially contribute to the improvement of therapeutic activities and, particularly, to decision making in the selection of therapy [11]. The *Ptah* (acronym for the description of the system in Slovene:" *P*odpora *t*erapevtskih *a*ktivnosti pri *h*ospitalnih infekcijah" - A Support of Therapeutic Activities at Hospital Aquired Infections) is based on a database of infections of surgical wounds, vein catheters and tracheal aspirate [14]. The data include:
- activity in which infection arose: operation, intubation, catheter insertion;
- infection: type and date of infection, successive day of treatment, date of specimen;
- microbiologic findings (antibiogram);
- therapy: prescribed antibiotics;
- general data, such as patient's temperature and local symptoms.

For the analyses of bacterial resistance and antibiotics' effectiveness, the most important data comes from antibiograms, which contain microbiologic findings on specimen taken from patients. For each isolated bacterium, an antibiogram displays a *resistance vector*; each element of the vector corresponds to a particular antibiotic and represents the resistance of the bacterium to that antibiotic. There are four possible levels of resistance: *Resistant*, *Intermediary*, *Sensitive*, and *Unknown*.

All analyses are based on time series of resistance vectors, which are constructed from the database using various criteria.

Bacteria resistance is important in selecting appropriate therapy. In Ptah bacteria resistance is graphically displayed as a number of R's (resistance) on the time axis. Considering most "dangerous" bacteria (Psedomonas spec, Meticillin resistant Staph.a,...) such diagram is early sign of alert zone. All procedures and therapy must be rechecked again including proper mesures and therapy (Figure 1).

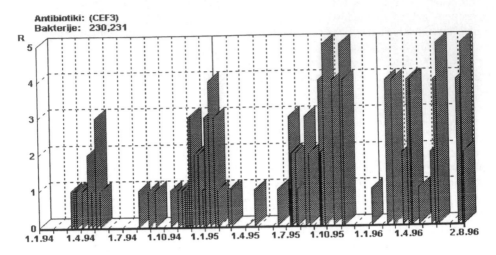

Figure 1. Resistance of Pseudomaonas species to Cephalosporins of III. Generation in time series. At the end of 1994 and 1995 there were obvious some epidemiological problems with Pseudosomonas sp.

Looking for transmission of such bacterias within the hospital Ptah offer graph of similarity of resistance vectors. Identification of such bacteria is based on the fact that these bacteria occur simultaneously at more patients and have similar resistance. Two vectors are similar when they differ in at most one element. "Clouds" of lines connecting such points present possibility of transmission of resistant bacteria (Figure 2).

Antibiotiki: (CEF3)

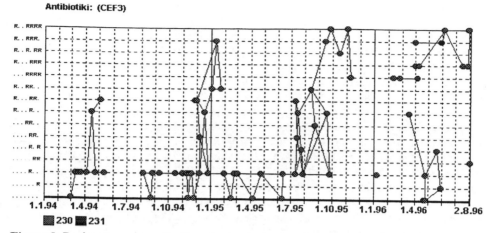

■ 230 ■ 231

Figure 2. Resistance vectors for Pseudomonas sp. regarding resistance on Cephalosporins of III. Generation

The prescription of antibiotics is essential in case of infection, especially nosocomial. Expected results are in close connection with the effectiveness of antibiotics. Effectiveness of antibiotic is not only antibiotic and patient related, but also doctor related. If the right therapy is prescribed in time, antibiotic can do its work. The ineffectiveness of antibiotics can be assessed statistically from time series as an average percentage of resistance in a given period. If effectiveness of antibiotic fall below threshold of 30%, its further use is no more suitable. After a longer period of non using such antibiotic, effectiveness can rise again (Figure 3).

Bakterije: 110,112,113

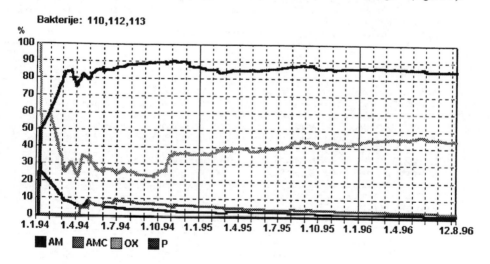

■ AM ■ AMC ▨ OX ■ P

Figure 3. Ineffectiveness of antibiotic (AM= ampicillin, AMX= amoxicillin and clavulonic acid, OX= oxicillin, P= penicillin) to Staphiloccocus species

3. Implementation problems

Despite of research and money used for research DSS is not in widespread use at the present time[15]. Probably DSS can begin to live only in established environment of integrated hospital information system. Information hospital system itself is composed not only of computers and nets, but also of demanding users. Doctors, nurses or managers with such interests are parts of integrated information systems. DSS can be fully implemented in such environment only. Probably new enthusiasm with electronic medical record will produce more DSSs also in important field of oncology [16,17,18] and other fields of medicine. Results of DSS are confirmed in very defined fields with very defined environment: (septicemia[19]), icterus (project Euricterus) and acute abdominal pain. DSSs are still supporting just a small part of medical problems. Nosocomial infections are part of side effects of medical treatment and are specially interesting for DSS. More precise treatments with fast and accurate answers are welcome. For better understanding presentations in DSS must be time related and possibly in graphic form. New generations of doctors with well established knowledge of computer usage will bring new enthusiasm.

References

[1]   Gardner P, Arnow PM: Hospital acquired infections. In Braumwald E (Ed): Harrison's Principles and Practice of Internal Medicine, McGraw-Hill, New York, 1987, 470-4.

[2]   Santamaria J: Nosocomial Infections. In: Oh TE (Ed): Intensive care manual, Butterworths, Sydney, 1990, 409-16.

[3]   Cercenado E et al.: A conservative procedure for the diagnosis of catheter related infections. Arch Intern Med 1990; 150: 1417-20.

[4]   Kamal GD, Pfaller MA, Rempe LE, Jebson PJ: Reduced intravascular catheter infection by antibiotic bonding; a prospective randomized controlled trial. JAMA 1991; 256: 2364-8.

[5]   Reed CR, Sessler CN, Glauser FL, Phelan BA: Central venous catheter infections concepts and controversies. Intens Care Med 1995; 21: 177-83.

[6]   Snowdon SL. Hygiene standards for breathing systems? Br J Anaest 1994; 72: 143-4.

[7]   Ryf C: Computerunterstutzte prospective Wundinfectionsuberwachung. Ideen und Prinzipien. Swiss Surg 1995; 1: 40-4.

[8]   Melcher GA: Computerunterstutzte prospective Wundinfectionsuberwachung. Erfahrungen und praktische Anwendung. Swiss Surg 1995; 1:45-7.

[9]   Hemmer M: Nosocomial pneumonia in mechanically ventilated patients. Critical Care Med 1993; 8:591-7.

[10]   Pestotnik SL, Classen DC, Evans RS, Burke JP: Implementing antibiotic guidelines through computer- assisted decision support: clinical and finacial outcomes. Ann Intern Med 1996; 124:884-90.

[11]   Bohanec M, Rems M, Urh B: Design of an information system for supporting therapeutic activities of hospital infections (in Slovene), In: Lavra~ N (Ed): Computer-based analysis of medical data, IJS Scientific Publishing IJS-SP-95-1, Bled, 1995, 64-75.

[12]   Kramar Z, Rems M: Computer evidence of hospital infections in General Hospital Jesenice (in Slovene). Medicinska informatika MI-92 Bled, 1992, 161-5.

[13]   Rems M, Kramar Z, Zupan~i~ M: Computer assisted surveillance of nosocomial infections in intensive care unit. Eight Anastaesia A-A Symposium, Portoro`, 1995, 165-7.

[14]   Bohanec M, Rems M, Slavec S, Urh B: Decision Support of Nosocomial Infection Therapy. Proceedings of 13th international congress of EFMI, MIE 96, Copenhagen, 1996.

[15]   Miller RA: Medical diagnostic decision support system - past, present and future: a threated bibliography and brief commentary. J Am Med Inform Assoc 1994, 1: 8-27.

[16]   McCormick KA: Including oncology outcomes of care in the computer-based patient record. Oncology, 1995; 9: 161-7.

[17]   Hammond P, Harris AL, Das SK, Wyatt JC : Safety and Decision support in oncology. Methods Inf Med, 1994; 33: 371-81.

[18]   Wigren T, Kolari P: Evaluation of a decision- support system for inoperable non-small cell lung cancer. Methods Inf Med, 1994, 33: 397-401.

[19]   Dybowsky R, Grandsen WR, Phillips I: Towards a statistically oriented decision support system for the menagement of septicemia. Artif Intell Med 1993; 5: 489-502.

Medical Informatics Europe '97
C. Pappas et al. (Eds.)
IOS Press, 1997

Human fluid balance modelling
and its treatment simulation with HIDION

Alexandru TRICA[1], Elena JITARU[1], George LITARCZEK[2],
Octavian TEODORESCU[3], Ioana MOISIL[4]

[1] Research Institute for Informatics. Bucharest. Romania (E-mail: trica@u3.ici.ro)
[2] Fundeni Clinical Hospital. Bucharest. Romania
[3] Clinical Hospital of Obstetrics and Gynecology Oradea. Romania
[4] National Centre for Health Statistics. Bucharest. Romania

Abstract HIDION is a tandem system composed of an expert system for diagnosis of the water and electrolytic balance disturbance and a modelling program for simulation and suggestion of the needed correction. The expert system attempts to make a diagnosis mainly based on clinical symptoms and on patient history, as they are generally available for most physicians. The treatment module assists the user to establish a right strategy for re-equilibration of the fluid balance. The first aim of the system is to achieve a correct diagnosis of the disturbances of the fluid balance and a choice of therapy tactics. The second aim of the system is an educational one for both physicians and nurses. The entire system, including the expert module as well as the modelling module is developed in Turbo Prolog.

1. Introduction

The disturbance of the fluid and electrolyte balance of a patient is one main reason for pathogenesis in many diseases. So a fast and right diagnosis of the fluid balance, as well as an early and correct therapeutical intervention are the crux of the patient's rehabilitation.

To make a qualitative diagnosis is a common task of an expert physician but it is not so easy to evaluate the quantitative deviation. Similar difficulties appear in the recovery measures needed for patient's re-equilibration. So a tool capable of modelling the patient's fluid balance and of simulating the effect of any interaction can be very helpful. A number of knowledge based systems have been developed for meeting this need [1,2].

HIDION is a knowledge-based system for diagnosis and treatment of fluid balance. The first objective of the system is to make a correct diagnosis of the disturbance of the fluid balance and a choice of therapy tactics, followed by the maintenance of an equilibrate fluid balance calculation. The second aim of the system is to be an educational tool for both physicians and nurses.

HIDION was meant to ease the task of making a qualitative and quasi-quantitative estimation of the state of fluid balance of patients in emergency and intensive care. It was designed for being used by physicians who have no computer knowledge.

2. General presentation of HIDION

HIDION uses a general flow of data and actions (Figure 1) as in the practice of the physicians:

- data / facts acquisition about the case;

- diagnosis of the patient;
- therapeutical measures establishing.

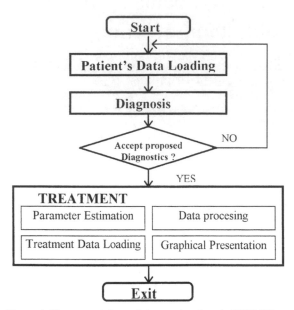

Figure 1 The general flow of data and actions in HIDION

HIDION uses a knowledge base, loaded by means of the knowledge acquisition module, which permits the loading and updating of the physicians' expertise in this area. As this module is not for clinical use it will not be presented in this paper.

HIDION consists of four main components:

1. HIDION Monitor,
2. Patient data management component,
3. Diagnosis component,
4. Treatment component.

The Patient data management module handles the facts concerning the patients' health state. It has a lot of lists of symptoms where the physicians can choose the adequate items from. It works with three kinds of *symptoms*: history data, clinical symptoms and lab results. Of course the lab results are not mandatory. After their handling the patient data are stored in a file to be used by diagnosis and treatment modules.

The Diagnosis module consists of an expert system. It attempts to make a diagnosis mainly based on clinical symptoms and on patient history, as they are generally available to most physicians. Rules for diagnosis and treatment are represented in the form of production rules. The system employs a combination of forward and backward reasoning [3,4,5].

The diagnosis module establishes a diagnostic that is expressed as a type of deviation (water excess or depletion, sodium excess or depletion) and approximate amplitude of deviation expressed in % from the normal value. As HIDION is an artificial diagnosis system it needs an acceptance from its user for the proposed diagnoses. A nonconfirmation leads to restarting the examination dialogue and to inquiring for more data especially in the lab category. After the confirmation, the program asks the physicians' appreciation on each disturbance of the water volume and Na concentration, while proposing itself a value. The received values are stored together with the patient data and will be used by the treatment module.

3. The treatment module

The HIDION treatment module main task is to assist the user in establishing a right strategy for reequilibration of the patient's fluid balance.

This module ensures the following activities:

- estimation of the parameters which define the fluid status;
- loading of the treatment data indicated by the physician;
- data processing for obtaining results with the proposed therapeutical measures;
- graphical presentation of the fluid balance.

The treatment program models the two main fluid compartments of the body: *extracellular* and *intracellular*.

The treatment program ensures a direct visualisation of the type and magnitude of the disorder indicating the amount of water and salt to be administrated or removed. The treatment module uses a graphical representation to show the fluid balance and its evolution according to medical advice. The model also permits interactive manipulation, simulating therapy and shows its direct results.

So it seems most interesting to have a means to visualise and appreciate the immediate impact of a therapeutical measure on the extracellular compartment of the body water. The final result after an equilibration with the intracellular compartment, which takes some time, will be present in a later phase.

It is surely difficult for any physician to exactly appreciate the dimension of the needed correction as it is difficult to appreciate the time during which this correction is to be made in order to avoid an excessive impact on the extracellular compartment. It would thus be of interest to dispose of a tool allowing to create a model of the fluid status of a patient and to permit a flexible step by step adjustment of the therapeutic measures.

The model of the fluid status is presented as a rectangle (Figure 2) with two compartments in which the height represents concentration and the basis the volume of the respective sectors [6].

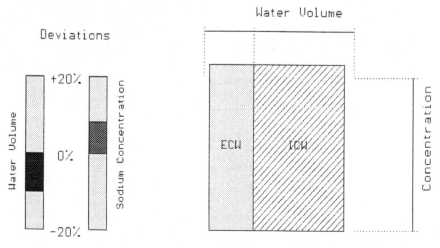

Figure 2 The screen layout of the water volume and salt concentration disturbances

The two compartments of the rectangle represent the extra and intracellular compartments respectively. For a better visualisation of the disturbances, two additional rulers are shown on the left of the screen. The initial rectangle presents the situation generated by the diagnosis section of the system.

The modelling module displays the volume and the osmolality of the liquid in either main compartment of body water. This ensures a direct visualisation of the type and magnitude of the disorder indicating the amount of water and salt to be administrated or removed. The treatment module uses a graphical representation to show the fluid balance and its evolution according to medical advice.

The next table shows the steps proposed by the physician and simulated by HIDION together with their results.

Table 1: Therapeutical steps towards the equilibration of water and electrolyte

Ste p	Starting Status		Therapeutical Intervention		Final Status	
	Water (%)	Salt (%)	Water (l)	Salt (mmol)	Water (%)	Salt (%)
1	90 %	109 %	+1.5	-	93 %	104.5 %
2	93 %	104.5 %	+1	-	94.5 %	103 %
3	94.5 %	103 %	+1.5	+200	97 %	102 %
4	97 %	102 %	+1.5	+100	100.2 %	100.5 %

A suggestive image of a step is shown in Figure 3 where the left picture shows the situation immediately after the therapeutical intervention and the right picture shows the equilibrated situation after a few hours. The steps described can be iterated as many times as necessary to achieve normalisation volume and concentration in both compartments of the body water.

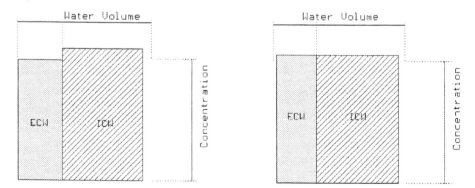

Figure 3 The equilibration between the two compartments

The trace of the therapeutical interventions is also presented synthetically on a square table divided into 9 equal sections (Figure 4). The base of the square represents volume variations ±15% body water, high Na concentration variations ±15% around the normal value of 140 mmol/l (119-161 mmol). The first point shows the initial situation, the next 4 points show the results of 4 therapeutical interventions presented in Table 1, the last one showing a very good situation: the disturbance close to 0.

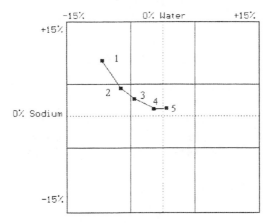

Figure 4 The trace of the therapeutical interventions

The status of fluid compartments can be figured on this picture and is very suggestive for the definition of the diagnosis - type and amplitude - as well as for the effect of the treatment.

4. Conclusions

HIDION is a useful system that can assist a physician in both diagnosis and treatment of the fluid balance disturbances. The treatment module, on which our attention has been focused in this paper, offers a powerful tool to support the physician in making his decisions concerning the therapy measures. It has been very well received by both clinicians and students and we hope that it will be used in the current activity.

Now we are working on transposing the HIDION system in MS Windows environment, using VISUAL PROLOG, and also on redesigning the graphical interface in order to put all images on the same screen and to offer a facility to resize any desired part.

References

1. Brelidze,Z., Nabakhteveli,N., Nanuashvili,A., Bokhua,A., Gonjilashvili,J. and Kuprava,R. : Clinical Information System of Fluid Acid-Base and Electrolytic Balance Estimation and Correction, *Proceedings of the 12-th International Congress of the European Federation of Medical Informatics*, Lisbon, 22-26 May 1994:104-8.
2. *** NANDA Diagnosis. http://www_son.hs.washington.edu/Fluid/page2.html.
3. Trica,A., Jitaru,E., Grosu,G.: Knowledge acquisition and management in SIRAM, *Proceedings of the National Symposium on Medical Informatics*, Constanta, CCSS-MS, 1989:304-6
4. Trica,A., Jitaru,E., Grosu,G.: The possibilities offered by SIRAM for building medical expert systems, *Romanian Workshop on Artificial Intelligence Applications in Medicine*, Baia Mare, CCSS-MS, 1991:112-20
5. Teodorescu,O., Litarczek,G., Trica,A., Jitaru,E., Diagnosis of Hydro-electrolytic Balance with HIDION, *Proceedings of The XIX-th National Conference on Medical Informatics*, Cluj-Napoca, 6-9 Nov. 1996:30-2.
6. Bland,J.: Clinical Recognition and management of disturbances of fluid balance, W.B. Saunders Company, Philadelphia, 1958.

Medical Informatics Europe '97
C. Pappas et al. (Eds.)
IOS Press, 1997

IDIS-KS: an Intelligent Drug Information System as a Knowledge Server[*]

I .Vlahavas, A. Pomportsis and I. Sakellariou
Dept. of Informatics, Aristotle University of Thessaloniki, 54006 Thessaloniki-Greece
e-mail: {vlahavas,pomportsis}@ csd.auth.gr, esakelar@athena.auth.gr

Abstract

Expert System technology in combination with other technologies such as Networks and Data Base systems can prove to be a valuable tool for medical experts, providing decision support and information services, and therefore facilitating and improving their everyday tasks. IDIS-KS described in this paper, is an consultation and information system dedicated to deliver drug information and suggestions about possible treatments to medical practicioners in the National area of Greece.

1. Introduction

Physicians and pharmacists confront in their everyday practice the problem of dealing with a large amount of information concerning medical compounds used in therapy. Not only this knowledge is large but also variable; new drugs are released and new clinical results are published. It is obvious that the distribution of this knowledge by "traditional" means (reference books, seminars, etc.) is both cost and time inefficient. The software packages developed so far dealing with this problem, are mainly data banks [6], which have little relation with the "expert system" philosophy and even less relation with the integration of all the embedded information, meaning interrelations, analysis and decision making.

This paper proposes the design and development of an Intelligent Drug Information System acting as a Knowledge Server (IDIS-KS) which will provide information and decision support services concerning drugs and medicines used in therapeutics mainly in Greece. The provided services will be available over a wide area network structure, enabling easy remote access to the interested pharmacists and medical practitioners, and can be especially useful in cases where immediate access to such information is costly or even impossible by other means.

2. Relevant Work

In most cases, medical information services are offered by data bases that provide easy access to the stored information. The Martindale[5] On-line/CD-ROM for example,

---

[*] This Work is partialy sponsored by EU under the TELEMATICS 2C project "Medical Emergency Aid through Telematics" (MERMAID), ref. no. HC 1034.

marketed by the Micromedex Inc., offers an easily accessible data base. Another example is Drugline[6], a drug information database, that offers problem-oriented drug evaluation comparable to a clinical consultation.

On the other hand, medical science has been also used as an area of application for the expert system technology before. The most well known example is MYCIN, is an expert system developed at Stanford University, which diagnoses and proposes a treatment for meningitis and bacteremia (blood infections) [1,4].

3. Our approach: the IDIS-KS Expert System

This proposed work, IDIS-KS, is a complement of a previous work done in our group concerning the development of IDIS, a prototype expert system that can suggest a possible treatment not only for a specific class, but for a wide range of diagnosed diseases [3]. This prototype system is in the rule base expert system mold; it contains a set of rules that incorporate all the information about drugs (indications, contra-indications, interactions, etc.) and the expert knowledge that enables to manipulate it. Its operation is simple; the user poses a query describing a diagnosed disease, interacts with the system providing information about the patient and receives as an answer a suggested treatment, in which possible contra-indications and interactions with other drugs that are prescribed to the patient have been considered. IDIS, being a prototype, includes only a small ammount of drugs and can deal with a small number of cases.

IDIS-KS extends significanlty the previous system by offering apart from decision support, conventional data base information services, multiple ways of presentation (multimedia, hypermedia), and network facilities.

4. Operation of IDIS-KS

The operation of IDIS-KS can be divided in two levels; the *information level* and the *consultation level* (figure 1).

In the *Information level* the system operates as a normal data base supplying information on drugs (nomenclature, indications, etc.) as well as relevant published material about new and existing compounds (clinical research and testing data, scientific articles and announcements, greek and foreign bibliography etc.). Additionally the system will inform the user of any recent changes to the stored knowledge and will incorporate hypermedia, multimedia data presentation and display tools.

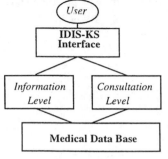

figure 1: Overview of the IDIS-KS Expert System

In the *Consultation level* the system operates as an expert system suggesting to the practicioner a proper treatment for her/his patient. The suggestecd treatment will be based on the information that is stored in the system's data base, and all possible interactions, contra-indications or other problems concerning the patient will have been dealt with and all necessary information like precautions, adverse effects, etc., will be presented in the system's output. The purpose of the second level is not, in any case, to substitute the medical expert, but to assist him in the decision making. Towards that direction the system will include explanatory facilities involving justification of the suggested treatment (*how queries*) and explanation

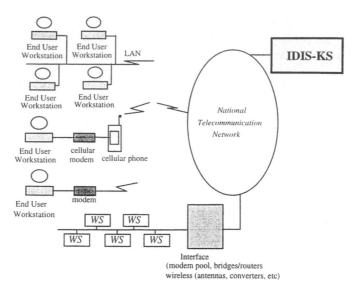

figure 2: Networking of the IDIS-KS

why a specific piece of information is requested *(why queries),* in order to provide the essential justification for the proposed treatment.

The IDIS-KS is an expert system that in its final form will provide the information and consultation services over a wide area network (using the existing telecommunications infrasrtucture), thus the expert system will act as an *intelligent knowledge server*[2]. Special consideration will be taken so that the system will be accessible through all possible offered networking protocols and services in the national area of Greece, (cellular communi-cations, IP networks, ISDN, GSM, ATM, etc.) making it available to everyone interested (figure 2).

5. Structure of IDIS-KS

IDIS-KS is comprised of three parts, the *Medical Data Base, Intelligent Tools* and finally the *Interface* (figure 3).

The *Medical Data Base (MDB)* is a conventional data base, dedicated to the storage of all relevant data concerning drugs and medical compounds. The knowledge contained in the data base will be created by medical experts, who will be responsible for its entry, update and verification.

The *Intelligent Tools* part consits of the information and consultation tools of the system and can be further devided in two subparts:

1. *The information management part* that provides the access facilities to all information stored in the MDB; it includes the knowledge discovery tools, data integrity and quality control, hypermedia and multimedia management tools, data presentation and display, etc.

2. The *decision support part* that implements the consultation level of the IDIS-KS. This part involves:

- The *System Controller* that handles the user query, by directing it to the appropriate module; either the *inference engine,* the *explanation facility* or the *library of past queries.*
- A *Rule Base* that incorporates the necessary expertise for deducing an answer to the specific user query, based on the data stored in the medical data base. The rules included

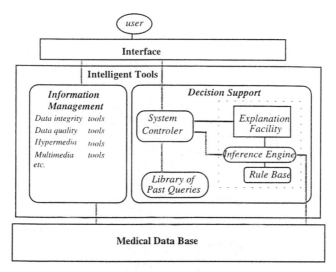

figure 3: The IDIS-KS Knowledge Server

will model the inference procedure of a human expert but will not contain drug specific knowledge about the medical substances; all necessary knowledge of the latter type will be retrieved from the MDB.

- An *inference engine* that is responsible for handling the above mentioned rule base, meaning inferences and rule firing.
- An *explanation facility*, that will be responsible for answering the *how* and *why* questions.
- A *library of past queries*, consisting of questions previously posed to the system. Any user query is matched against this library and if it has been posed earlier then the answer will be retrieved directly without the need of reconstructing it. This will improve the system performance and minimise unnecessary computation.

3. The *Interface* that provides a *user friendly graphical* environment in which the user interact with the IDS-KS. The interface will be easy to use and will not require previous computing experience from the end user. It will be able to adjust to the particular needs, interests and authorisation levels of the user. A number of interfaces will be developed to support the network connections to all platforms proposed above.

6. Simple Cases Drug Consultant

Currently, the above described decission support architecture has been applied to the development of an expert system that will assist the user, by providing a safe procedure to follow in order to supply medication in most common conditions . This system, called SCDC (Simple Cases Drug Consultant), has been developed as part of the Mermaid [8] Eurpean funded telemedicine project. The latter aims to the provision of multilingual medical emergency service around the world by using state of the art satellite and terrestrial communications to transfer the expertise to seafarers when necessary. SCDC is intented for use on board when communication with one of the land bases is considered unnecessary. It interracts with the user obtaining all the necessary input and then retreives from the database all the information required in order to provide him with the necessary advice and information concerning the drug treatment of the patient in need. It has been developed in

Prolog (LPA Prolog [9]) while all the information needed has been stored in a relational data base (Paradox [10]).

7. Conclusion

The technologies involved in this project are neither new nor experimental if examined on their own. What we believe to be of both scientific and practical interest is the combination of them that will enable the offering of high quality services to the medical community. The aim is to improve the quality of offered services in the area of Greece and be of valuable help to all interested parties.

As an extension of the above, a specialised Drug Information Centre (DIC) [7] can be founded for recording all drugs and medicines used in therapeutics mainly in Greece and for supporting the expert system, i.e. knowledge verification and maintenance. This center could also provide off-line access (by phone or fax) to users unable to consult IDIS-KS via a network connection offering services to a larger number of users.

8. References

[1] Buchanan, B. G. and Shortliff, E., H. eds. 1984. *Rule Based Expert Systems: The MYCIN Experiments of the Stanford Heuristic Programming Project.* Reading, MA: Addison-Wesley.

[2] Erikson, H., *Expert Systems as Knowledge Servers*, IEEE Expert & Their Applications, June 1996, IEEE Computer Society, pg 14 - 19.

[3] Karakolidou, V. *Development of an Expert System for Providing Pharmaceptical Information*, BSc Thesis, Dept. of Informatics, Aristotle University of Thessaloniki, Greece, July 1996.

[4] Luger, G.,F., and Stubblefield, W., A., 1993. *Artificial Intelligence*, The Benjamin/Cummings Publishing Company, Inc. Second Edition.

[5] Martindale Online, Royal Pharmaceutical Society of Great Britain, Lambeth High Street, London, SE1-7JN.

[6] Öhman,B., Lyrvall, H., Törnqvist, E., Alván G., Sjöqvist, F. *Clinical pharmacology and the provision of drug information*, European Journal of Clinical Pharmacology, Springer-Verlag, 1992, pp 563-568

[7] Mamzoridi K., Pirpasopoulos K., Vlahavas I. and Pomportsis A., *Towards a Drug Information Center: The Aesculapius Project*, In proceedings of the 1st EURO DURG Conference, Karolinska, Sweden, 1996.

[8] MERMAID is the acronym for the project "Medical Emergency Through Telematics", sponsored by the EU programme TELEMATICS 2C, ref. no. HC1034.

[9] LPA Win Prolog is a trademark of Logic Programming Associates Ltd.

[10] PARADOX is a trademark of Borland International Inc.

Medical Informatics Europe '97
C. Pappas et al. (Eds.)
IOS Press, 1997

Five steps from a simple data base to an expert system in nutrition

Claudia Vicol[1], Dipl. Eng, Ioana Dobre[1], Dipl. Eng and
Constantin Ionescu-Tirgoviste[2] MD, PhD

1 - Institute for Computers, 167 Calea Floreasca, 72321 Bucharest, Romania, Phone:
(+40.1)2321948, Fax: (+40.1)2307845, e-mail: ioana@itcgate.itc.ro
2 - Institute for Nutrition and Metabolic Diseases, 5-7 I. Movila, Bucharest, Romania,
Phone: (+40.1)2107100

Abstract: The paper describes the experience from the Medical Informatics
Department - ITC in the field of the human nutrition. The informatic systems
were developed staring from a minimal data base and simple programs. The
final versions are expert systems running within complex medical informatic
products.

The first step: the beginning - a simple data base for dietetic purposes

Human nutrition is a very important medical field.

The aim of our work is to ensure nutritional supervision with the help of the computer. The estimated result is the efficient assessment and improvement, as much as possible, of the human nutritional behaviour. This will lead to the decreasing of the number and consequence of nutritional mistakes.

The main factors which affect the human nutritional behaviour, and can lead to an inadequate nutritional state, malnutrition or better said mis-nutrition, can be classified in three categories: ·

- food-related factors, such as daily food intake and food composition
- non-food-related factors, such as infections and metabolic diseases
- social factors: cooking technologies, traditions, family income, personal tastes.

All these factors have been taken in view in all the stages of the elaboration of our information system, which allows its possibility of being used by a wide range of specialists: nutritionists, physicians of all specialities, sociologists, chemists, food manufacturers.

Our work in the field of human nutrition begun five years ago. We have started by gathering data about most ordinary nutrients. The result was the first version of our food data base. Its size was rather small, less than one hundred records. At that time the hardware in our department was prehistoric, IBM PC2 with 286/8Mhz and 30 or 40 MB HDD. The DB management system used was FoxPro 1.02 under DOS 4.02.

The food data base indicated the proportion of protein, carbohydrate, fat, water, vitamins, trace elements and total caloric value contained in a food. Since then, the information has been permanently enriched or modified, regarding the new scientific findings. The values were taken primarily from the work of the Alimentation Chemistry Institute and the Public Health and Alimentation Hygiene Institute from Bucharest. These nutrients are the most frequently used in our country and their values correspond to the specific food sources of our country (such as different fruit and vegetable varieties and animal breeds) [1].

In this first stage, the program ensured the classification of nutrients and the complete nutritional description of basic foods. For each food item in the data base the following information are provided: amount of energy, proteins, carbohydrate, fats, water, vitamins and trace elements, along with the number of grams of a standard serving, cost, serving size, manufacturer, source of information, date of the most recent updating. We take into account the interaction between foods and human body by the mean of digestibility coeffi-cients. The economic aspect is taken into account by providing the food price and a score which assesses its availability on the market. The program also provided the classification of foods after the criterion of their belonging to one of 10 main categories (such as meat, dairy products, fruit, vegetables a. s. o.) on nutritional or economical criteria.

Second step: a more complex data base

Our data base increased in size to hundreds of items. We added new tables aiming to help a wider range of users of the data base [2].

Adding new fields to the food data base

For each food of our data base, we provide a guidance score, which reflects the suitability of using it at different meals within a day: breakfast, mid-morning snack, lunch, afternoon snack, dinner, evening snack. This is useful for the diet generator module. For some special nutrients, which are indicated or forbidden in certain diseases, we also provide a suitability score.

The dietetic library

A new feature of the program is the description usual and simple dietetic meals. We are adding every day new recipes to the composite foods database. They are characterised by the type and amount of their ingredients and the cooking indications and they can be used as an eventual ingredient food for another recipe or a meal component.

Step 3: The diet analyser

As the food data base grew, we found new fields of interest in using it as a stand-alone informatic product: a diet analyser.

The nutritional inquiries

The first use was to perform nutritional inquiries among social or professional groups in order to establish correlation between alimentary behaviour and the incidence of different diseases, especially metabolic diseases.

As an example, here there are the results of a nutritional assessment made the last year at the Diabetes Centre from Bucharest. The nutritional data was calculated on the base of three days diet intake. A number of 140 insulin dependent diabetes mellitus 15-60 years patients were investigated. The group was stratified according to the sex, age at the onset and the duration of the disease. The mean, standard deviation, minimum and maximum intake in energy, proteins, fats, carbohydrates, fibres, alcohol, are given in the following table:

	Mean	SDV	Minimum	Maximum
Energy (kcal)	2426.03	581.88	1112.83	4005.81
Protein (g)	103.39	24.94	41.92	178.55
Animal proteins (g)	70.18	21.96	20.81	142.71
Vegetal proteins (g)	33.09	6.55	19.10	55.22
Fat (g)	111.85	40.34	32.21	217.36
Saturated fats (g)	44.66	15.79	14.26	89.50
Polyunsaturated fats (g)	21.55	10.36	2.67	49.36
Cholesterol (mg)	447.74	199.03	80.92	1022.42
Carbohydrate (g)	252.97	41.98	172.10	377.75
Fibre (g)	13.08	3.51	6.55	24.08
Alcohol (g)	1.53	3.85	0	22.00

The first rules for the knowledge - based system in nutrition

At this stage, our system was still a data base system but we started to gather experience in the field of human nutrition and to describe it as simple rules, which became the core of a simple knowledge - based system.

Step four: Diet generator

We were lucky and got more powerful computers, with 486 processors and lots of RAM. Our programs ran under Windows 3.11 and we had a significant experience in human nutrition and in medical informatic systems development [3].

Nutritionally balanced diet generator

It was time to leap to a new generation of products. We used the simple knowledge-based system issued at the previous step in conjunction with Prolog language and we elaborated our first expert system, meant to guide the nutrition for healthy people. The system provided the capability to create nutritionally balanced diets for individual needs and preferences and also supplies several versions of daily menus. It is this new quality of our program that makes it useful both to physicians specialised in other domains of internal medicine and to the patients themselves. If the patient has a home computer, he is enabled to establish by himself the diet considered the most adequate, according to his own tastes and food supplying possibilities.

Step five: More expert systems

As we found out that unfortunately sick people are much more frequent than healthy people, we started to develop expert systems which purpose is to assist their nutrition.

COMPEDIET

The first product of this kind is a customised program that assists the therapy in diabetes mellitus for children aged of 3 to 15 [4] : it is named **COMPEDIET**, it is meant to assist the medical activity in a children's antidiabetic centre and its main possibilities are:

- takes over, stores and processes the information resulted after the clinical and paraclinic investigations on the diabetic child, as well as the personal data and the pathological and physiological heredocolateral records, risk factors and social factors.
- displays and updates the information contained into the antidiabetic drugs database for each drug (composition, way of administration, indications, reactions, adverse effects, s. o.);
- selects from the food database the primary foods and recipes which are appropriate for the diabetic child.
- calculates the insulin doses to be administrated within treatment scheme according to the daily food intake, weight, corporal surface or age;
- generates adequate treatment scheme and evaluates the pharmacological risk according to: pharmacological effects, adverse reactions, side effects, interactions and incompatibilities between drugs.
- analyses the child's usual diet prior to the diabetes onset.
- generates every day and weekly diets from basic aliments or dietetic food, based on a file of recipes of dietetic food.

This program will be soon improved, in order to allow its use in the nutritional therapy of the adult with diabetes.

OBEZINF

The food data base and the enriched knowledge-base were used to develop another applied informatics product, which was destined to supervise the treatment of children with obesity. It's name is **OBEZINF** and is meant for computer aiding various phases of medical activities of treating obesity in a section of infantile endocrinology: patient's identification, behaviour inquiry, records registering, efficient following of the obese patient through a specialised medical record.

OBEZINF accomplishes the following functions :

- manages the relevant medical information about the obese child: personal data, clinical and laboratory data, antropometric data. Each patient has a personal data file, from the beginning of the monitorization (or hospitalisation).
- draws the shape of the body of the obese child and allows comparing with the shape of a normal's child body.
- performs a nutritional inquiry, along with taking into account their physiological and pathological characteristics, the level of physical activity, food preferences and social status. This is the step when the program analyses the diets and compares the results with the correct values. Statistics are also generated.
- suggests diagnosis
- generates a therapeutical diet, which takes into account the large amount of data collected previously and the facts from the knowledge data base.

The result is a diet suggestion for 7 days, 5 meals a day, as well as an extra physical activity level suggestion and, if necessary, the doses of eventual drugs. We found very useful to store pictures of the obese patients, at different moments of their evolution and also picture of normal weight children, in a data base that allows the physician to compare them more efficient.

A rise of the efficiency of physicians' and nurses' activity is accomplished by elaborating the dietetic prescriptions in a short time, taking into account the patient's preferences, by following the obese patient's evolution on a long term.

These systems are developed under Windows95.

Conclusions and further development of our systems

As we have noticed several improvements in the quality of medical activity :

- the medical staff are saved a lot of time by getting an operative diet analysis or generation
- diets can now be more diverse, including nutrients that are not used in standard diets, but are allowed or preferred by the patient
- medical expertise of high level professionals in nutrition can be transferred to every person interested in this problem.

We decided to expand our work to new medical fields and new information technologies.

We shall soon implement an expert system for the nutrition of elderly people and a smart-card based monitoring system as well as an expert system for the nutritional assessment of the athletes.

References
1. Favier J.C.: **Elaboration d'une banque de donnees sur la composition des aliments. Cahiers de nutrition et de dietetique** - 1983, vol.18, Nr..3, pag. 137 - 143.
2. Claudia Vicol, Ioana Dobre, C. Ionescu-Tirgoviste: **NUTRITIONIST, a data base for dietetic assistance** in HC96 Proceedings
3. Abbot, J. R. Bryant, B. Barber: **Information Management in Health Care**, The Institute of Health Services Management
4. IULIAN MINCU : **Alimentatia rationala a omului sanatos si bolnav** -Ed Medicala - 1975.

Medical Informatics Europe '97
C. Pappas et al. (Eds.)
IOS Press, 1997

Is Neural Network Better than Statistical Methods in Diagnosis of Acute Appendicitis?

Erkki Pesonen

Department of Computer Science and Applied Mathematics, University of Kuopio,
P.O.Box 1627, 70211 Kuopio, Finland

Abstract. Three statistical classification methods: discriminant analysis, logistic regression analysis and cluster analysis were compared with the back-propagation neural network algorithm in the diagnosis of acute appendicitis. The differences in the classification accuracy, which were evaluated with the receiver operating characteristic (ROC) curve were small, though discriminant analysis and back-propagation showed slightly better results than the other methods. The agreement of the methods on the diagnosis increased the accuracy of the classification, so that the number of misclassified cases reduced. The back-propagation neural network offers a good choice for statistical classification methods, but it was not found to be better than them. The use of several methods and their agreement as the basis of the diagnosis seems to give the best results for this diagnostic classification problem.

1. Introduction

The computer-aided diagnosis of acute abdominal pain has been widely studied during the last 20 years. The accuracy that has been achieved with different methods has varied between 50% - 90% [1-9].

We have been investigating the use of neural networks in medical decision making problems, especially with acute abdominal pain. In these studies we have found that neural network algorithms can classify the patient cases from databases nearly as well as a trained surgeon [9].

To see how well neural networks perform in comparison to statistical methods, we chose three statistical classification methods: discriminant analysis, logistic regression analysis and cluster analysis, and compared them with the back-propagation neural network algorithm in the diagnosis of acute appendicitis.

2. Materials and methods

Our data material consists of 1333 patients who had been admitted to University Hospital of Tampere and to Savonlinna Central Hospital in Finland and had been suffering from acute abdominal pain. Altogether 43 parameters were recorded from these patients. In this study we selected a subgroup of parameters, that consisted of 17 clinical signs and age and sex of the patient. This parameter group has been found in our previous studies to present the most confident parameters in predicting the acute appendicitis diagnosis. These parameters are presented in Table 1. A detailed description of the data can be found in [10]. We used only those patient cases where the data from all these parameters was available with no missing values, so the number of patients reduced to 1064 cases.

All the values on the parameters were normalised and recoded suitable for neural network inputs. The smallest value was made equal to 0.1 and the largest value equal to 0.9, and other values equally between those. The location of tenderness was converted to two-dimensional location coordinate values.

The data was divided at random into two sets: a training set that consisted of 717 patients and a test set that consisted of 347 patients. The training set was used to develop classification models and the test set was used to evaluate the classification accuracy of these models.

The three statistical analyses, discriminant analysis, logistic regression analysis and quick cluster analysis, were computed by the SPSS statistical program package. Discriminant and logistic regression analysis were used with forward stepwise method, so that only those parameters that were found to be statistically significant were included in the resulting models [11].

The back-propagation neural network algorithm of the Matlab Neural Network Toolbox program package was used. A network with two layers: six nodes in the first hidden layer and two nodes in the second layer was used [12].

These four classification methods were compared separately and also as combined classification methods. By combined methods we mean that the class was defined as acute appendicitis when all combined methods agreed on the diagnosis.

The results of the classification were compared with receiver operating characteristic curve (*ROC*) analysis, especially by the area beneath the *ROC*-curve [13]. The value of this measure varies from 0.5 to 1.0. When the area is 0.5 no discrimination exists and when the value is 1.0 then the discrimination is perfect.

The combined methods were compared with the *diagnostic accuracy* (defined as the percentage of the cases correctly classified to a class from all the cases that really belong to that class) and the *predictive value* (defined as the percentage of the cases correctly classified to a class from all the cases classified to that class).

3. Results

In the discriminant analysis and logistic regression analysis only those variables that were found statistically significant were chosen to the model. These parameters are presented in Table 1. The parameters that were found to be statistically significant in both analyses were: location of tenderness, rebound, guarding, rigidity and leukocyte count.

The results of the comparison of the classification accuracy of the four methods by the ROC-analysis are presented in Table 2. The area under the ROC-curve is presented for both the training data set and the test data set. The differences between the training set of patients and test set of patients were small. The best two methods were the discriminant analysis and the back-propagation neural network.

Table 1. The parameters used in this study, and the parameters that were selected significant in the discriminant and logistic regression analyses.

Parameter	Discriminant analysis	Logistic regression analysis	Parameter	Discriminant analysis	Logistic regression analysis
Age	x		Rebound	x	x
Gender			Guarding	x	x
Mood			Rigidity	x	x
Colour		x	Murphy's positive	x	
Location of tenderness	x	x	Bowel sounds	x	
Scar		x	Renal tenderness		
Distension		x	Rectal digital tenderness		
Abdominal movement			Leukocyte count	x	x
Mass		x			

Table 2. The comparison of the classification accuracy of three statistical methods: discriminant analysis, logistic regression analysis and cluster analysis, and the back-propagation neural network algorithm by the ROC-analysis in the diagnosis of acute appendicitis.

Analysis	Area under ROC-curve	
	Training set	Test set
Discriminant analysis	.9163	.9393
Logistic regression analysis	.9000	.8944
Cluster analysis	.8748	.8755
Back-propagation neural network	.9554	.9281

In addition to the comparison of the four individual tests, also combinations of these tests were examined. The results of these comparisons are presented in Table 3. Here the accuracy of the tests was evaluated by the diagnostic accuracy and predictive value. Also these estimates for the individual tests are presented in the table. The use of combined tests increased the predictive values and so less false positive cases were found.

Table 3. The comparison of the classification accuracy of three statistical methods: discriminant analysis, logistic regression analysis and cluster analysis, and the back-propagation neural network algorithm, and their combinations in the diagnosis of acute appendicitis.

Analyses	Diagnostic accuracy	Predictive value
Discriminant analysis	.91	.65
Logistic regression analysis	.93	.56
Cluster analysis	.75	.62
Back-propagation neural network	.93	.62
Discriminant & Logistic regression	.90	.68
Back-propagation & Discriminant	.88	.71
Back-propagation & Logistic regression	.90	.70
Back-propagation & Discriminant & Logistic regression	.88	.71

4. Discussion

The ROC-analysis offers a good way to compare different methods when the choice of the decision border is not predetermined. It also evaluates the classification properties more generally than if the accuracy is compared with specific decision borders.

The differences that were found in the comparisons were considerably small. Two of the four methods: discriminant analysis and back-propagation neural network seem to work with equal accuracy. With these methods a useful model was found for the prediction of acute appendicitis in patients suffering from acute abdominal pain.

Often the training set of data is classified better than test set, but here the situation was opposite when discriminant analysis was examined. With cluster analysis the results were almost equal. This shows that these models fit very well also to the patients of the test set and only very few cases were misclassified in the analysis.

The combination of the methods increased the predictive values, and therefore it would be preferable to use these combined models in addition to the individual models. The accuracy of the diagnosis would increase and less false positive results would occur. The combination of the models seems to evaluate the border line cases more accurately than the individual models.

One challenge for the future is to investigate in detail the cases that were difficult for these models. Why are they difficult? Do they have something in common? Could they be identified and treated separately with some other models? This in one of the things we are going to investigate in future.

The back-propagation neural network algorithm managed well in the comparisons. The classification results were about as good as was achieved with the statistical methods. This result can be interpreted in two ways. The back-propagation does not offer any magic to this decision making problem, because it is only as good as statistical methods. On the other hand, back-propagation should not be disqualified, because it offers as good results as the statistical methods. The latter opinion is what we think, and therefore we shall use neural networks also in our future studies on building decision support systems for the diagnosis of acute appendicitis.

References

[1]   FT de Dombal *et al.*, Computer-aided diagnosis of acute abdominal pain, *Br Med J* **2** (1972) 9-13.
[2]   I. Teicher *et al.*, Scoring system to aid in diagnosis of appendicitis, *Ann Surg*, **198** (1983) 753-759.
[3]   E. Arnbjörnsson, Scoring system for computer-aided diagnosis of acute appendicitis. The value of prospective versus retrospective studies, *Ann Chir Scand* **155** (1985) 185-189.
[4]   I. Adams *et al.*, Computer-aided diagnosis of acute abdominal pain, *Br Med J* 293 (1986) 800-840.
[5]   R. Eberhart *et al.*, Neural network paradigm comparisons for appendicitis diagnoses. In: Computer-based medical systems. Proceedings of the fourths annual IEEE symposium, IEEE Computer Society Press, Los Alamitos, California, 1991, pp. 298-304.
[6]   S. Phillips *et al.*, A comparison of three classification algorithms on the diagnosis of abdominal pains. In: Proceedings of the Second Australian Conference of Neural Networks (ACNN91), Sydney University Press, 1991, pp. 283-287.
[7]   M. Eskelinen *et al.*, A computer based diagnostic score to aid in diagnosis of acute appendicitis, *Theor Surg*, **7** (1992) 86-90.

[8]   C. Ohmann *et al.*, Evaluation of automatic knowledge acquisition techniques in the diagnosis of acute abdominal pain, *Art Int Med* **8** (1996) 23-36.

[9]   E. Pesonen, M. Eskelinen and M. Juhola, Comparison of Different Neural Network Algorithms in the Diagnosis of Acute Appendicitis, *Int J Biomed Comput* **40** (1996) 227-233.

[10] E. Pesonen, J. Ikonen, M. Juhola and M. Eskelinen, Parameters for a Knowledge Base for Acute Appendicitis, *Meth Inform Med* **33** (1994) 220-226.

[11] M. Norusis, SPSS for Windows Professional Statistics Release 6.0, SPSS Inc., Chicago, 1993.

[12] H. Demuth and M. Beale, Neural Network Toolbox. User's guide. Math Works Inc., Natick, Massachusetts, 1993.

[13] K-P. Adlassnig and W. Scheithauer, Performance evaluation of medical expert systems using ROC curves, *Comp Biomed Res* **22** (1989) 297-313.

382

Medical Informatics Europe '97
C. Pappas et al. (Eds.)
IOS Press, 1997

Neural network analysis of biochemical markers for early assessment of acute myocardial infarction

Johan Ellenius[*], Torgny Groth[*] and Bertil Lindahl[#]
From the [*]Department of Biomedical Informatics and Systems Analysis,
and the [#]Department of Cardiology, University of Uppsala, Sweden

Abstract. Neural network analysis was applied for early diagnosis/exclusion of acute myocardial infarction and prediction of infarct size. Eighty-eight patients admitted with onset of chest pain within 8 hours were included. Frequent blood samples for measurement of myoglobin, CK-MB and troponin-T were obtained and used in the development of a set of neural network components of a decision support system. The results indicate that this approach could provide useful support for assessment of patients with suspected AMI.

1. Introduction

Early diagnosis is essential for the appropriate handling and optimal treatment of patients with suspected acute myocardial infarction (AMI) [1]. In most of these patients the 12-lead ECG is nondiagnostic on admission, and the rule-in and rule-out of AMI has to be based on repeated measurements of biochemical markers [2]. Artificial neural networks have previously been applied for AMI diagnosis based on clinical data including ECG [3] and biochemical markers [4, 5].

The aim of the present investigation was to develop and evaluate artificial neural network methods, based on frequent measurement of selected markers of AMI, for (i) early diagnosis/exclusion of AMI; (ii) early prediction of infarct size; and (iii) to compare the performance of neural networks with experienced physicians.

2. Material and methods

2.1 Patients and laboratory investigations

The investigation was part of a swedish multicenter study [6]. All patients admitted to the participating coronary care units with chest pain, and with onset within the previous 8 hours and, in case of AMI, not given thrombolytic treatment were included; in total 88 patients. The study was approved by the local ethics committees.

Blood samples were drawn from an indwelling forearm venous catheter; the first sample on admission and thereafter every 30 minutes during the first 3 hours and then at 4, 6, 9, 12, 18, 24 and 48 hours after admission. The mass concentration of myoglobin, CK-MB and troponin-T were measured in plasma. The coefficients of total analytical variation were estimated to 6.1%, 8.4% and 6.3% for myoglobin, CK-MB and troponin-T, respectively.

AMI was considered present if at least two of the three WHO-criteria were fulfilled [7]; Number of AMI and non-AMI patients were equal to 29 and 59, respectively. The infarct size was arbitrarily labeled "major" (n=19) if the peak plasma CK-MB mass concentration was >80 µg/L and "minor" (n=10) if peak CK-MB mass concentration was $\leq$ 80 µg/L.

2.2 Computational methods

The measured concentration levels of biochemical markers were *normalised* and expressed in units of the respective upper reference limits. The normalised values were further *fuzzified* to the range (0; 1) with the use of *piecewise-linear membership functions*, adjusted individually for the input variables to achieve separation between the actual classes of classification. These pre-processed measurement values were first taken as input to computational modules used for the detection of AMI. If AMI was detected, the system made a prediction of the infarct size. If AMI was not detected after a predefined optimal period of monitoring (2 hours), AMI was excluded. The method was implemented on a Macintosh computer with use of MATLAB 4.2 and the Neural Network Toolbox 2.0 (The Mathworks, Inc. Natick, Mass, USA).

Three single-layer perceptrons (Multi-SLP), trained on normalised and fuzzified measurement values of myoglobin and CK-MB, were used for classification of AMI/non-AMI. Each individual single-layer perceptron (SLP) was trained to detect AMI based on measurements from a specific time interval (<6 h; 6-8 h; or >8 h) since onset of infarction. Prediction of infarct size was performed with use of a single-layer perceptron using normalised, but not fuzzified , measurements of myoglobin and CK-MB, and their respective two-point derivatives, as input variables. This structure is identical to the linear logistic model.

The single-layer perceptrons are all using sigmoidal transfer functions and were trained with use of the Levenberg-Marquardt method to minimize a cost function (sum of squared residuals) as implemented in the Neural Network Toolbox. Recognizing that the phenomenon known as "overtraining" does not occur in models of sufficiently low complexity, the single-layer perceptrons were trained until the training set was classified with a minimum error.

2.3 Selecting neural network architecture

The so called *cross-validation method* [cf. 8] was used to select an adequate neural network architecture for each classification problem; data from all 88 patients were randomly partitioned into a training set (67%) and a cross-validation set (33%) while preserving the prevalences of major AMI, minor AMI and Non-AMI, in the two sets. Neural network architectures of varying complexity were trained and evaluated on the cross-validation set. The performance was assessed by calculating the diagnostic sensitivity, specificity and positive and negative predictive values in addition to the mean time to diagnosis. The procedure was repeated one hundred times for each architecture and the mean and standard error of the mean (SEM) were calculated. By comparing these measures of diagnostic performance using ROC-analysis, a 'best architecture' could be selected.

2.4 Evaluation method

Three clinicians with several years of working experience in the emergency department and the coronary care unit, were presented with the series of measured values of biochemical markers set by set in time order, simulating the clinical situation. They were asked to classify the patients in a test set of 11 AMI and 27 non-AMI patients. In case of 'AMI' classification, the clinicians were asked to continue measurements until able to make a prediction of the size of the infarction as either 'minor' or 'major'. By following this procedure, the assessments put forward by the clinicians could be compared to the assessment by the computer method on the same test set.

3. Results and discussion

Single-layer perceptrons and feed-forward neural networks with one hidden layer consisting of a varying number of units are often used for medical classification problems. Our classifier for AMI/non-AMI uses an approach combining a robust linear technique (the single-layer perceptron) with non-linear fuzzification of input variables (cf [9]). The fuzzification membership functions in our case were selected by inspecting the frequency distributions of measured variables for the diagnostic classes in the training set.

As expected, the Multi-SLP resulted in a better classifier than a multi-layer perceptron MLP (with two units in the hidden layer) for classification of AMI/non-AMI. The training of the MLP was stopped (in order to avoid overtraining) when the performance of the network was optimal, as measured by the sum of squared residuals on the *cross-validation set*. The performance of the MLP thus approximates an upper bound of what is attainable using the technique of early stopping for maximizing generalization. The performance of this "optimal" MLP was considered inferior to the Multi-SLP with its significantly higher diagnostic sensitivity. In fact, the MLP had a performance comparable to a simple logistic regression model. The troponin-T measurements were found not to add to the diagnostic performance of networks for early detection/exclusion of AMI.

The computer system correctly detected AMI on the first measurement in 90% of the cases, to be compared to 70% for the clinicians. For the remaining cases, the computer system required one more measurement (additional 30 minutes) for correct diagnosis, while the clinicians required on the average two more measurements (additional 60 minutes). The falsely diagnosed myocardial infarctions were classified as 'minor AMI' when the system performed infarct size prediction. The clinicians excluded AMI within the range 0-540 minutes, compared to 120 minutes in all cases for the computer method.

The computer method needed approximately half an hour of monitoring time (2 sets of measurements), to make a correct prediction of major/minor infarct size while the clinicians required two and four hours (5 and 9 sets of measurements) on the average. Examples of the time curves for the biochemical markers and time points when AMI was detected and size was predicted by the computer and the three clinicians are shown in Figure 1 for a minor AMI.

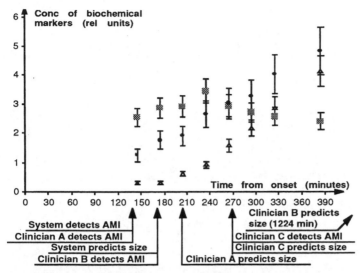

Figure 1. Time series measurement results with 95% confidence intervals of infarct markers for a patient with a minor acute myocardial infarction. Time points are noted when the computer and the three clinicians, respectively, detected the infarction and predicted the infarct size.

▨ = myoglobin; ● = CK-MB; Δ = troponin-T

Relative concentration = plasma concentration in µg/L divided by 90/57 (men/women), 8 and 0.2 µg/L for myoglobin, CK-MB and troponin-T, respectively.

Conclusions

Neural network analysis of serial measurements of markers could provide useful support for the early assessment of patients with suspected acute myocardial infarction. With the limited number of patients, the present results must be interpreted with caution and regarded as indicative of the potential benefit of neural network analysis for early assessment of patients with acute chest pain.

References

[1]   Acute myocardial infarction: pre-hospital and in-hospital management. The task force on the management of acute myocardial infarction of the European Society of Cardiology. Eur Heart J 1996;17:43-63.

[2]   Newby LK, Gibler WB, Ohman EM, Christenson RH. Biochemical markers in suspected acute myocardial infarction: the need for early assessment [editorial]. Clin Chem 1995;41:1263-5.

[3]   Baxt WG. Analysis of the clinical variables driving decision in an artificial neural network trained to identify the presence of myocardial infarction. Ann Emerg Med 1992;21:1439-44.

[4]   Furlong JW, Dupuy ME, Heinsimer JA. Neural network analysis of serial cardiac enzyme data. A clinical application of artificial machine intelligence. Am J Clin Pathol 1991;96:134-41.

[5]   Pedersen S, Jorgensen J, Pedersen J. Use of neural networks to diagnose acute myocardial infarction. II. A clinical application. Clin Chem 1996;42:613-17.

[6]   Lindahl B, Venge P, Wallentin L. Early diagnosis and exclusion of acute myocardial infarction by biochemical monitoring. Coronary Artery Disease 1995;6:321-328

[7]   Gillum RF, Fortman SP, Prineas RJ, Kottke TE. International diagnostic criteria for acute myocardial infarction and stroke. Am Heart J 1984;108:150-158.

[8]   Ripley B. Pattern recognition and neural networks. Cambridge University Press 1996.

[9]   Forsström JJ, Irjala K, Selén G et al. Using data preprocessing and single layer perceptron to analyze laboratory data. Scand J Clin Lab Invest 1995; 55, Suppl. 222:75-81

386

Medical Informatics Europe '97
C. Pappas et al. (Eds.)
IOS Press, 1997

Application of Neural Networks to the Follow-Up of AIDS Patients

Mauro Giacomini[a,d], Carmelina Ruggiero[a], M. Maillard[b],
Flavia B. Lillo[c], Oliviero E. Varnier[d,e]
[a]DIST, Department of Communications Computer and System
Sciences, University of Genova, Via All'Opera Pia 13,
16145 Genova, Italy
[b]Division of Infectious Diseases and [c]Laboratory of Virology, AIDS
Centre S. Luigi, Hospital H. S. Raffaele, Milano
[d]Molecular Virology Unit, Advanced Biotechnology Center,
Genova, Italy
[e] Department of Clinical and Experimental Oncology, School of
Medicine, Genova, Italy

Abstract: The present work aims to obtain groups of patients with similar profiles of p24 antigen concentration and of CD4+ cell counts. These two markers were chosen because their evaluation represents a significant step in the clinical follow up of HIV-1 infected subjects. The classifications were obtained by a Kohonen neural net trained in three ways: with p24 antigen profiles only, with CD4+ cell count profiles only and with both sets of profiles. The results show that the clustering fashion of the two parameters closely resembles the clustering fashion of CD4+ only rather than the one of p24Ag, both with reference to cluster formation and with reference to distance among clusters.

1. Introduction

The Acquired Immune Deficiency Syndrome (AIDS) is caused by a retrovirus (HIV-1), which preferentially attacks some specific cells of the human immune system. These cells contain a surface molecule, called CD4+, which is also used by the virus as an entry door. After entry of the virus in the target cell its RNA (proviral RNA) activates the mechanism of retrotranscription, which causes the insertion of a couple of virus DNA (virionic DNA) within the cell DNA. After a latency period, whose extension is not known, and for reason which are also unknown, the virionic DNA activates an intense replication of the virus. The new virus capsides produced aim to leave the cell in order to find new cells in which a new replication process can take place. This cause the break of the cell membrane and the consequent death of the cell. This phenomenon causes the progressive decrease of CD4+ cells with severe impairment of the immune function, which is the key feature of AIDS.

One of the methods to evaluate the amount of virus present in a patient is the measurement of viral particles in peripheral blood and its variation during a specified period; for this purpose a structural protein of HIV-1, called p24, has been chosen as a marker and its concentration quantified as pg/ml [1]. Generally the higher this value the worse the patient prognosis.

The immune system function is monitored through the quantification of peripheral blood mononuclear cells, particularly the ones showing the CD4+ receptor. As already mentioned these are the preferential target of HIV-1 infection and measurement of their progressive loss is directly related to the infauste disease progression [2].

2. Clinical samples

The number of patients considered in the present study was 176. For all patients the following data was available: date of blood collection and serum concentration (pg/ml) of the p24 antigen. For a limited number of patients (38) and at different time intervals, the CD4+ cell count was also available. The detection range for the p24 antigen was from 10 to 500 pg/ml. In the present study values below 10 pg/ml was considered equal to 0 and those above 500 pg/ml equal to 500.

3. Neural network based elaboration

We have grouped patients with similar profiles both for p24 and for CD4+. We have chosen to use the Kohonen neural net [3] because of its self-oraganizing capabilities, since non initial information is available about the presence of groups, both for p24 and for CD4+. The Kohonen neural net has an output matrix whose dimension can be chosen by the user. Each matrix element contains the input vectors, which have been found to be similar, therefore considered as members of one class.

3.1. Supervised neural learning pre-processing

The time interval and the number of blood collections available are not the same for each patient so a pre-processing phase was necessary because the Kohonen network requires homogeneity of the elements to be grouped. In order to set up a suitable input data set, we obtained a continuous function for each patient fitting the data using a back-propagation neural network [4, 5]. The main reason for this choice is the high generalisation properties of neural networks, which originate fitting capabilities better than those of other curve fitting procedures [5]. Also, this choice allowed us to use the very weights (real coefficients) generated by the neural back propagation net as an input vector to the Kohonen neural net, avoiding further processing for change of parameters. This number is the same for all patients, independent by the number of observations.

The parameters of the neural back-propagation net as follows:

output threshold	0.5
learning threshold	0.01
input nodes	1
hidden nodes	20
output node	1
learning rate	0.6
momentum	0.9

The choice of the 0.01 learning threshold value (the maximum error between the observed value and the corresponding value of the approximated function) represents a trade off between precision requirements on one side and computational speed and need to limit the influence of small data variations possibly due to noise and quantization errors. The number of hidden nodes has been set to 20, which is the average number of observations for each patient. All other parameters have been set to standard values for all neural nets.

3.2. *Kohonen neural net classification*

One input vector has been obtained for each of the available cases. This vector contains: the bias value of the output node of the backpropagation network used for data fitting, 20 weights of the connections between the input and the hidden node of the same network and 20 weights of the connections between the hidden and the output node of the same network. Moreover one element has been added which is the average of all p24 observations in order to retain information on the values of the data (since the information deriving from the neural backpropagation network focuses on trend in data series). As a result a 42 element vector has been set up and used for the input of Kohonen neural net. Similarly, a 42 element vector has been set up for CD4+ profiles.

Since the number of cases analyzed must be greater than the number of elements of the matrix, the Kohonen network output has been chosen to be: a 12x12 matrix for the p24 classification, a 6x6 matrix for CD4+ classification (in which the number of cases is smaller) and a 6x6 matrix for joint p24-CD4+ classification.

We have found that 100 iterations allow to reach a low analogic cost which indicates that the classification process has taken place without difficulties and that the classification obtained is reliable.

The Kohonen network provides information about the number of input vector present in each matrix element and about the Euclidean distance among each vector and the centre of gravity of the set of vectors contained in that element; the lowest value gives the best result.

4. Results

The three classification processes which have been carried out allow to singled out low and high observation values, moreover in each matrix similar profiles are near to each other and are grouped mainly according to the average value.

The analysis of the results by the combined p24 and CD4+ classification shows that the cases with low P24 concentration and high CD4+ cell count are grouped in one element. Near elements contain cases with high CD4+ values, but different P24 values. Similar profiles are grouped in one element.

The clustering fashion of combined classification closely resembles the clustering fashion of CD4+ classification rather than the one of p24 both with reference to cluster formation and with reference to distance among clusters.

To verify the correctness of the clustering obtained by the Kohonen algorithm in the combined classification, the Centre for Disease Control (CDC) classification for case definition of AIDS [6] for each patient present in the output matrix was considered.

The progression of the HIV infection (fig. 1) moves from the lower left area (CDC II patients) to the lower right (CDC III and IV C2 patients) and to the higher part of the matrix (CDC IV C1).

5. Conclusion

The distribution obtained by the Kohonen algorithm clearly parallels the clinical relevance of the analysed data: the study of the p24 profile during patient follow up provides important information about the viral replication and therapy efficacy, but does not necessarily reflects disease stage and progression. This is better defined by the impairment of the immune function and measured by the CD4+ cell count.

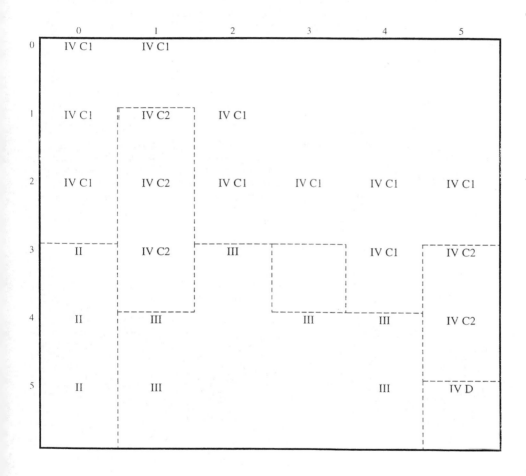

Fig. 1

Distributions of AIDS patients class, as Kohonen matrix output

The clustering fashion of the two parameters resembling that of CD4+ rather than the one of p24Ag might be due to the absence of noise in the CD4+ cell count, while the p24 data suffer from the analytical interference due to the presence of antibodies masking the antigen itself.

6. Acknowledgements

Partially supported by "Istituto Superiore di Sanità - Progetto di Ricerche sull'AIDS Grant N° 9302-07" and by "Ministero dell'Università e della Ricerca Scientifica e Tecnologica - Progetto: Informatica Medica; Unità operativa: Metodi informatici e telematici per l'integrazione dell'assistenza primaria, secondaria e terziaria". Mauro Giacomini is supported by a study grant (N° 25670/SAP 7.2) of the 'Istituto Superiore di Sanità programme entitled 'Lotta all'AIDS'.

7. References

[1]   Lillo FB, Cao Y, Concedi DR, Varnier OE. (1993) Improved detection of HIV p24 antigen after acid dissociation of immune complexes. *AIDS,* **7**, 1331-1336.
[2]   Tsoukas CM, Bernard NF. (1994) Markers predicting progression of human immunodeficiency virus-related disease. *Clin Microbiol. Rev.*, **7**, 14-28.
[3]   Kohonen T. (1989) Self-Organisation and Associative Memory, 3rd ed. (Heildelberg, Springer)
[4]   Rumelhart, D.E., Hinton, G.E., and Williams, R.J. (1986) Learning internal representations by error back propagation, in Rumelhart, D.E. and McClelland J.L. (Eds.), Parallel distributed processing: Explorations in the microstructure of cognition - Chap. 8 - (Cambridge MA, MIT Press)
[5]   Nabhan, T. M., and Zomaya, A. (1994) Toward generating neural network structures for function approximation. *Neural Networks* **7** (1), 89-99.
[6]   *Mortality Morbility Weekly Report* (1987) **36**, 3-15 1987

Medical Informatics Europe '97
C. Pappas et al. (Eds.)
IOS Press, 1997

Removing Irrelevant Features in Neural Network Classification using Evolutionary Computations

I. Ciuca*, J.A. Ware**, A. Cristea***
*Research Institute for Informatics, Bucharest, Romania
**Glamorgan University, Pontypridd, UK
***Institute of Virology "Stefan S. Nicolau", Bucharest, Romania

Abstract-Evolutionary artificial neural networks (EANN) are a new paradigm that refers to a special class of artificial neural networks (ANN) in which evolution is another fundamental form of adaptation in addition to learning. Evolution can be introduced at various levels of ANN. It can be used to evolve weights, architectures and learning parameters. Evolutionary computations are population-based search methods that have shown promise in many similarly complex tasks. This paper presents an application of evolutionary programming for simultaneously inducing the input structure and weights evolving for multilayer feed-forward perceptrons (MLP) with standard sigmoidal activation function.

1. Introduction

In its complete form, neural network induction involves both structural and parametric learning [15], that is learning both an appropriate topology of nodes and links in addition to weight values. Current connectionist methods to solve this task fall into two broad categories: constructive algorithms and destructive methods. Constructive algorithms initially assume a simple neural network and add nodes and links [1,2], while destructive methods start with a large network and prune off superfluous components [3,4,5,6,9,10,11,12]. Although both techniques address the problem of network optimization they limit the available architectures, investigating only restricted topological subsets rather than the complete class of network architectures.

Evolutionary computing comprises a promising collection of algorithms for structural and parametric modification of neural networks. They are population-based search methods - inspired by Darwin's theory on natural selection - which include genetic algorithms, evolution strategies and evolutionary programming [20].

Genetic algorithms [14] are a popular form of evolutionary computing that rely chiefly on the reproduction heuristic of crossover. This operator forms offspring by combining representational components from two members of the population.

Evolution strategies and evolutionary programming [16] emphasize the behavioral link between parents and offspring, rather than genetic link. They rely chiefly on the reproduction heuristic of mutation.

Designing ANN through simulated evolution has been investigated for many years [15, 19, 21, 22]. These investigations have looked at evolving weights [22], evolving weights and architectures simultaneously[15], [17], and even evolving weights, architectures and node transfer functions simultaneously [19] for both full and partially connected ANN.

When evolving a neural network, the best approach seems to be evolutionary programming [15, 19] although genetic algorithms [21] and hybrid techniques have also proved effective [20].

As an alternative to normalized sensitivities for reducing the number of irrelevant features in an input vector [13], an evolutionary programming technique will now be presented which simultaneously facilitates weight evolution.

2. An Evolutionary Computation Algorithm for Input Structure and Weight Evolving

Irrelevant feature discarding in neural network classification can be regarded as a specific structure evolution - where techniques from evolutionary computing can be used to solve the problem. Evolutionary computations can facilitate - simultaneously - structure and parametric (weight) evolution.

Using the arguments that mutation operator is the most suitable for neural network structure and parametric (weight) evolution [15], the following presents an evolutionary programming technique that is a form of evolutionary computation to network induction. This algorithm will simultaneously perform the irrelevant feature discarding and neural network learning for full connected feed-forward neural networks used in classification applications.

Let $S = \{\eta | \eta$ is a neural network with real-valued weights and bias and a given maximum input space size$\}$.

Let a population of P feed-forward neural networks from S with a single hidden layer having the maximum input space size n, the output space size m and the hidden layer size h.

All non-input nodes employ the standard sigmoid activation function $f(x) = \dfrac{1}{1 + e^{-\lambda x}}$, with λ a parameter.

Let d be the number of all the elements (all weights, bias and all the inputs) submitted to mutations

Then the EP method will be implemented as follows [15]:

1. Define the problem as finding the real-valued d-dimensional network η that is associated with the extremes of a function $F(\eta) : R^d \to R$, where F is the output error function (also referred to as the fitness function).

2. Select at random an initial population of parent networks, η_i, $i = 1,...,P$ from a feasible range in each dimension. The distribution of initial trials is typically uniform.

3. Create an offspring network η_i', from each parent η_i

4. Selection then determines which of these networks to maintain by comparing the errors $F(\eta_i)$ and $F(\eta_i')$, $i = 1,...,P$. The P networks that posses the least error become the new parents for the next generation.

5. The process of generating new trials and selecting those with least error continues by going to the step 3 until a satisfactory solution is reached or the available computation time is exhausted.

This algorithm is presented in Fig. 1

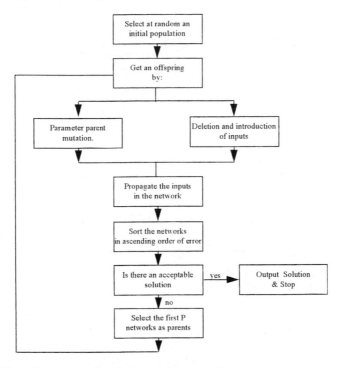

Fig. 1 Structure of evolutionary programming

The acceptable solution is the network with the maximum number of removed input nodes but with the output error smaller than a pre-defined threshold.

The mutations were executed in order: weight and bias mutations followed by input component mutations. The weight and bias mutation operator alters the values of parameters w currently in the network by the expression:

$$w = w + N(0, \alpha E(\eta)) \qquad \forall w \in \eta$$

where w is a weight or bias, $E(\eta)$ is output mean square error (fitness function) given by

$$E(\eta) = \frac{1}{T.m} \sum_{p=1}^{T} \sum_{i=1}^{m} (y_i^{(p)} - t_i^{(p)})^2$$

with $y_i^{(p)}$ = the computed i output component for input selected pattern p

$t_i^{(p)}$ = the desired i output component for input pattern p

T = number of input patterns in training set

m = output space size

α is a user defined proportionality constant and

$N(\mu, \sigma^2)$ is a Gaussian variable with mean μ and variance σ^2.

The input mutations alter the number of input components to a network. They consist in deletions and introductions of input components and must be executed in the order - deletions followed by introductions - on a uniform distribution basis.

This order is imposed because of the necessity to have no network with zero input components in a propagating cycle. The number of deletions and introductions can vary uniformly over a shrinking interval based on the parent network's fitness. In the experiments below, the maximum number of nodes deleted and added was three and the minimum was one. Also α was considered as being equal to 1.

For every network the state of every input node (feature) - either active or removed - was recorded in a vector of size n.

3. Experiments and Results

The experiments were conducted on a medical classification application using meningitis disease data set [13]. The data set was randomly partitioned into a training set, a testing set and a generalization set. The size of these sets was respectively of 19, 10 and 17. The testing set was used to avoid the over training. When the testing set error has started to increase the evolving process was stopped.

The population size in EP algorithm was of $10 + 10$ neural networks (10 as parents and 10 as offspring). The input space size was of 29 features. After applying the both normalized input sensitivities Jacobian (JNS) and logarithmic (LNS) [13] and EP algorithm , the removed features and elapsed time were as presented in Table 1.

For JNS and LNS the elapsed time includes the time for training the neural network using an evolutionary programming algorithm. While for EP the elapsed time obviously includes the training time and time for removing the irrelevant features. To keep a good generalization capability, removing irrelevant features was performed in the final part of the training procedure.

Table 1- Comparing results

Method	No. of removed features	Evolving time in %
JNS	10	100
LNS	11	110
EP	10	130

The proportion of removed features using the EP algorithm was 85%, that is the same as for LNS but the time taken was a little longer. For EP algorithm the output error initialy decreases very quicky but then more slowly, therefore the evolving time was a little longer.

4. Conclusions

Removing irrelevant features in parallel with training a neural network using a evolutionary computation paradigm is an option that fascinates. The paper presents a simple evolutionary programming algorithm chiefly based on the mutation operator. The neural network architecture was a feed-forward multilayer perceptron (MLP) with a standard sigmoid activation function. The EP results were compared with the normalized input sensitivity results for the meningitis disease data. The EP algorithm achieved similar results as other techniques with respect to the removing irrelevant features but the evolution time was a little longer.

References

[1] T. Ash, "Dynamic node creation in backpropagation networks", *Connection Science*, Vol. 1, no. 4, 1989, pp. 365-375.

[2] M. R. Azimi-Sadjadi, S. Sheedvash and F. O. Trujillo, "Recursive dynamic node creation in multilayer neural networks", *IEEE Trans. On Neural Networks*, Vol. 4, no.2 1993, pp. 242-256.

[3] M. Mozer and P. Smolensky, "Skeletonization: A technique for trimming the fat from a network via relevance assessment", in *Advance in Neural Information Processing Systems 1*, D. Touretzky, Ed. San Mateo, CA: Morgan Kaufmann, 1989, pp. 107-115.

[4] C. A. Omlin and C. L. Giles, "Pruning recurrent neural networks for improved generalization performance", *Tech. Report No. 943-6, Computer Science Department, Rensselaer polytechnic Institute*, April 1993.

[5] E. D. Karnin, "A simple Procedure for Pruning Backpropagation Training Neural Networks", *IEEE Trans. On Neural Networks*, June Vol. 1, No. 2, 1990, pp. 239-242

[6] R. Reed, "Pruning Algorithms-A Survey", *IEEE Trans. On Neural Networks*, Vol. 4, No. 5, Sept. 1993, pp. 740-747.

[7] F. M. Frattale Mascioli, G. Martinelli, G. Lazzaro, "Comparison of Constructive Algorithms for Neural Networks", *Proc. of ICANN'94; Intl. Conference on Artificial Neural Networks*, Sorrento, Italy, 1994, pp. 731-734.

[8] T. M. Nahban, A. Y. Zomoya, "Toward Generating Neural Network Structures for Function Approximation", *Neural Networks*, Vol. 7, No. 1, 1994, pp. 89-99.

[9] Q. Xue, Yu Hen Hu, W. J. Tompkins, "Structural Simplification of Feed Forward, Multi-layer Perceptron Artificial Neural Networks", *Proc. of ICASSP'91*, Toronto, Canada, 1991.

[10] M. Cottrell, B. Girard, Y. Girard, M. Mangeas, C. Muller, "SMM: A Statistical Stepwise Method for Weight Elimination", *Proc. of ICANN'94; Intl. Conference on Artificial Neural Networks*, Sorrento, Italy, 1994, pp. 601-604.

[11] S. Y. Kung, Yu Hen Hu, "A Frobenius Approximation Reduction Method (FARM) for Determining Optimal Number of Hidden Units", *Proc. of the IEEE Intl. Conference on Neural Networks*, Seattle, Vol. 2 July 1991, pp. 163-168.

[12] H. H. Thodberg, "Improving Generalization of Neural Networks through Pruning", Intl., *Journal of Neural Systems*, Vol. 1, No. 4, USA, 1991, pp. 317-326.

[13] I. Ciuca and E. D. Hord, "On the Irrelevant Feature Discarding in Neural Networks and its Application in Medicine", *MIE'96; Medical Informatics Europa*. Copenhagen 1996, pp. 965-969.

[14] J. H. Holland, **"Adaptation in Natural and Artificial Systems"**, *Ann Arbor: University of Michigan Press*, 1975.

[15] P.G. Angeline, G. Saunders and J. Pollak, "An Evolutionary Algorithm that Constructs Recurrent Neural Networks", *IEEE Trans. On Neural Networks*, Vol. 5, No. 1, 1994, pp. 54-65.

[16] D. B. Fogel, "An Introduction to Simulated Evolutionary Optimization" *IEEE Trans. On Neural Networks*, Vol. 5, No. 1, 1994, pp. 3-14.

[17] D. Thierens, "Non-Redundant Genetic Coding of Neural Networks", Proc. of IEEE ICEC'96; *Intl. Conference on Evolutionary Computation, Nagoya University*, 1996, pp. 571-575.

[18] X. Yao, Y. Liu, "Ensemble Structure of Evolutionary Artificial Neural Networks", *Proc. of IEEE ICEC'96; Intl. Conference on Evolutionary Computation, Nagoya University*, 1996, pp. 659-664.

[19] Y. Liu and X. Yao, " Evolutionary Design of Artificial Neural Networks with Different Nodes", *Proc. of IEEE ICEC'96; Intl. Conference on Evolutionary Computation, Nagoya University*, 1996, pp. 670-675.

[20] J. M. Yang, C. Y. Kao, "A Combined Evolutionary Algorithm for Real Parameters Optimization", *Proc. of IEEE ICEC'96; Intl. Conference on Evolutionary Computation, Nagoya University*, 1996, pp. 732-737.

[21] X. Yao and Y. Liu, "Evolving Artificial Neural Networks for Medical Applications", *Proc. of the 1st Korea-Australia Joint Workshop on Evolutionary Computation*, 1995, pp. 1-16.

[22] D. B. Fogel, L. J. Fogel and V. W. Porto, "Evolving neural networks", *Biological Cybernetics*, Vol. 63, 1990, pp. 487-493.

Medical Informatics Europe '97
C. Pappas et al. (Eds.)
IOS Press, 1997

From Natural Language to Formal Language: when MultiTALE meets GALEN

Ceusters W [a, b], Spyns P [b], De Moor G [b]

a Office Line Engineering NV, Hazenakkerstraat 20, B-9520 - Zonnegem, Belgium
b RAMIT VZW, University Hospital, De Pintelaan 185, B-9000 Gent, Belgium

In the GALEN project, the syntactic-semantic tagger MultiTALE is upgraded to extract knowledge from natural language surgical procedure expressions. In this paper, we describe the methodology applied and show that out of a randomly selected sample of such expressions, 81% could be analysed correctly. The problems encountered are summarised and areas of further investigation identified.

1. Introduction

The purpose of the GALEN project is to develop language independent concept representation systems as the foundations for the next generation of multilingual coding systems [1]. At the heart of the project is the development of a reference model for medical concepts (CORE) supported by a formal language for medical concept representation (GRAIL) [2]. A particular characteristic of the approach is the clear separation of the pure conceptual knowledge from other types of knowledge, including linguistic knowledge [3], in order to arrive in the future to application-independent medical terminologies [4]. Although on a theoretical basis the feasibility of these objectives is debatable [5], actual work within the GALEN-IN-USE project shows that on a relatively concise domain such as surgical procedures, distributed collaborative modelling can be achieved over linguistic borders. As could be expected, the process is however extremely slow. Formal "naming" and subcategorisation of new concepts at the one hand, and (in)consistent modelling of natural language expressions using the building blocks of the CORE that already are available, turn out to be the most frequent reasons for discussion. Given the very promising results of the MultiTALE semantic tagger for neurosurgical procedure reports [6, 7, 8], it was investigated whether or not this manual modelling work could be speeded up by using MultiTALE as an automatic modelling device.

2. Material and methods

100 English surgical procedure expressions were randomly selected from the SNOMED International V3.1 procedure, excluding generic (codes P1-0xxxx) and anaesthetic (codes P1-Cxxxx) procedures. These expressions were then processed by the original MultiTALE tagger. The results were analysed to identify possible shortcomings at the level of the lexicon, the syntactic-semantic grammar and the desired format of the output, i.e. GALEN templates [9, 10]. Based on this analysis, a stepwise lingware refinement methodology was adopted, until a satisfactory number of expressions could correctly be processed.

The purpose of this study was then to investigate 1) whether the high level ontology of GALEN and the representational power of the GALEN surgical procedure templates were sufficiently elaborated for use in natural language understanding, 2) to identify what additional linguistic knowledge was needed to improve the results, and 3) to investigate whether the SNOMED expressions themselves could unambiguously be understood using the available conceptual and linguistic knowledge.

3. From MultiTALE to MultiTALE II

Prior to any modification, MultiTALE analysed the expression *P1-11E52: closed reduction of fracture of zygoma or zygomatic arch* as an action of type repair which has as direct object a pathology, namely a fracture of zygoma or zygomatic arch (fig.1). The semantic links discovered (action and do), as well as the semantic types (repair, path, anat) have their origin in CEN/ENV 1828:1995 [11]. In addition, for the individual concepts discovered, the SNOMED International code is given.

```
(1)  action  repair  noun     closed reduction > P1-10E30
(2)    -       -     prep     of
(3)  do      path    sg       fracture of zygoma or zygomatic arch
(4)   -      path    sg               fracture of zygoma
(5)   -      path    sg                 fracture > M-12000
(6)   -       -      prep                of
(7)   -      anat    sg                  zygoma > T-11168
(8)   -       -      coor     or
(9)   -      anat    adjnoun  zygomatic arch > T-11167
```

Fig. 1: MultiTALE analysis of the sentence "closed reduction of fracture of zygoma or zygomatic arch"

Notice that the correct final results given in lines 1 and 3 originate from an erroneous intermediate processing at lines 8 and 9 where the coordination is attributed at the wrong constituents. This is entirely due to the tagging nature of MultiTALE (as opposed to traditional parsers) according to which only the segmentation at the highest level matters. With the objectives of GALEN in mind, this approach was no longer feasible as a more detailed analysis was required. MultiTALE was upgraded to MultiTALE II which produces the output of the same sentence as given in fig. 2 and fig. 3.

```
np    {{Closed reduction} of {fracture of {zygoma or zygomatic arch}}}
np         { Closed reduction }
adj            Closed
noun           reduction
prep       of
np         { fracture of { zygoma or zygomatic arch } }
noun           fracture
prep           of
np             { zygoma or zygomatic arch }
noun               zygoma
conj               or
noun               zygomatic arch
```

Fig. 2: MultiTALE II syntactic output of the expression "Closed reduction of fracture of zygoma or zygomatic arch"

```
RUBRIC "Closed reduction of fracture of zygoma or zygomatic arch"
MAIN reduction
     ACTS_ON fracture
         HAS_LOCATION zygoma / zygomatic_arch
     HAS_APPROACH closed
```

Fig. 3: MultiTALE II semantic analysis of the expression "Closed reduction of fracture of zygoma or zygomatic arch", presented in GALEN-template format

In order to achieve these results, the following changes to the original system were needed.

3.1 Implementation of a refined model for surgical procedures

ENV 1828:1995 recognises only four semantic links: *deed, direct object, indirect object* and *means.* Especially the links *indirect object* and *direct object* turned out to be underspecified for being useful within a natural language understanding environment, and lead to "non-monotonic like" semantic analyses. See for instance:

(1) Injection (*deed*) of antibiotic (*direct object*)
(2) Injection (*deed*) of cyst (*direct object*)
(3) Injection (*deed*) of antibiotic (*direct object*) in cyst (*indirect object*)
(4) Irrigation (*deed*) of cyst (*direct object*) with antibiotic (*means*)

For this reason, more refined links are foreseen such as *has_location, has_source, has_target, has recipient.* As internally in MultiTALE II these links stand in a n-to-1 relationship to the original links, output can still be given according to the specifications of the ENV. However, in order not to duplicate the work of the modellers in the GALEN-IN-USE project, the conceptual model was not more enhanced than needed for an unambiguous interpretation of the expressions, leaving out the details required for generation purposes. In addition, only that part of the GALEN ontology that surfaces grammatically in the expressions, was incorporated [12].

3.2 Implementation of a concept hierarchy

The MultiTALE tagger was directly based on the "flat" concept model of ENV 1828:1995, lexemes being encoded directly as *surgical_deed, anatomy, pathology* or *instrument.* To resolve certain linguistic ambiguities, a hierarchical model was needed. The relevant parts of the hierarchy needed to analyse the sentence of figure 3 , and the restrictional constraints on how some concepts may be linked, are outlined in figure 4.

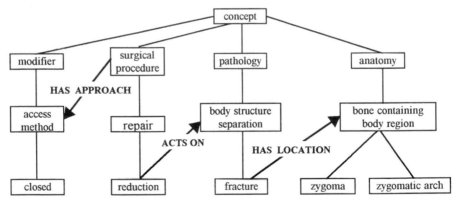

Fig 4: Relevant part of the concept hierarchy for the sentence *closed reduction of fracture of zygoma or zygomatic arch*

3.3 Implementation of mechanisms for knowledge discovery

As MultiTALE II is designed to enrich the GALEN CORE and linguistic annotation modules (semi)automatically, mechanisms had to be foreseen for dealing with unknown words in the input. This was achieved using a bottom-up parsing strategy where both syntactic and semantic configurations limit each others possible interpretations. In fig 5, the sentence "injection of xyz" (were xyz obviously is an unknown word) is analysed by MultiTALE II with one possible syntactic solution (xyz being a noun), and four possible semantic interpretations. First, xyz might be a body part, body region or pathology in which a not specified chemical is injected, as in *P1-10542: injection of ligament.* In these three cases, the HAS_DESTINATION semantic link applies. Next, xyz might be the chemical itself, with no destination specified, as in *P1-05027: injection of gas.*

np	{ Injection of xyz }	RUBRIC "Injection of xyz"
noun	Injection	MAIN injection
prep	of	ACTS_ON xyz : chemical
noun	*xyz	

RUBRIC "Injection of xyz"
MAIN injection
ACTS_ON chemical
HAS_DESTINATION xyz : body_part / body_region / pathology

Fig 5: Syntactic and semantic analysis of the sentence "injection of xyz"

4. Results

Out of the 100 randomly selected expressions, 10 could not be processed by MultiTALE II. For 7 of them, the required concepts or links were not yet available in the GALEN template-formalism, clearly a reason for failure outside the responsibility of MultiTALE. Of the remaining three, two showed peculiar (a)grammatical configurations while the other one contained deictic references and ellipsis, linguistic phenomena for which no grammar rules are currently implemented (*P1-B9846: Bilateral repair of inguinal hernia, one direct and one indirect*). Of the 90 expressions that could be processed, 73 (81%) were analysed correctly, giving the only one possible interpretation, 58 of which by using exclusively the links foreseen in the GALEN template formalism (an intermediate representation developed in order not to confront the domain modelling experts with the complexity of the GRAIL language), while for the remaining 15, additional semantic links were introduced. It would have been possible to map these extra links to the "garbage"-link HAS_-OTHER_-FEATURE that is allowed in the templates, but we choose deliberately for not doing so in order to preserve the depth of the interpretation. 17 expressions led to multiple interpretations, 48 all together. Of those 48, 75% could be judged being correct.

5. Discussion and conclusion

The results presented in this paper reflect not the final desired outcome of MultiTALE II, but are rather to be seen as a first evaluation of the actual stage of the system, with further improvement in mind. Ambiguities in the input phrases was the most important reason for multiple interpretations. E.g. *P1-A1122: Decompression of orbit only by transcranial approach*, where "only" can refer to the orbit (nothing else being decompressed), to the decompression (nothing else than a decompression being done on the orbit), or to the approach (no other approach allowed for giving this code). Coordination also led often to multiple interpretations, though the semantic constraints prevented all possible syntactic combinations, as can be seen in fig 2, where syntactically a possible bracketing would have been: *{{Closed reduction} of {{fracture of zygoma} or zygomatic arch}}*. This possible syntactic solution is however not retained on semantic grounds. Failure to reach an adequate interpretation was due to one of three reasons. For few sentences, the representational power of the GALEN-templates was not sufficient. It is for instance not yet possible to represent coordination amongst different semantic links that apply at the same time to one concept, e.g. *P1-2682B: repair of internal or complex fistula of trachea*, where "internal" and "complex" specify two different features of "fistula". Also, the GALEN templates allow numbers to be linked to concepts using the HAS_NUMBER link, but quite often, an exact number cannot be deduced from the expression, as just a plural is given. See *P1-7AC34:*

Lysis of adhesions of spermatic cord, where one can only infer that there must be more than one adhesion. For some other sentences, specific surface linguistic constructs turned out to be problematic. E.g. in *P1-19B05: Primary suture of ruptured ligament of ankle, collateral*, "collateral" obviously specifies "ligament", but no grammar rule could yet be implemented in such a way that this sentence would be analyzed correctly without introducing erroneous output for other sentences such as *P1-40141: Incision and drainage of hematoma, complicated*. Similar difficulties are caused by coordinated multiword units upon which ellipsis is applied, as in *P1-21A08: ... rhinoplasty with lateral and alar cartilages ...*. A third reason for incorrect results, is the lack of detailed anatomical knowledge such as the one required for correctly parsing *P1-17A26: Tenodesis for proximal interphalangeal finger joint stabilization*, where the system must know that "interphalangeal" refers to "joint" and not to "finger", in contrast with "abdominal wall mass" were "abdominal" refers to "wall".

The main conclusion of this work is that it is indeed feasible to develop a syntactic-semantic parser that quite satisfactorily translates natural language expressions into a predefined formalism for further processing. However, in order to be able to extract new knowledge from texts, a certain amount of background knowledge, both conceptual and linguistic, must be available. The precise boundaries of each of them are not yet clear, what requires further investigations.

6. References

1. Rector AL, Nowlan WA, Glowinski A. Goals for Concept Representation in the GALEN project. In Safran C. (ed). *SCAMC 93 Proceedings*. New York: McGraw-Hill 1993, 414-418.
2. Rector AL, Glowinski A, Nowlan WA, Rossi-Mori A. Medical concept models and medical records: an approach based on GALEN and PEN&PAD. *Journal of the American Medical Informatics Association* 1995, 2: 19-35.
3. Rector AL, Nowlan WA, Kay S. Conceptual Knowledge: the core of medical information systems. In Lun KC, Degoulet P, Piemme TE, Rienhoff O (eds.). *MEDINFO 92 Proceedings*. Amsterdam: North - Holland 1992, 1420-1426.
4. Rector AL. Compositional models of medical concepts: towards re-usable application independent medical terminologies. In Barahona P & Christensen JP (eds.) *Knowledge and decisions in health telematics*. Amsterdam: IOS Press 1994, 133-142.
5. Ceusters W, Deville G, Buekens F. The chimera of purpose- and language-independent concept systems in healthcare. In Barahona P, Veloso M, Bryant J (eds.) *MIE 94 Proceedings* 1994, 208-212.
6. Ceusters W, Deville G, De Moor G. Automated extraction of neurosurgical procedure expressions from full text reports: the Multi-TALE experience. In Brender J, Christensen JP, Scherrer J-R, McNair P (eds.) *MIE 96 Proceedings*. Amsterdam: IOS Press 1996, 154-158.
7. Ceusters W, Deville G. A mixed syntactic-semantic grammar for the analysis of neurosurgical procedure reports: the Multi-TALE experience. In Sevens C, De Moor G (eds.) *MIC'96 Proceedings*, 1996, 59-68.
8. Ceusters W, Lovis C, Rector A, Baud R. Natural language processing tools for the computerised patient record: present and future. In P. Waegemann (ed.) Toward an Electronic Health Record Europe '96 Proceedings, 1996:294-300.
9. GALEN Consortium. *Guidelines and Recipes for Completing templates.* Internal document VUM02/96 version 1.0.
10. GALEN Consortium. *Links and Templates Summary.* Internal document VUM/03/96 version 1.0.
11. CEN ENV 1828:1995. Medical Informatics - Structure for classification and coding of surgical procedures.
12. Ceusters W, Buekens F, De Moor G, Waagmeester A. The Distinction between Linguistic and Conceptual Semantics in Medical Terminology and its Implications for NLP-Based Knowledge Acquisition. In: *Proceedings of IMIA WG6 Conference on Natural Language and Medical Concept Representation*. Jacksonville 19-22/01/97, 71-80.

Medical Informatics Europe '97
C. Pappas et al. (Eds.)
IOS Press, 1997

Browsing and Querying Multimedia Report Collections[1]

F. Consorti[†], P. Merialdo and G. Sindoni[‡]

[†]IV Clinica Chirurgica, Policlinico Umberto I, Università di Roma "La Sapienza"
Viale del Policlinico, 5 00161 Roma, Italy

[‡]Dipartimento di Informatica e Automazione, Università degli studi di Roma Tre
Via della Vasca Navale, 84 00146 Roma, Italy

Abstract. In this paper a system and new methodologies that enable efficient exploration of distributed collections of multimedia reports are described. A conceptual model for the report and a method to semi-automatically create a hypermedia report network have been defined. The main issues addressed in this project were to exploit the textual component of a report to give a more evident semantic meaning to the data produced during the relative exam and to provide users with new interaction paradigms based on Internet technologies.

1. Introduction

MR BRAQUE (Medical Report BRowse And QUEry) is an implemented prototype system that allows physicians to compose diagnostic reports in an assisted environment [5] and to consult a report collection in a hybrid way, using both browsing and querying. In order to provide services to a Global Health Care System, Web technologies have been used to implement the human-computer interaction features.

In this work we focus on the modalities of interactive exploration of the document collection: new modalities for multimedia document retrieving have been investigated in order to provide physicians with efficient tools for exploring the source of knowledge represented by a medical reports collection. The paper is organized as follows: in Section 2 an overview of our multimedia report model is presented; in Section 3 we introduce the proposed modalities of interaction with the report collection; conclusions and future directions are discussed in Section 4.

2. Multimedia Report Modeling

We consider the medical report as a complex multimedia document [5] that is composed by two main elements: a textual component and a non-textual component. The textual component provides (textual) information about patient, about responsible diag-

1 This project has been supported by MURST, Università degli studi di Roma Tre Consiglio Nazionale delle Ricerche and Hewlett Packard.

nostician, about exam conduction methods and a sharp description of data produced by
the exam (images, bio-signals). Data produced by the exam represent the non-textual
component of the document. At the moment we are considering only still image reporting. Hence, in the following of the paper we will refer to a set of still images as the

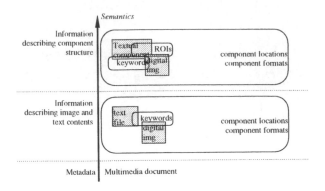

Figure 1 Enhancing Multimedia with the Use of Metadata

non-textual component of a report.

We think that the main objective of a report management system is to effectively
transfer all the knowledge that can be extracted from the images by the diagnostician to
the physicians who must take their decisions according to this knowledge. To achieve
this goal an effective management of multimedia documents is needed. In particular it is
necessary to make the images *semantically self-explaining*. To do that we make a mas-
sive use of *meta-information* [1], [6].

Fig. 1 shows two schematic solutions for the management of distributed multimedia
documents in the WWW environment. Text component and image component are
stored in flat files located in (possibly) different sites. To allow querying about the
document as a whole, metadata about document composition (e. g. *URL* and *media type*
of each component) and metadata about the whole document storage (e. g. *last modification date of the last modified component*) are needed. Moreover, data about the format and compression technique of the images must be provided in order to allow presentation. Besides, multimedia systems should be able to support querying on component
content. This can be achieved only adding information describing component contents.

Our solution is to describe the report by means of a conceptual model [5] and to
manage its structure by means of a OODBMS. Moreover, information about relationships between textual component objects referring to Regions of Interest (ROI) on the
image component is managed. A ROI is a zone of an image that delimits the edges of
some interesting feature of the image. In the hypermedia context, it is possible to define
anchors on ROIs into images, allowing to attach links to ROIs. The concept of ROI can
be easily extended to texts (a ROI is a sequence of characters) and to other type of multimedia objects: ROI descriptors depend on the media-type. We consider this as meta-
information, that is data that describe the content of the textual component and of the
images at the same time.

With this kind of management the system allows to describe the content of the components and permits to locate the objects inside the components. For instance, it is possible to locate the remarks inside the images and, if more than one remark is detected, it
is possible to distinguish them.

3. Querying and Browsing the Report Collection

Querying is the main interaction modality to retrieve information from a database. The user specifies a set of properties to be satisfied by the target documents and the system gives back the documents corresponding to these properties. If the result of a query consists in a set of documents, a common way to present them to the user is to provide an index whose items represent hypertext links to each document.

Three different modalities of presentation of hypertext indices are presented in literature [4]: guided tour, indexed tour and indexed guided tour. They are represented in fig. 2. Anyway, in many contexts this paradigm may not be effective. For example, if the physician is interested in a patient's clinical history and, while analyzing each one of the patient's reports, he/she discovers some interesting remarks, relative, for example, to a specific pathology, he/she could be interested in analyzing the clinical histories of other patients with the same pathology. Hence he/she ought to go on at first with a

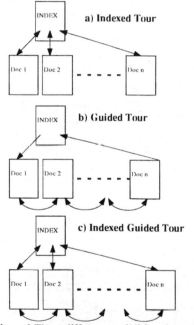

Figure 2 Three different modalities of presentation of hypertext indices

query to retrieve all the reports referring to the given pathology, and then analyzing the clinical histories (or part of them) of all the patients the retrieved reports belong to. In practice, the querying paradigm is used iteratively to create a browsing path through the report database (fig. 3).

In the MR BrAQue system, the main intuition is that the querying process has to be as transparent as possible to the user. The system allows to dynamically create an *orthogonal browsing network*, that is an hypermedia network such that, every time interesting information is found into a document, the physician can change the seeking criterion, choosing from the current document which properties are to be maintained constant in the prosecution. We call *orthogonal browsing* this kind of interaction because, if we represent all the query properties in a *n*-dimensional discrete space, we see how, keeping constant $m<n$ of these properties corresponds to constrain browsing into a ($n-m$)-dimensional space. In fig. 4 a 2-dimensional example of this concept is depicted.

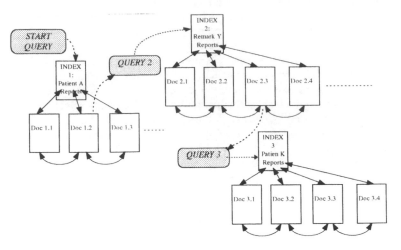

Figure 3 A Browsing Path through the Report Database

When all the query properties are set, the query is proposed to the system and the relevant documents are re-organized as a guided tour.

A suitable graphic interface shows the user a sort of navigation map organized into horizontal paths and steps: each step corresponds to a query submitted to the system,

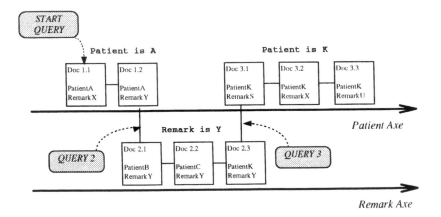

Figure 4 A 2-dimensional Orthogonal Browsing Path

while the following horizontal path corresponds to the fetching and browsing of a set of result documents.

4. Conclusions and Future Work

In this paper a mixin of the database and hypermedia paradigms for managing multimedia collections of diagnostic reports has been presented. The concepts of meta-information and orthogonal browsing have been illustrated: they are the main features of the MR BRAQue system, a hypermedia report management system developed at the Policlinico Umberto I of Rome.

The future directions of the project will be turned to generalize the system to support every kind of report, in particular reports for functional exams. For this purpose, we will explore the use of ontology in the requirements engineering area, to verify if it is possible to define and organize domain ontology able to represent the different kinds of reporting contexts and to be used as reference frameworks for setting up different system configurations. Besides, at the moment, we are exploring the DICOM standard [2] [3] structured report data model in order to make our system DICOM-compatible.

References

[1] F. Consorti, P. Merialdo, G. Sindoni *"Metadata Reference Model for Medical Documentation: a Hypermedia Proposal"* in Proc. Of the First IEEE Conf. on Metadata 1996. Available at
http://www.nml.org/resources/misc/metadata/proceedings/sindoni/ieee.html

[2] P. Merialdo, G. Sindoni, B. Spalluto *"Conceptual Abstractions over Standards"* Extended abstract submitted to the II IEEE Metadata Conference.

[3] D. Bidgood *"Digital Imaging and Communications in Medicine (DICOM)"* - Supplement 23 *"Structured Reporting"* ACR-NEMA Available at:
http://nelle.mc.duke.edu/standards/HL7/sigs/image-management/HTML/dicom-home.html

[4] T. Isakowitz, E. A. Stohr, P. Balasubraamanian *"RMM: Methodology for Structured Hypermedia Design"* in Comm. ACM 38,8: 34-44 Aug. 1995.

[5] F. Consorti, J. Di Prospero, P. Merialdo, G. Sindoni *"A method to Define and Design Tools for Hypermedia Medical Reports Management"* in Proceedings of the MIE 96 Conference. Part A 489-493 Aug. 1996.

[6] P. Merialdo, G. Sindoni *"Using Metadata to Enhance Multimedia Query Semantics"* in Proceedings of the XIII ERCIM-DG Workshop on Heterogeneous Information Management. Prague Nov. 1996.

[7] A. L. Rector, A. Gangemi, E. Galeazzi, A. J. Glowinski, A. Rossi Mori *"The GALEN CORE model schemata for anatomy: towards a re-usable application-independent model of medical-concepts"* in Proceedings of MIE94: 229-233.

[8] P. Agnello, A. Gangemi, E. Galeazzi, J. Niinimäki, V. Pakarinen, A. Rossi Mori *"What is a medical term? Terms and phrases in controlled vocabularies and continuous discourses"* in Proceedings of MIE94: 234-239.

[9] M. Agosti, M. Mellucci, F. Crestani *"Automatic Authoring and Construction of Hypermedia for Information Retrieval"* in Multimedia Systems (1995) 3:15-24.

[10] S. Brunati, A. Dezi, A. Fratton *"Dati obbligatori del referto: identificazione e motivazioni"* in Giornale Italiano di Endoscopia Digestiva 16,3: 39-51, 1993.

Medical Informatics Europe '97
C. Pappas et al. (Eds.)
IOS Press, 1997

ADM-INDEX: An automated system for indexing and retrieval of medical texts

SEKA L.-P.[a], COURTIN C.[a], LE BEUX P.[a]

[a] *Laboratoire d'Informatique Médicale, faculté de Médecine, Université de Rennes I, Avenue du Professeur Léon Bernard, 35043 Rennes cedex, France*

Abstract : ADM-INDEX is a system for indexing and retrieval of Patients Discharge Summaries (PDSs) by using linguistic methods (morphologic, syntaxic and semantic processing). The ADM-INDEX knowledge base is a restructuring of a diagnostic aid knowledge base (ADM) in order to allow the linguistic analysis of medical texts. The ADM system is a comprehensive medical knowledge base which has been developped since 1972 at the University Hospital of Rennes and which has been the first professional videotex medical diagnostic aid in France. After linguistic analysis, ADM-INDEX build the index table with thesaurus wording, medical words, concepts and phrases, unknown words contained in each PDS. The benefit of using those different elements is to improve information retrieval. Although our system is constructed with the ADM dictionary, it can be easily applied to other medical nomenclature or thesaurus. In this paper, we present on the one hand the ADM-INDEX knowledge base which is constituted by rules, a dictionary and a thesaurus, and on the other hand, the process of indexing and retrieval information.

1. Introduction

The semantic field of medicine is very wide and complex. A large number of its activities consists in producing medical reports written in natural language (Patients Discharge Summaries or PDS). PDSs describe the patients state of health. They are important documents in so far as they are firstly used for the patient's medical follow -up, and secondly as synthesis and self-teaching tool and also documents for communication, clinical research, epidemiological studies, evaluation of medical care.

Considering the abondance of information contained in each PDS, it is necessary to store and access them in a selective and judicious way through a quick and efficient system. This system will provide a significant help to physicians in accomplishing their task.

Elaborating such a system implies not only to solve problems concerning medical language (paraphrases, ambiguities..) [1] for this system must select the judicious concepts which would enable to represent the document's content, but also the use of medical nomenclature. The knowledge bases of medical decision systems such as INTERNIST [2], DXPLAIN [3], QMR [4], ADM [5] may be used as a starting point to build a corpus of entity and concepts.

We chose A.D.M. base (Diagnostic Medical Aid) as the core of our system because on one side it was developed in the Medical Informatics Laboratory, University of Rennes and on the other side it is both qualitatively and quantitavely rich (12.000 diseases, syndroms, undesirable effects and clinical forms by a 130.000 entities nomenclature, a 60.000 words dictionary). In spite of this abondance in terms, the ADM base does not lend itself to the analysis of medical texts (lack of syntactic and semantic information) which are written in natural language. ADM-INDEX is a restructuration of ADM base entity dictionary in order to adapt it to linguistic analysis of documents. We will show how we can detect concept and/or medical phrases, how we build index register and how we use it for information retrieval. We will end with the implementation and one of the applications of such a system which is necessary to have an automatic indexing and cross reference between our information and knowledge bases on a web server.

2. Material and methods

The knowledge base is composed of a dictionary. rules and a thesaurus. In a system as ours, the dictionary plays an essential role because it contains morphological, syntactic and semantic information. These information are useful to the different stages of analysis for the exact recognition of phrases. Besides, it must be a springboard for the inference and the deduction in so far as it will provide the necessary elements for starting the deduction and/or inference process. Inference and deduction are two important process for an indexing system using linguistic technics [6].

The dictionary : ADM-INDEX dictionary (around 60.000 words) essentially aims at detecting medical concepts and phrases whatever form it has in the text. Our dictionary inludes the ADM one in which words are classified by families (around 24.000 families). The links between the different words of a family are based on synonymy and inflexion. There are two categories of words : simple words and complex words which are subdivided into compound words and associated words.

• Simple words (around 45.000) : Among them, there are meaningless words (determiners,....) and non essential words (mostly adverbs).

• Complex words : they are composed by a group of simple words. There are two types of this kind of word.

. The Compound words (around 900) were created to avoid the dissociation of words. It enables to express a very strong link between its components on one side and on a other side to deal with synonymies between, for instance "Fievre jaune" (compound word) and "Amaril" (simple word). A compound word is very rigid. It neither accepts partial synonymy (synonymous of its components), nor allows a permutation in the order of its components.

. The Associated words (around 750) are like compound words but they are less rigid. Indeed, associated words enable to take into account synonymies between components.

We add syntactic and semantic information to the different constituents of ADM dictionary in order to make them more qualitative.

Constituents definition : There are three types of constituents which are concept[1]. expressions and simple words. Each constituent will be defined according to the group of following elements.

. CODE_SIG	: code associated to the constituent
. CATEG	: indicates whether the constituent is a word, a concept or a expression,
. TYPE	: indicates whether the constituent is a void word or not
. [MEDIC]*[2]	: indicates whether the constituent is a medical term or not
. [CATEGRAM]*	: grammatical category of the constituent
. [CAT_SEM]*	: semantic category of the constituent
. [PERHIERAG]*	: hierarchical fathers according to the generic link
. [PERHIERAP]*	: hierarchical fathers according to the partitive link
. [MOT]	: constituent's word
. [LOC]*	: localization of the constituent in comparison with the others
. [PREC]*	: specified concepts categories
. [DEF]*	: definition of the constituent if necessary
. [OPP]*	: concepts or words to which it is opposed
. [IMP]*	: implied concepts
. [CAUSE]*	: causes that generates it

Figure 1 : Representation of ADM-INDEX dictionary constituents

We also use the operators /// and // to represent the different meanings and possible cases. The symbol /// represents the different cases which are mutually exclusive and the symbol // represent the different possibilities within each case. They are useful to take into account the different contexts in which a concept, an expression or simply a word is used. This makes the concept belong to several families at the same time although it is registered in only one.

---

[1]. A concept is a scientific or linguistic term which definition is well specified and which represents a group of objects or ideas.
[2]. * means that the rubric is optional

Their use prevent from having several inputs for a same word in the dictionary if there are several meanings for it. For instance, in French, the word "Secretaire" (Secretary) can have 3 meanings : *boss assistant, writing desk* and *of secretary bird*. This word will only be registered once in the dictionary. It will be represented as follows :

. CODE_SIG	: 27139000
. CATEG	: Concept
. TYPE	: non avoid
. CATEGRAM	: Substantive
. CAT_SEM	: human_being 1/// Animal 2/// Object 3
. PERHIERA	: human_being 1/// bird 2 /// furniture 3
. MOT	: Secretary
. LOC	: Administration 1
. DEF	: boss assistant 1/// see: secretary bird 2/// writing desk 3

What follows is the translation of this representation : when SECRETARY is used in the administration field, then it means the boss assistant; when it is used in an animal context, then it is the synonymous of "Secretary bird"; when it is used in a furniture context, then it means "writing desk". The numbers link the different characteristics with the concept according to the semantic category considered.

The dictionary's elements attribute to a given term in the dictionary, Morphological, syntactic and semantic information. *Morphological information* is considered within the families (a family contains each form of a word). The CODE_SIG links a word with a family. *Syntactic information* is indicated in the field CATEGRAM (substantive, verb, adjective, prefix, ...). *Semantic information* is taken into account for the use of compound and associated word, the links existing between the different concepts (CAT-SEM, CAUSE...), the explicit definition of some concepts, the use of /// and // operators.

This way to represent words and concepts will make it possible to better identify them in the texts. Moreover, using syntagms (compound and associated words) makes it possible to well specify the idea or notion which is expressed and to reduce the cases of polysemies. Besides, structuring the dictionary with the family system gives all the inflexion forms of a word. We do not need to make a special lexical treatment to identify the words. This has the advantage of accelerating the process.

We will detect the different terms through rules and transformations. Fives rules and three transformations (Permutation, Reduction and Substitution) will accomplish the appropriate treatments to detect the good terms. The definition and use of these three transformations can be justified by the fact that constituents of the dictionary are mainly in their minimal form.

The thesaurus : ADM-INDEX thesaurus wording are hierarchically organised. This organisation is mainly based on generic "IS_A " and partitive "PART_OF" relations. This term hierarchy is based on the definition of the different concepts. Wording hierarchy is very important in an indexing process in so far as it not only makes it possible for sons to inherit their fathers's properties but also to prefer exact concept to broad concept. Besides, within the thesaurus, similarity between terms is a necessary element because it reduces the silence[L1][1] risks when searching for information.

3.   Implementation and results

Indexing : It is based on a certain number of process. Presentation of these process will be made according to the way they follow each other.

• The process of cutting and recognizing words. It enables to divide the text into sentences. Each sentence is then divided into words in order to carry out the recognition of each word. At this stage, the spelling of unknown words may be corrected.

• Syntactic and semantic analysis : this unit is composed of two secondary units
   - The syntactic "segmentor" which divides the sentences into parts (nominal groups) comparable to the dictionary headword. As regards medical texts, trying to use complete

---

[1] . Silence : the fact that nothing is proposed or not enough relevant answers are proposed when the base is consulted

syntactic analyser is illusive because texts often do not comply with natural language's grammar. Hence, the necessity to use a syntactic "segmentor". This segmentor is based on strong markers which are Verb, conjunction, preposition, predicative expression and punctuation sign. The benefit of using a syntactic "segmentor" is to reduce the unnecessary trials and avoid false concept recognition.

- The semantic conceptual analyser, from the sentence segmentation, detects concepts or phrases. Compound words are firstly identified, then associated words. Terms identification comes in this order because the links between the constituents of a compound word are stronger than those of associated words.

. compound word recognition : this stage will begin with the choice, within each nominal group, of a particular word called "*Principal*". The *Principal* belongs to the category of Substantive, Prefix or Adjective because these three categories are most likely to be in the first place in an expression. If there are several *Principals* in one group, priority depends on the rank of the *Principals* . The *Principals* accelerate the recognition process of compound words. They are used to consult the dictionary. Consulting aims at providing all headwords of compound words beginning with a given *Principal* or one of its inflexions. We will apply the compound word rule to this phrases list in order to only select the good terms.

. Associated word recognition : this recognition consists in consulting the dictionary with all words and compounds words (already detected) of the sentence. The result of the consulting will be composed of all associated words containing the word considered or one word of its family. We apply the different associated word rules to this phrases list in order to only select the good terms. When there are still isolated concepts, these latter will be replaced by their fathers in the sentence through generic and partititve link of the thesaurus in order to search for other possible associated words.

However, when two compounds or associated words are detected and if one of them is lexically contained in the other, the longest is selected because it is in general the most precise and it reflects better what has been expressed.

Once compound and associated words are detected, we will search for A.D.M. terminology[1] wording. Their detection will happen the same way as in the associated words detection because we consider wording as associated words.

• Index generation : The creation of index table will occur according to a method which results from an association of methods that already exist [7]. It consists in only keeping, as elements which could belong to the index table, concepts and/or medical terms, medical words, unknown words and very precise wording of the thesaurus ("son wording" are more precise than "father wording"). This not only compresses the index table but it also make far more significant matching. Including unknown words index table will produce "noise"[2] but we would rather have noise than silence. Each index is linked to a list. The list includes the text reference, the number of sentences in which the index appears with its nature.

Retrieval process : This process fistly capture the user's request and extracts all concepts, medical terms and thesaurus wording. Secondly, we create for each concepts and thesaurus wording a complete semantic consultation set through the similarity links in the thesaurus. We will consult the index table with these sets which allow to select all documents semantically close to each other through the consultation wording. Once documents are selected, they are given a rating according to the number and the nature of each index contained in each of them.

4 . Applications and results

ADM-INDEX knowledge base representation is based on RDBMS ORACLE relational model. The system has been developped in PRO C. The actual system is used in ICONOWEB project [8] which contains around 3.500 clinical cases. ADM-INDEX is considered as the heart of the indexing-retrieval engine of the multimedia ICONOWEB project. ICONOWEB's main objective is to build multimedia clinical case documents and to put them at the disposal of medical students so that they can exploit them at best.

---

[1] . Terminolgy wording is in the thesaurus

[2] . Noise means proposing too many non judicious answers as solution when the base is consulted.

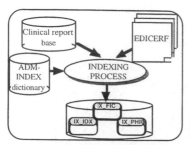

Fig 2: Indexing process in Iconoweb

ADM-INDEX is used for indexing two kinds of texts : the book of medical imaging references (EDICERF) and clinical cases with images and descriptions (ICONOCERF); each case is structured in chapters (History, Author, Context, Diagnostic....) and stored in a relational database. ADM-INDEX makes links between clinical reports and A.D.M. database, EDICERF books and A.D.M. database, clinical reports and EDICERF books. These links are very useful. Indeed, when you search information, the query process analyses conceptualy the request and shows (after a matching process) all clinical cases (by chapter : Diagnostic, Context ...), EDICERF books (by chapter : Pediatry ....) and ADM deseases which contain the query concepts. Thus, you can navigate easily on the Web server.

If a concept is present in the Context chapter, the system may present the report without diagnosis and commentaries and allow the user to propose a diagnosis. In this case, ADM-INDEX plays an important role. In fact, it makes a parallel between the user's answer and the concepts in the diagnostic and then gives an answer and a correction.

5.   Discussion

Starting with an existing ADM entities dictionary has the advantage of covering pratically all medical fields and being complete. It takes into account the particularities of medical language and common sense language. Besides, the system is not only linked with A.D.M. terminology. It is possible to replace this terminology by another thesaurus or medical terminology. We have developped a tool which translate a terminology in ADM-INDEX formalism. Thus, we can adapt easily the system to the ICD9 and ICD10 (International Classification of Diseases), to SNOMED (Systematized NOmenclature of MEDecine) and to the MESH (MEdical Subject Headings), which all have french translation. Although, the system is based on french language, the translation of concepts given in the most important terminologies may give a powerful indexing and retrieval system on english texts.

In the extraction unit, the selection method reduces silence as much as possible. That is very important because the lack of document can be a great disadvantage if these documents contain judicious information. On the other side, it may increase the noise for general queries, which does not matter because the user may refine his queries with more precise concepts.

References

[1].   Ghazi Joseph: Vocabulaire du discours médical, structure, fonctionnement, apprentissage. Edition Didier Eudition, 1985
[2].   Miller R. A., M.D., Pople H. E., Jr., Ph.D., Myers J. D., M.D. : *INTERNIST-I, an experimental computer-based diagnostic consultant for general internal medicine.* The New England Journal of Medicine. 1982; 307: 468-477.
[3].   Miller R. A., Masarie F. E., Myers J. D. : Quick Medical Reference (Q.M.R.) for diagnostic assistance MD Comput. 1986; 3: 34-48
[4].   Barnett G. O., M.D.; Cimino J. J., M.D.; Hupp ꞌ. A., M.D.; Hoffer E. P., M.D. : *DXPLAIN An evolving diagnostic decision-support system* JAMA, July 3, 1987 (vol 258, N° 1)
[5].   Lenoir P., Riou C., Fresnel A.: *L'aide au diagnostic médical (ADM). Modalités et perspectives.* Médecine de l'homme N° 135.
[6].   Jayez Jacques: *L'inférence en langage naturel.* Ed. Hermès, Paris, 1988
[7].   Hersh W. R., Hickam D. H., Leone T. J.: *Words, concepts or both: optimal indexing units for automated information retrieval.* In Proceedings SCAMC 93, pp. 644-648, 1993
[8].   Duvauferrier R., Rambeau M., André M., Denier P., Le Beux P., Coussement A., Caillé J. M., Robache P., Morcet N. : *Iconothèques et ouvrages multimédia sur serveur et cd-rom en imagerie médicale (l'expérience française).* J. Radiol 1995; 76 (12) : 1079-85.

Medical Informatics Europe '97
C. Pappas et al. (Eds.)
IOS Press, 1997

411

On Different Roles of Natural Language Information in Medicine

György Surján' László Balkányi
Haynal University of Health Sciences H 1389 PO.B 112 Budapest, Hungary

Abstract In this paper the authors analyze the main different function types of language in medical environment in different communicative situations and descriptive tasks. These functions are categorized as knowledge transfer, documentation, directive function, expression of emotions. The computer representation of the information have to be different according to the different tasks. The paper highlights the most important differences and concludes that further research is necessary in the details.

1. Introduction

For its outstanding universality, natural language is a unique powerful tool which may serve many different purpose at the same time in medical environment.. While considering representation of natural language information in computer systems, we have to decide, which roles have to be handled by computers. The aim of this study is to present the most important function types of language in health care environment and highlight the differences in the representation methods needed for the different function types. E.g. language is able to express emotions. Do we want to do it by computers? At first, we have to see which are the cardinal functions of language in medical or health care environment, and then we have to select the functions which are the reasonable tasks for computer representation.

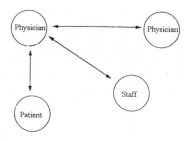

Figure 1
Main communication situations
- the viewpoint of a physician-

2. Analysis of traditional use of language in health care environment

Somewhat arbitrarily we would like to overview this topic from the point of view the physician. Basically language is used for communication and description. But these functions are neither independent nor sharply distinguishable. (See the "database" and "mail-box" paradigm of information).

2.1 Communicative situations

Figure 1 illustrates some of the important roles in health care, which whom the physician has to communicate. Let us see the most important functions in them.

Patient (patient's relatives) <-> physician communication
Main functions: querying (obtain important information about the case history)
        empathy (understanding emotions and intents of the patient)
        emotional lead (dissolving anxiety of patient)
        education (explaining the existing disease, the possible outcomes, treatments etc.)
        instructive (giving instruction how to use medicines, to give dietetic
                        restrictions etc.)
Staff <-> physician communication
Main functions: informative (giving information about patients, etc.)
        educative (passing certain part of medical knowledge)
        instructive (managing the work of the staff)
Physician <-> physician communication
Main functions: informative (giving information about result of examinations, etc.)
        educative (passing medical knowledge obtained from personal experience)
        operational (requesting examinations etc.)

2.2 Descriptive situations

An other kind of usage of language is the medical documentation, which is mainly in written form. All of these are descriptions of some experiences related to a single patients.

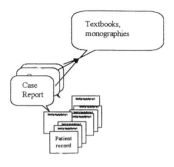

Figure 2
Descriptive information objects

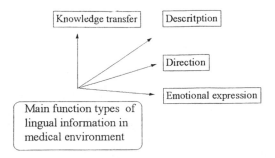

Figure 3
Main function types

Scientific publications, monographs, medical textbooks contain the essence of thousands of such individual observations, while case reports are some kind of intermediary forms: they contain essential information about a single case. (Figure 2) A more detailed description of this organization of medical information object is given in [1] This is obviously not an exhaustive list of all possible use of medical language, but we can see, that all these functions can be assorted into four main groups.(Figure 3)

Main function types are not independent and not always separable from each other. This functions are usually not separable clearly form each other: a certain information or message might serve all of these functions at the same time.

3. Characterization of the main functions

⇒ *Knowledge transfer*   This function of language is well known. What sometimes might be forgotten, is the fact, that this purpose is deeply different from the descriptive function. If I want somebody to understand something it is not sufficient simply describe the given topic. I might have to use parallelisms, examples etc. This difference might cause lexical and syntactic differences.

⇒ *Description*   Most frequently research in natural language processing and concept representation deals with the descriptive function of language. However there is no pure description. All the descriptions are made for some audience, real or virtual. This might be the descriptor itself. Therefore descriptions will differ according to the target audience. However this is mostly subconscious for the descriptor, in spite of communicative situations. In descriptions the semantic and grammatical correctness is a usual requirement.

⇒ *Direction*   In this function the emphasis is on the intention of the locutor to influence the behavior of an other actor (staff member, patient etc.) Semantic and syntactic correctness is not strongly required, and frequently sacrificed because of shortage of time. It is an special but certainly not exclusive feature of medical language.

⇒ *emotional expression*   This is a more or less subconscious feature of human language, which is present in written language also, but more characteristic to verbal communications. Emotions are detectable for intelligence, and such detection might be subject of descriptions. ("Patient's fear from cancer"), but this is very different from direct expressions of the emotions of the locutor, which is dominantly syntactic. (Repetition of terms, irregular order of words etc.)

4. Natural language information in computerized environment

In this chapter we would like to show, which of these functions are subject of computerization, and what computers should do in each field.

4.1 Knowledge transfer and descriptions

Knowledge and descriptions representable in computers as complex structures built from concepts and relations. Concept representation is one of the widely researched area of medical informatics. The quickly evolving multimedia tools will have deep influence to this area: more and more information will be stored in graphics, pictures, sounds. The future patient records perhaps will contain e.g. video picture of the ear-drum instead of textual description of its position, shape, perforation etc. Such documents will contain much more information and offer the possibility of the exact comparison along the curse of a disease, etc. What never should not be missed from the documentation is the judgment of the physician on the detected object. (E.g. a round shaded spot on the tympanic membrane is thought to be a perforation or an atrophic site?) This secondary or interpreted information is the situation as it is understood by the physician. This kind of information remains conceptual, but not necessarily verbal information. It is possible that in certain parts of this area formal or semi-formal representations will be effective in the future. Today it is only a research area and language possibly never will be entirely replaced by any kind of formal notations.

As a first step toward it some verb phrases could be eliminated from the texts. E.g. in a surgical operation report the sentence: *"A postauricular incision was made"* - says nothing more than the simple noun phrase: *"Postauricular incision."* The latter is grammatically incomplete but fully intelligible.

4.2 Direction

The governing or directing function of language in medical environment is sometimes disregarded. Descriptions are static, the directing function needs a dynamic, procedural approach. Here the question is not "what syncope means?" but "what to do if syncope occurs?" While human locutors often scarifies grammatical and semantic correctness for the quickness and effectiveness of such operational correctness, in computers probably we should not follow this manner. Human intelligence has the property of subconscious correction of small mistakes. Our computers are not so good in this sense. E.g. they do what we instruct them not what we would like to be done.

4.3 Emotional expression

Yet emotions of the locutor have some influence on the structure of lingual expressions, natural language processing systems are not able and not intend to capture emotions. Medicine can not be acceptable without emotions and empathy, and some important decisions might depend on emotional aspects, the problem can not be avoided. Humans i.e. members of medical staff have to act as emotional detectors, they have to formulate the emotional situation and express the emotions explicitly as far as possible by language [2].

5. Conclusions

Natural language has more function in medical environment, than just represent certain data about patients. These functions in traditional environment are not always clearly separated or separable. However computers are not able to handle all these functions. From those which presumably will be computationally tractable in the not too far future, two main type of functions have to be emphasized: the descriptive and operative. Systems designed for manage operational knowledge (the Arden syntax shows such examples [4]) have to be combined with those approaches designed for managing terminological knowledge like GALEN [5]. Large amount of natural language messages should have been analyzed to get a sufficiently detailed picture, but this was not our aim here. We are convinced that deeper research is necessary here.

References

[1] L Balkányi, Explorations on the nature of medical information. Ph.D. thesis University of Leiden
[2] Baud R.H, et al, Representing Clinical Narratives Using Conceptual Graphs, *Meth Inform Med.* 1995; **34**:176-86
[3] Z Harris, A theory of Language and Information - a mathematical approach. Clarendon Press Oxford, 1991
[4] Prokosch, H.U., Kamm, S. Wieczorek, D., Dudeck, J., Knowledge Representation in Pharmacology -A Possible Application Area of the Arden Syntax. Proceedings of the 15th SCAMC, MCGRAW-HILL Inc New York 1992
[5] Globe, C. Bechhofer, S. Solomon, D. Rector, A. Nowlan, A. Glowinsky, A., Conceptual, Semantic and Information models for Medicine. Information Modeling and Knowledge Bases IV. (Proceedings of the 4th European-Japanese Seminar on Information Modeling and Knowledge Bases 31st May-3rd June 1994, Stockholm) IOS Press, Amsterdam, 1995

Medical Informatics Europe '97
C. Pappas et al. (Eds.)
IOS Press, 1997

The Read Thesaurus - Creation and Beyond

C D G Stuart-Buttle, P J B Brown, C Price, M O'Neil, J D Read
NHS Centre for Coding and Classification, Woodgate, Loughborough, England

Abstract. The creation of the Read Thesaurus was a unique undertaking, involving over 2000 clinicians. This clinically-led, multidisciplinary enterprise posed many organisational and professional challenges. The process of term collection and integration and the problems encountered are described. A brief account is given of the large task of maintenance and refinement. This paper looks at the practical and cultural aspects and describes how problems were tackled by good organisation, clear guidelines and much goodwill.

1. Introduction

One notable feature that sets the Read Thesaurus [1] apart from other terminologies is the national scale on it was created. This paper describes the process of its creation from the point of view of the practicalities, the problems encountered and how they were overcome, not the terminology problems. It briefly describes the way in which the thesaurus continues to be maintained.

2. Background

The Read Codes [2,3] were developed in the early 1980s by Dr. James Read to record clinical summaries in General Practice. This version, still in use today, is known as the Four Byte Set. By the late 1980s a new version was developed, Version 2, to create hospital summaries. This was structured to be compatible with and to carry maps to the International Classification of Diseases, 9th Revision [4] (ICD-9) and the Office of Population Censuses and Surveys Classification of Surgical Operations and Procedures, 4th Revision [5] (OPCS-4).

3. Philosophy

The initial proposal for a set of clinical terms for use by clinicians came from the medical profession. With the National Health Service Centre for Coding and Classification (NHS CCC) the Clinical Terms Project [6,7] was set up based on the existing versions of the Read Codes, followed by similar projects for the professions allied to medicine and for nursing, midwifery and health visiting, collectively known as the Terms Projects. From the outset the initiative had professional ownership and leadership. At its height, between 1992 and 1995, the work involved over 2000 clinicians from all disciplines, working together in a spirit of co-operation never seen before. Different professions were getting together, sometimes for the very first time, to discuss clinical terms for topics of common interest.

Insulin dependent diabetes mellitus
IDDM
Type 1 diabetes mellitus
Juvenile onset diabetes mellitus

Figure 1: Synonymous terms

The creation of a thesaurus of this nature had to have clear limits. The emphasis was on natural clinical terms as found in written records. This meant the relegation of classification categories, such as "Asthma not otherwise specified", to an optional status so that they do not appear on initial picking lists for data entry. No attempt was made to capture the context in which a term might be used, for example as a complication. This has to wait for further work. No clinical term was disallowed. Figure 1 illustrates the retention of older terms which might be considered to be out of date, in this case as synonyms for the concept of *Insulin dependent diabetes mellitus.*

4. Project Organisation

The project was managed, using PRINCE methodology (Projects IN Controlled Environments), by the NHS CCC which also provided training, terminological expertise, computer equipment and financial control.

A total of 55 Specialty Working Groups (SWGs) were set up, covering all medical, profession allied to medicine and nursing specialties. Each nationally recognised SWG chairperson had the official approval of the relevant professional body. Each recruited six to ten SWG members, usually with expertise in sub-specialties, or representatives from other specialties with a shared interest, and a full-time researcher.

Each SWG put together a proposal for the work, with clear time-scales, and funds were allocated to pay for the researcher, equipment, regular meetings, travel expenses and an honorarium for the chairman in recognition of the extra work entailed in the rôle. Every SWG had a Specialty Assurance Team, an independent group of three peers which reviewed the work to ensure completeness and that the terms were not idiosyncratic.

An invaluable quarterly forum of all chairpersons and researchers met to exchange views and debate issues. A panel of chairpersons rules on any inter-professional disputes. Only once has this been invoked to settle a question of terminological style.

5. Guidelines

The SWGs were given some broad guidelines. The new set of natural clinical terms had to include those in existing versions of Read Codes. The results had to be mapped to ICD-9, ICD-10 [8] and OPCS-4 in order to allow generation of data in these formats for statistical purposes. Detailed guidance on the development of hierarchical lists was also given.

6. Term collection

The initial task was to collect a list of acronyms and abbreviations. This gave the SWGs time to get used to each other and to new computers, software and ways of working. The NHS CCC took several hundred headings from Version 2 of the Read Codes and ICD-10. Each SWG indicated a major, minor or no interest in each topic. Prime responsibility for each was assigned to only one SWG, which had the responsibility for creating the initial list of terms for the topic and for consulting all those others with a major interest. They were then supplied with electronic lists of Version 2 terms upon which to base their lists. They also had copies of ICD-10 in order to help ensure compatibility.

Microsoft Word© was used to develop hierarchical lists of terms because of its outline facility and its annotation facility was used to record extra detail in the form of qualifiers [9] (see later). NHS CCC macros automated some of these processes. Initial lists were imported into a relational database (Oracle©) where they are maintained. For many SWGs the lists were exported into a simple browser, developed in house, and piloted by their peers. Further modifications were made as a result of feedback.

7. Integration

Once delivered, the final files were processed into a standard format, again using macros. Duplicate concepts were identified using customised software and eliminated manually. The lists were restructured to achieve as much consistency as possible. The integration of Version 2 terms was checked using customised software. During this period a single editor - the Read Code Processor - was built in house to maintain the thesaurus. Once finalised, the lists were manually and individually mapped to ICD-9, ICD-10 and OPCS-4, checked by a classification expert and subsequently independently validated. This brief description of integration does not reflect the enormous human effort on the part of a dedicated team authors and technical staff at the NHS CCC.

8. Problems

An enterprise of this scale inevitably had its problems. These were, however, fewer than might be expected. Only those relating to organisational and cultural issues are described here. Where difficulties were encountered, whether terminological or cultural, the solution was always found by getting together the parties involved.

There was a significant training requirement for the SWGs. Many were unfamiliar with computers. Training was needed in basic file housekeeping, in Microsoft Word© and the NHS CCC software. Significant time was invested to try to create a good understanding of terminology among the SWGs, in order that the submitted work was of a consistent standard. Naturally this was not always successful, and submitted lists sometimes required many hours of reworking by NHS CCC authors.

The NHS CCC had initially anticipated that the new terms could be accommodated within the structure of Version 2. It soon became apparent from the volume and complexity of the terms that this was not possible. A different structure was proposed, known as Version 3 [10]. This had new features, notably a directed acyclic graph and a system of core terms and qualifiers [9] consisting of attributes and values (Figure 2). Considerable

Core term	Attribute	Value
Appendicectomy	*Approach*	*Laparoscopic*

Figure 2: Version 3 qualifier structure

discussion and education was required to ensure that the clinical professions understood the need for the change and fully supported it.

Despite the strict division of topics, SWGs drifted into others' domains, because of worry that terms important to them would be omitted. This required the NHS CCC to ensure either that the overlap was removed or that it was picked up during integration. The SWGs also placed far more and varied information into qualifiers than had been intended. Management of their expectations of when these would be released has been difficult.

There were a few disputes (all settled amicably) over who should have prime responsibility for a topic. For example, who should have first claim on the topic of cleft lip and palate - the Ear Nose and Throat, Maxillo-facial or Dental SWGs? Other SWGs were reluctant to share their lists with those who had declared a major interest until very late in the process. Prompting by the NHS CCC usually ensured that the sharing occurred.

Some SWGs simply did not recognise commonly used generalist phrases (e.g. *Chest infection*) as valid terms because they were regarded as too vague or outdated. The usefulness of such terms was understood when specialists saw that they too are generalists in every other area than their own. The creation of a General Practice SWG also helped here.

Version 3 is built as a *type-of* hierarchy (Figure 3), where each concept is a *type of* the concept above it. This created difficulties for SWGs who wished to see all terms relating to, for example, diabetes under a single heading. There was concern that rigid enforcement of such a model would devalue the terms. Significant educational input was necessary in order to create an understanding of the need for a consistent structure for analysis and for accurate placement of new terms.

The medical SWGs had a relatively straightforward task. Terms already existed in the Read Codes and there were other sets of terms to refer to. For most of the nursing and profession allied to medicine SWGs this was a completely new exercise, involving both the identification and recording of their vocabluary.

The level of detail in the submitted lists varied from superficial and classification-like to very detailed. The rule of thumb applied to the level of detail was not to go beyond what the creator would want to retrieve and analyse.

Ensuring that busy clinicians, who were mostly donating their time, kept to agreed delivery dates was extremely difficult. This resulted in some delays as integration could not start until all files for a particular section were received.

9. Maintenance and refinement

Creation was an enormous and complex task. Maintenance requires a substantially larger effort as has been reported by others [11]. This is because the thesaurus is updated every quarter (monthly for drugs and appliances); semantic definitions [12] are being applied to concepts to support retrieval and placement of new terms; forward compatibility between versions is maintained; and maps to the classifications require constant maintenance. All this work is still done largely manually by a team of clinically trained authors and classification experts. As more of the thesaurus is semantically defined there will be greater

```
📂 Read thesaurus
  └📂 Operations and procedures
    └📂 Eye procedure
      └📂 Eye muscle operation
        └📂 Combined operation on eye muscles
          └📄 Bilateral medial rectus recession
```

Figure 3: Version 3 sub-type hierarchy

scope for automation of some of these processes.

The main database contains all terms so far integrated. Those marked as experimental or developmental are not released for live use. Released and developmental concepts are combined in browsers to enable users to see what will be available.

A major challenge in maintaining the thesaurus is keeping the clinical professions engaged with the process. The maintenance phase has seen an almost total shift of responsibility for the thesaurus to the NHS CCC authors, with relatively little involvement by the professions who created it. They still wish to "own" it and be consulted on changes but this takes time and is in conflict with a dynamic product. Currently changes are made to the thesaurus by the NHS CCC authors with reference when necessary to the SWGs. The SWGs receive retrospectively every quarter a report of changes made. This allows changes to be made at the request of users who expect a rapid response, while still giving the creators of the thesaurus a say in developments and changes.

It is not possible to subject a terminology to a true test of fitness for purpose except in operational use. Testing outside real implementations can only show part of the picture. The value of the full thesaurus in practice has yet to be demonstrated. Feedback from operational testing has already been extremely valuable and of a different nature to that received from early piloting in browser software. The NHS CCC is attempting to involve the SWGs in those sites that are operationally testing the thesaurus in order that its creators and users gain a shared understanding of the nature and requirements of a computerised clinical terminology.

10. Summary

The creation of the Read Thesaurus was a vast and unique undertaking, made possible only by the nature of the NHS and the goodwill of the clinical professions. Its operational testing and maintenance are a greater task and one which will take considerable time, effort and patience.

References
[1] O'Neil MJ, Payne C' Read JD. Read Codes Version 3: A User Led Terminology. *Meth Inform Med* 1995; **34**: 187-92
[2] Chisholm J. The Read Clinical Classification. *British Medical Journal* 1990; **300**: 1092
[3] Read JD, Benson T. Comprehensive Coding. *British Journal of Healthcare Computing* May 1986; 22-5
[4] International Classification of Diseases. 9th Revision. Geneva: WHO, 1975
[5] Classification of Surgical Operations and Procedures. 4th Revision. Office of Population Censuses and Surveys. London: HMSO, 1990
[6] Severs MP. The Clinical Terms Project. *Bulletin of Royal College of Physicians* (London) 1993; **27**(2): 9-10
[7] Stannard CF. Clinical Terms Project: a coding system for clinicians. *British Journal of Hospital Medicine* 1994; **52**(1): 46-8
[8] International Statistical Classification of Diseases and Related Health Problems. 10th Revision. Geneva: WHO, 1992
[9] Read Codes File Structure Version 3.1 - The Qualifier Extensions. Version 1.2. Loughborough. Information Management Group, 1995
[10] Read Codes File Structure Version 3.1. Loughborough. Information Management Group, 1995
[11] Cimino JJ, Clayton PD, Hripsack G, Johnson SB. Knowledge based Approaches to the Maintenance of a Large Controlled Medical Terminology. *JAMIA* 1994; **1**: 35-50
[12] Price C, Bentley TE, Brown PJB, Schulz EB, O'Neil MJ. Anatomical Characterisation of Surgical Procedures in the Read Thesaurus. In Cimino JJ (Ed). Proceedings of the 1996 AMIA Annual Fall Symposium. Philadelphia: Hanley & Belfus: 1996; 110-114

Medical Informatics Europe '97
C. Pappas *et al. (Eds.)*
IOS Press, 1997

Semi-Automatic Coding with ICPC: The Thesaurus, the Algorithm and the Dutch Subtitles

Rudolph S. Gebel, general practitioner
Staff member Dutch College of General Practitioners
Lomanlaan 103, P.O. Box 3231, 3502 GE Utrecht, The Netherlands

Abstract

In the ICPC Thesaurus Project, which ran from 1990 to 1992, the Dutch translation of the English version of the ICPC-components 1 and 7 was made available for automated coding by structuring and improving the thesaurus and by developing an algorithm for selecting possible ICPC-codes from a set of medical terms given as input to the program. The thesaurus and algorithm are available to the developers of GP information systems and are at present incorporated in all Dutch GP-systems. This paper brings you up to date with the semi-automatic coding system and the so called Dutch subtitles, an extension to the ICPC.

1. Introduction

In the Netherlands, the International Classification of Primary Care (ICPC) [1] is accepted as the standard for coding and classification in general practice.

The ICPC classification system consists of two axes. One axis consists of the different body systems, the chapters, including a general chapter and a chapter on social problems. Each chapter is represented by a letter (for example F for the eye). The other axis consists of seven different components of ICPC. In this paper we only deal with the first (complaints and symptoms) and seventh (diagnosis) component. Each component contains several titles, represented by two digits (for example, the diagnostic component runs from 70 through 99). Thus, each so called Short Title is represented by a letter and two numbers, for example D88 APPENDICITIS.

In 1988, the Dutch translation of the Short Titles and of the so called inclusion terms (a rudimentary thesaurus) was ready for use. [2]

2. The ICPC Thesaurusproject

At the beginning of the ICPC Thesaurusproject in 1989, the ICPC-thesaurus was barely structured, mainly due to the fact that the thesaurus consisted of nothing more than a translation of the inclusion terms. An example of the inclusion terms of the Short Title K80 ECTOPIC BEATS ALL TYPES is:

ICPC-code	inclusion term no	inclusion term
K80.	1	ECTOPIC RHYTHM
K80.	2	ECTOPIC HEART BEAT
K80.	4	PREMATURE BEAT
K80.	5	ECTOPIC HEART RHYTHM
K80.	8	PREMATURE HEART BEATS
K80.	9	NON-SPECIFIC PREMATURE BEATS
K80.	10	SUPRAVENTRICULAR PREMATURE BEATS
K80.	11	VENTRICULAR PREMATURE BEATS

Due to the structure of the inclusion terms, many general practitioners believed them to be a subclassification, which led to much confusion. As you can see from the example above, the different inclusion terms do not exclude each other, which is the basis of a good classification. So, the first task of the project was to structure the thesaurus in such a way, that it could be easily automated and maintained.

This was done by grouping terms into so called word clusters. Word clusters are groups of terms that all mean the same: synonyms, spelling variants, lay terminology etcetera. Each cluster is linked to one or more Short Titles. With each Short Title, the importance of each word cluster for that specific Short Title is expressed as either 'Essential' or 'Non-essential'. Only essential clusters are used to select candidate codes, non-essential clusters are only used to influence the order in which the candidate codes are displayed.

An example of a word cluster, translated into English, is VARICELLA, which contains two words: VARICELLA and CHICKENPOX. Another example is the cluster APPENDIX, which contains the words APPENDIX and APPENDICULAR. After a first testphase, the clusters were revised, using the comments we received from the GP's that participated in the testing, and adding terms from the ICD-10, using the existing conversion table between ICD-10 and ICPC. [3]

Secondly, we had to handle the fact that the ICPC was developed as an international classification for epidemiological research, and not as a coding tool for Dutch general practice. As a result, some diseases which are extremely rare in Dutch general practice, have a separate Short Title (like malaria, A73), whereas more common diseases, like bursitis, have their place in the so called ragbags, i.e. L99. This formed a barrier for many GP's to use the ICPC. To meet the demands, we developed the so called Dutch subtitles. [4]

Subtitles form an extension to a Short Title and contain frequently assessed diagnoses in Dutch general practice. For example, the Short Title 'F99 Other diseases eye/adnexa' is divided into the following subtitles:

F99.01	Ectropion/entropion/blepharochalasis eyelid
F99.02	Dry eyes
F99.03	Pterygium
F99.04	Scleritis/episcleritis
F99.05	Occlusion retinal artery or vein
F99.06	Diplopia
F99.07	Anopsia all forms
F99.08	Color blindness
F99.99	Other diseases eye/adnexa

In developing the subtitles, we used data about prevalence and incidence of the different Short Titles derived from the Transition Project [5], and the conversion table between ICPC and ICD-10, as mentioned before.

Through the subtitles, more specific coding is possible which makes it more satisfactory to the Dutch GP, because he is now able to use the ICPC-codes as a tool for preventive activities, for prescribing medication etcetera. Epidemiological research at the level of the Short Titles is still possible by discarding the last two digits. In 1997, a new edition of the subtitles is presented.

Over 300 Short Titles from a total of 691 have two or more subtitles:

Tabel 1: Number of subtitles per Short Title

no. of subtitles per Short Title	no. of Short Titles	percentage of Short Titles
0	380	55,0
2	118	17,0
3	99	14,3
4	41	5,9
5	27	3,9
6	10	1,5
7	5	0,7
8	2	0,3
9	7	1,0
10	1	0,2
11	1	0,2

3. The semi-automatic coding program

The semi-automatic coding program works as follows:

During the consultation, the GP enters the symptom, complaint or diagnosis he wishes to encode in the journal of the GP information system he uses. The word(s) used will point to the corresponding word clusters. As explained earlier, these clusters are coupled with one or more Short Titles. The Short Titles are represented in order of likelihood. The GP chooses a Short Title. He can then choose one of the subtitles that belong to the Short Title (when available). The symptom, complaint or diagnosis is then encoded with the correct ICPC-code and stored into the database.

For example, the doctor types:

HEADACHE

The system presents the doctor with the following options:

```
N01   HEADACHE [EX. N02,N89,R09]
N02   TENSION HEADACHE
N89   MIGRAINE
N90   CLUSTER HEADACHE
R09   SYMPTOMS/COMPLAINTS SINUS [INCL.PAIN]
```

At first glance, the presentation of the last possibility, R09, seems illogical. We have chosen to display the exclusion codes as well, as presented at code N01 in this case. That way, the doctor can make a responsible choice.

After choosing N89 MIGRAINE, the following subtitles are presented:

```
N89.01    CLASSIC MIGRAINE
N89.02    MIGRAINE WITH NEUROLOGICAL SYMPTOMS
N89.99    OTHER/NON SPECIFIC MIGRAINE
```

As you can see, in this case the last code is a so called ragbag. We have given the ragbag-subtitles the extension 99, so that it is possible to add other subtitles without having to change the numbers.

The doctor decides that the right code is N89.01. Now he can make a choice. By toggling with the TAB-switch, he can either store his own text (N89.01 HEADACHE) or he can store the text of the subtitle (N89.01 CLASSIC MIGRAINE).

In retrospect, it would have been better if he had typed 'MIGRAINE' instead of the less specific term 'HEADACHE'. First of all, the computer can't interpret the fact that the doctor means 'migraine' if he types 'headache'. Secondly, the outcome of the search with 'MIGRAINE' would have been limited to one Short Title, i.e. N89.

4. Further developments

Since 1995, a helpdesk is available at the Dutch College of General Practitioners to help solve coding problems encountered by the GP. The comments we get are used to improve the thesaurus and the algorithm. Most comments are concerned with not finding the correct code despite correct input.

The old ICHPPC-2-Defined criteria [6] will be replaced by the international ICPC inclusion criteria. As soon as the WONCA Classification Committee approves of these criteria, Dutch inclusion criteria based on the international standard will be developed to ensure better classification.

In 1997, a stand-alone version of the semi-automatic coding program will be developed, mainly for educational and scientific purposes.

Finally, a layman 'translation' of the Short Titles and subtitles will be developed as part of the promotional research of the author. One of the tasks that will be performed is a total review of all word clusters.

5. Conclusions

Through the semi-automatic coding system, the ICPC has become easier to use. This is demonstrated by the fact that the use of ICPC has significantly increased since the introduction of the coding system (from 33% of all general practitioners in 1993 [7] to over 60% in 1997 (preliminary results of the NUT-III-project)). The Reference Model 1995 (the blue print of all GP information systems in Holland) can cause a dramatical increase of the use of ICPC in the electronic patient record increases dramatically because of the introduction of the episode oriented registration. The ICPC will be an anchorpoint for episode oriented registration and be the link to prescribing medication, related consultations, other information sources, printing patient information leaflets etcetera.
Maintaining the ICPC and the coding system is a continuing process. The introduction of ICPC-2 forms a great challenge in the near future.

Acknowledgements

The author wishes to thank Dorry Cox, Henk Westerhof and Han van Overbeeke of the Dutch College of General Practitioners for their comment on the manuscript.

References

[1]   Lamberts H, Woods M, eds. International Classification of Primary Care. Oxford, Oxford University Press 1987

[2]   Kanter JS de, Lamberts H, Mulder JD. ICPC International Classification of Primary Care, Thesaurus, Dutch translation. Part I Systematic list. Part II Alfabetic list. Leiden, January 1989

[3]   Lamberts H, Wood M, Hofmans-Okkes IM (ed.). The International Classification of Primary Care in the European Community with a multi-language layer. New York, Oxford University Press 1993

[4]   Boersma JJ, Gebel RS, Lamberts H. ICPC with Dutch subtitles. Utrecht, Dutch College of General Practitioners 1995

[5]   Lamberts H. In het huis van de huisarts. Verslag van het Transitieproject. Lelystad, Meditekst 1994

[6]   WONCA. ICHPPC-2 Defined. Oxford, Oxford University Press, 3rd edition 1983

[7]   Westerhof HP, Van Overbeeke JJ (red.). Report of the NUT-II-project, part II. Utrecht, Dutch College of General Practitioners, Utrecht, 1994

Medical Informatics Europe '97
C. Pappas et al. (Eds.)
IOS Press, 1997

A Formal Model of Diabetological Terminology and Its Application for Data Entry

C. Birkmann[*], T. Diedrich[§], J. Ingenerf[*], J. Rogers[+], W. Moser[*], R. Engelbrecht[*]

[*]medis - Institut für Medizinische Informatik und Systemforschung, GSF - Forschungszentrum für Umwelt und Gesundheit, Ingolstädter Landstraße 1, D-85764 Neuherberg, Germany

[+]Medical Informatics Group, Depart. of Computer Science, University of Manchester, Manch. M13 9PL, UK

[§]DFI - Diabetes Forschungsinstitut Düsseldorf, Auf'm Hennekamp 65, D-40225 Düsseldorf, Germany

Abstract. This paper summarises the developmental activities for an electronic patient record system in diabetology based on GALEN technologies. It focusses on the modelling of primarily terminological medical knowledge of this subspecialty and describes its application for predictive data entry.

1. Introduction

A formal model of terminological knowledge and a corresponding structured data entry system as part of an electronic patient record system (EPR) are being developed for the subspecialty diabetology and will lateron be integrated into a GP-diabetes management system. The final clinical workstation is intended to support clinicians in their care and management of diabetes and will allow to enter and manipulate administrative and medical patient data. The current developments based on GALEN technology are part of the EU-funded Galen-In-Use project, which establishes Terminology Servers for medical applications based on a computer-supported model of medical terminology.

The GALEN-based structured data entry system is to demonstrate that the GALEN technology improves the quality and consistency of the captured data and further enhances the maintainablility and scalability of medical record systems. It will thereby profit from a semantically sound representation of medical terminology. The data entry system will enable the user to enter data in a structured and standardised manner and in some cases as free text also. The GALEN approach inherently supports the generation of dynamic, context-relevant forms and thus enables intuitive, quick, and easy entry of detailed clinical data. In a later phase of the project the diabetes management system will furthermore demonstrate the added functionality the GALEN approach offers: multilingual appearance, report generation, retrieval of data, and data driven decision support.

2. Data Entry in Electronic Patient Record Systems

The demand for electronic patient record systems in Germany is increasingly met. Therefore it is now important to offer high-quality electronic systems with improved medical conten' and functionality. Data entry by commercially available electronic patient record systems i: not as easy and consistent as desirable. Research in electronic patient record systems attempt:

to find practicable and convincing solutions to improve data entry [1, 2]. The GALEN project aims to permit easy and consistent data entry by tackling the problem of terminology [3].

Terminology is considered by GALEN as software. Terminological services (e.g. the conversion between natural languages) will be provided based on a centrally shared, semantically valid model of clinical terminology. This terminological model which forms the heart of the Terminology Server supports computer-based systems and allows detailed clinical information to be captured, represented, manipulated, and displayed.

3.   Diabetes Model

3.1   GALEN Technology

The diabetological terminology is represented with the representation language of the GALEN project, the Galen Representation And Integration Language (GRAIL), resulting in the diabetes model. GRAIL allows to represent medical concepts compositionally with elementary clinical concepts, attributes combining these elementary concepts, and resulting complex concepts [4]. In addition a constraint mechanism with several levels of sanctioning allows to construct only sensible complex concepts [4].

The Terminology Server combines separate modules each of which serves a different aspect of the provided terminological services [3]. The concept module organizes terminological knowledge, whereas the extrinsic module links non-terminological to terminological knowledge [3]. The other modules are the code conversion module and multilingual module which are mapping concepts to codes or natural languages and vice versa [3].

3.2   Modelling Terminological Knowledge

The diabetes model has been developed systematically extending the concept module and specifically for the diabetological data entry system. It is based on the terminological knowledge of the standardised DIABCARD dataset version 2.0 [5]. This dataset contains medical information concerning signs and symptoms, findings, diagnoses, and the therapy of diabetes and other relevant diseases. Tool was the Knowledge Management Environment integrated Terminology Server (KiT) [6]. The non-terminological knowledge of the dataset has been added to the extrinsic module or the application model which is integrated in the concept module.

The modelling process was characterised by different ways of proceeding: Basic structures and constructs had to be proposed, consolidated or revised. A consistent model based on the source characterised above was developed rapidly. Special solutions were found for quaint details required by the source and not easily fitted into the preexisting terminological model.

The terminological diabetes model includes a dictionary of concepts and a grammar. Nearly 1200 items of the data source have been modelled including their relationship to each other as provided by the data source.

A number of elementary concepts relevant for general medical applications as well as specific diabetological applications has been added to the preexisting concept structure. Clean taxonomies were kept and created, existing structures extended, and new structures either created in analogy to existing ones or frequently from scratch after profound analysis. Examples of new elementary concepts are kinds of body parts (fig. 1), roles (e.g. AntigenicRole, AllergicRole), units (e.g. mg/dl, IU), drugs, and enzymes.

BodyPart
    NAMEDSensoryOrgan
       EyeOrgan
    NAMEDSensoryOrganSubPart.
      NAMEDEyeOrganSubPart
        Macula
        OcularLens
        OpticPapilla
        Retina

Fig. 1   Newly created taxonomy showing elementary concepts of the eye anatomy.
The levels of indenting denote the subsumption hierarchy. The taxonomy presents is-a-kind-of relations.

Tab. 1   Attributes introduced and their usage

attribute	usage
hasDiagnosisProbability	how reliable is the diagnosis of a pathological phenomenon?
hasDiseaseStage	which stage is a pathological phenomenon in?
hasDosage	in which dosage is a drug applied?
hasImmediateComplication / hasLateComplication	which pathological phenomenona occurring after a short / long period of time are complications of pathological phenomenona?

New attributes were added. These enable the representation of details of e.g. pathological phenomena and drug therapies (tab. 1).

Complex concepts (tab. 2) are frequently necessary to represent the items of the data source. Modelling conventions once established simplify modelling. The sanctioning mechanism is carefully applied in order to prevent nonsense compositions. A secondary structure is frequently superimposed on the primary conceptual hierarchy to rearrange the conceptual hierarchy as needed in the diabetological context. Central medical concepts are frequently modelled as general and heterogeneous GRAIL concepts.

The data source contains non-terminological knowledge which is represented in the extrinsic module. Linking extrinsic knowledge to terminological knowledge is done by application attributes (fig. 2). These are hierarchically organised in the application model, subsumed

Tab. 2   Examples of complex concepts

item of dataset	complex concept

goal of therapy	Feature which <
	     isFeatureOf [Feature GeneralisedProcess GeneralisedSubstance]
	     hasQuantity (Quantity which <
	         hasMagnitude PrimitiveValueType
	         hasUnit Unit >)
	     isGoalOf TherapeuticAct >.

visual symptom	Vision which <
	     hasAbnormalityStatus nonNormal
	     hasPersonReporting Patient >.

cataract	(OcularLens which
	     hasOpacity (Opacity which
	         hasAbsoluteState opaque)) name Cataract.

visual acuity	(Vision which isActedOnSpecificallyBy Glasses) name VisualAcuity.

by the ApplicationAttribute, designed conceptually, and arranged semantically thus permitting navigation.

(DrugPreparation which isMadeOf Drug)
extr. <u>hasBrandName</u> DrugBrandName;
extr. <u>hasGenericName</u> DrugGenericName.

Fig. 2   Application attributes (underlined) and their usage.
Extr. - extrinsically.

4.   Application

The application will adopt the medical record architecture developed by the German MED-WIS-project DIADOQ which implements a procedure-based and problem-oriented approach to the EPR [7]. The application will enable structured data entry for current patient data. It will also record the measures together with their results and medical reasons of examinations and therapies. In its content the application like the diabetes model is based on the DIABCARD dataset version 2.0.

Starting point and presently focus of the application is the German Diabetes Passport (fig. 3, center; adapted from the German by the authors). Edited by the *Deutsche Diabetes-Gesellschaft (DDG)* the Diabetes Passport contains the measures internationally recognised as minimally necessary to prevent diabetic complications. It aims to achieve the goals of the St. Vincent Declaration. The Diabetes Passport presents a miniature EPR ideally suited to demonstrate the benefits of the GALEN technologies.

The application allows to enter clinical data of the Diabetes Passport right away. These data are values for therapeutical goals and actual values of several clinical parameters used to monitor diabetics. For the laboratory parameters the user can choose a unit from a list of adequate units (fig. 3, left). Explanations can be displayed for the clinical parameters and how these are measured. Further dialogues enable the user to enter detailed medical data (fig. 3, right) to be stored in the patient's overall medical record. A summary of these detailed data is transferred to the corresponding input field of the Diabetes Passport. Additional functionality is offered: The entered actual values are compared with the corresponding normal range and the given therapeutic goal. The therapeutic goal in some cases is preset with a value, usually the upper limit of the normal range. The present application as outlined with e.g. normal ranges and unit selection (fig. 3) is supported by the present diabetes model (3.2).

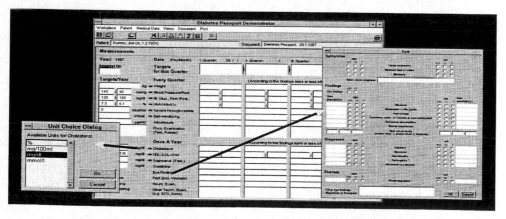

Fig. 3 Aspects of the Application: Diabetes Passport, unit selection and detailed input of eye findings

5.   Discussion and Conclusion

The modelling activity has extended the terminological model to support a data entry system for diabetic management. About 2000 elementary and complex concepts and 20 attributes are added by the diabetes model. These are covering general and specialised medical knowledge. Numerous constraints added allow to automatically generate many further sensible composites. Considering the kind of modelled knowledge, the potentially generated concepts, and the clean taxonomies of the structured knowledge, we feel that our terminological diabetes model will be useful for other medical applications - general and diabetological.

Modelling in GRAIL is demanding, because representing terminological knowledge has to be precise and unambiguous. The difficulty of modelling terms depends on the regularity of the necessary structures and atoms, the coverage of the existing model, and the length of the items. Exquisite concepts are considerably more difficult to represent than common concepts. Modelling according to established conventions whenever possible is convenient and produces a regularly structured model more easily projected to the application.

Some information has been deliberately included in addition to the medical knowledge of the data source. It is intended to complete corners of the preexisting model or the represented medical context. Terms denoting two or more concepts are frequently modelled in every possible form. Concepts are frequently presented in two alternative nominalisations. Metalanguage like „other" residual in the data source is referred to the application to be dealt with there.

The verified diabetes model will be quality checked according to various criteria: modelling structure; central reconciliation; verification against the application; clinical correctness of the information presented in the user interface; subjective satisfaction of the user; intuitive interaction with the application; reusability.

The system currently implemented as an offline version reflects the present diabetes model. It thus does not automatically adapt to changes in the model, which is a future aim. Further technical implementations to be realised in the near future are the application programming interface and filter of the EPR. As these technical features progress, the diabetes model will be modified according to the needs of the technical implementation. The application will be extended to cover all of the medical knowledge included in the DIABCARD dataset. It is furthermore planned to integrate technologies for speech recognition, report generation, and clinical guidelines.

6.   References

[1] van Ginnecken AM. The structure of data in medical records. Yearbook of Medical Informatics. Stuttgart. 61 - 70. 1995.
[2] Moorman PW, van Ginnecken AM, Siersema PD, van der Lei J, van Bemmel JH. Evaluation of reporting based on descriptional knowledge. Yearbook of Medical Informatics. Stuttgart. 199 - 207. 1996.
[3] Rector AL, Solomon WD, Nowlan WA, Rush TW. A Terminology Server for medical language and medical information systems. Proceedings of IMIA WG6. Geneva. 1 - 16. May 1994.
[4] Rector AL, Gangemi A, Galeazzi E, Glowinski AJ, Rossi-Mori A. The GALEN CORE Model schemata for anatomy: Towards a re-usable application-independent model of medical concepts. Proceedings of Medical Informatics Europe. Lisbon. 186 - 189. 1994.
[5] Engelbrecht R, Hildebrand C, Blecher M. Improving patient care by the use of smart cards. Proceedings of AMICE 95. Amsterdam. 227 - 233. 1995.
[6] Solomon D, Toft C. The GRAIL KnoME. GALEN Documentation, July 1996.
[7] Böhm V, Moser W, Diedrich T, et al. A computer-based patient record system for diabetes outpatient clinics - the conceptual model and its implementation. In: The future of health information management. Eds. Hoffmann U, et al. Munich: MMV. 27 - 33. 1996.

Medical Informatics Europe '97
C. Pappas et al. (Eds.)
IOS Press, 1997

Integration of a Knowledge-based System and a Clinical Documentation System via a Data Dictionary

H.-P. Eich, C. Ohmann, E. Keim, K. Lang

Theoretical Surgery Unit, Department of General and Trauma Surgery,
Heinrich – Heine - University, Düsseldorf, Germany,
[eich, ohmannch]@uni-duesseldorf.de

Abstract. This paper describes the design and realisation of a knowledge-based system and a clinical documentation system linked via a data dictionary. The software was developed as a shell with object oriented methods and C++ for IBM-compatible PC's and WINDOWS 3.1 / 95. The data dictionary covers terminology and document objects with relations to external classifications. It controls the terminology in the documentation program with form-based entry of clinical documents and in the knowledge-based system with scores and rules. The software was applied to the clinical field of acute abdominal pain by implementing a data dictionary with 580 terminology objects, 501 document objects, and 2136 links; a documentation module with 8 clinical documents and a knowledge–based system with 10 scores and 7 sets of rules.

1. Introduction

Computer-aided decision-support has rarely been introduced into clinical routine. The existing programs are not user-friendly and often there is no linkage between clinical documentation and knowledge base.

The data dictionary approach is used to guarantee the consistency of clinical and terminological data. This has become a standard to documentation in clinical routine, but not to knowledge-based systems (hereafter referred to as KBS). However, a data dictionary is necessary for the integration of clinical documentation and KBS [1]. KBS are often island systems which can only be linked to a clinic-wide documentation system, if both systems use the same vocabulary. One of the most positive effects of such a linkage is the on-line application of the KBS directly to clinical data.

In this paper we describe design and realisation of a KBS and a clinical documentation system linked via a data dictionary. The system is exemplarily applied to the diagnosis of acute abdominal pain.

2. System description

The aim of our project was to develop a documentation program and diagnostic support module for acute abdominal pain. We used object-oriented analysis, design and programming methods corresponding to the notation of Coad & Yourdon [2,3]. The program modules were developed with Borland C++ and Borland Database Engine under WINDOWS 3.1 and WINDOWS 95 on an IBM-compatible PC. The whole KBS [4] consists of three sub-modules: a data dictionary, a KBS and a documentation program (Fig. 1).

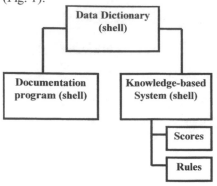

Fig. 1 : Informatical Conception

The data dictionary is a controlled vocabulary by which the integration of a knowledge base and documentation component can be achieved. In our approach it contains terminology objects and document objects, a difference which is not made in the majority of existing systems [1]. On the one hand we have definite clinical terms which meanings do not change, and on the other hand we have clinical parameters which can differ in the way they are measured. Terminology objects are described by their ID, name, definition, by internal relations to other terminology objects and by links to external classifications (e.g. SNOMED). We use five internal relations ("is a", "is part of", "is equivalent to", "is associated with", "is located in") to build up a semantic network. Document objects are terms which are usually used for clinical documentation. These objects are medical terms, possible answers, sub-documents or documents. Each document object is described by its ID, name and definition. In addition to that, a clinical parameter is described by its type, scale and unit. Each document object is linked to a terminology object. The data dictionary is developed as a shell. This conception gives the opportunity to handle terminological knowledge from different medical fields only by changing the data base. The user can easily enter new terminology and document objects.

Our documentation program is designed to collect clinical data. We use a form-based data-entry for each document (e.g. history). To reach a high acceptance rate the documentation was designed in collaboration with physicians of our surgery unit. With this documentation program we have carried out several prospective evaluation studies, in which our aim was to build up a quality-controlled prospective database on which knowledge-based methods can be applied.

The third component of our system is the KBS. It is used for diagnostic support. We have integrated rule-based systems which consists of automatically generated rules from prospective databases and diagnostic scores. Different knowledge acquisition techniques were evaluated [5]. Sets of rules in the clinical field of acute abdominal pain were generated with inductive rule-generating algorithms such as CN2 [6] and C4.5 [7]. Set of rules have a simple structure which gives the physician an inside-view why a specific diagnosis is preferred by the system. Also, different scoring-systems [8] were analysed concerning their structure and way of application. Each set of rules or score is integrated as one knowledge module. This module can be applied to patient data or the user can see its definition. The application of knowledge modules is controlled by the KBS. The user can set a filter with several criteria to find an appropriate module to his problem. These criteria are clinical problem (e.g. diagnosis, prognosis, treatment), specification (e.g. appendicitis), population (e.g. acute abdominal pain, suspected appendicitis) and method (e.g. scores, set of rules). The KBS has its own graphical human interface and can be used as a stand-alone system.

To establish such a system two forms of integration have to be taken into consideration: the terminological integration and the functional integration. The terminological integration can be achieved by the data dictionary. It guarantees that both documentation and KBS use the same vocabulary. Both components handle only IDs of clinical parameters, possible values or documents. For a functional integration the documentation component has to be extended with a trigger function which executes the KBS. Also data-entry or report modules should be adapted to achieve a user-friendly graphical human interface.

The interaction of the components and flow of information is shown in figure 2. The documentation component gets information about IDs of parameters, values and documents from the data dictionary (i). If the physician wants decision support, he calls the KBS (ii) from documentation. By this call information about the current patient (e.g. ID, sex, existing documents and duration of hospital stay) is given to the KBS. The KBS is responsible for selection and display of different knowledge modules. Information how to display terminology comes form the data dictionary, too (i). If the user has selected a specific knowledge module that should be executed, the KBS has information about which parameters are needed and requests their values from the database interface (iii). The KBS has a read-only access to the database.

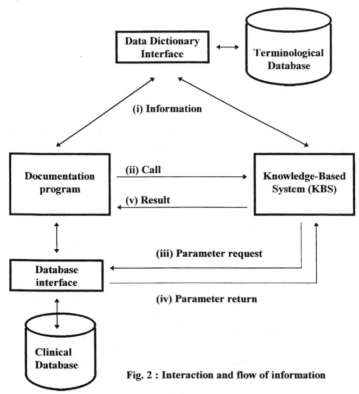

Fig. 2 : Interaction and flow of information

The database interface returns all found parameter values to the KBS (iv). The selected score or set of rules is then executed. The decision support result is sent back from the KBS to documentation (v) where it is displayed to the user. If a result should be stored to patient data, this can be done in the documentation module.

3. Results

According to the methods presented above a data dictionary for the clinical field of acute abdominal pain was created. It consists of 580 terminology objects and 501 document objects. Between these objects 2136 different links were established. Also the interface to KBS and documentation program was developed.

So far, ten diagnostic scores were integrated in the KBS. For the integration of scoring-systems a score description module was developed which allows the definition of a score with an arbitrary structure and the storage to our relational database. The parameters of the score have to be selected from the data dictionary to guarantee a correct application to clinical data. Furthermore, seven sets of rules were generated with C4.5 and integrated in the KBS. The rules were developed from an European database for acute abdominal pain. One of these sets of rules has 13 different diagnostic outcomes. The other sets have two diagnostic outcomes to strengthen or to exclude a specific diagnosis found by the first set.

Eight different documents were integrated in the documentation program so far. These are documents for history, clinical investigation, laboratory investigation, ultrasound, x-ray examination, operation, diagnosis and discharge. To store this data a database interface was programmed.

Figure 3 shows a screen shot of our KBS for acute abdominal pain. In the foreground the KBS with a set of rules is presented. The user has specified his problem, specification, population and method. The KBS found one set of rules of which two rules are displayed in the middle of the screen. In the background the documentation program with a form-based entry for the history of acute abdominal pain is presented.

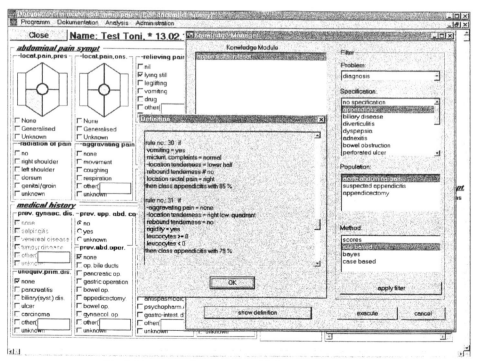

Fig. 3: Documentation program with knowledge manager

4. Discussion

The results above show that an integration of a clinical documentation system and a KBS can be established, if terminological and functional integration is achieved via a data dictionary.

Under consideration is now the linkage of KBS to a commercial clinical information system. In this case the terminological data has to be mapped with data from the information system. The whole process of mapping terminology should be done by a meta-data dictionary. The data dictionary used by the KBS is left untouched not to violate the integrity of the knowledge base. If no data dictionary is present on side of the clinical information system the correct terms with its IDs have to be identified directly out of documentation. For functional integration a trigger is needed to execute the KBS.

5. Acknowledgements

The work was supported by grant of the German Ministry of Education, Science, Research and Technology (MEDWIS – program, project A 70).

6. References

[1] R. Linnarson and O. Wigartz, The data dictionary - a controlled vocabulary for integrating clinical databases and medical knowledge bases, *Methods of Information in Medicine* **28** (1989) 78-85.
[2] P. Coad and E. Yourdon, Object-oriented analysis and object-oriented design. Yourdan Press, Englewood Cliffs, 1991.
[3] P. Coad et al., Object models, strategies, patterns applications. Yourdan Press, Englewood Cliffs, 1995.
[4] C. Ohmann et al., Expertensystem zur Unterstützung von Diagnosestellung und Therapiewahl bei akuten Bauchschmerzen. *Informatik, Biometrie und Epidemiologie* **26** (1995) 262-274.
[5] C. Ohmann et al., Evaluation of automatic knowledge acquisition techniques in the diagnosis of acute abdominal pain. *Artificial Intelligence in Medicine* **8** (1996) 23-26.
[6] The Turing Institute, CN2 Software Systems, George House, 36 North Hanover St., Glasgow G1 2AD, UK, 1993.
[7] J. R. Quinlan, C4.5 Programs for Machine Learning. Morgan Kaufmann, San Mateo, CA, 1993.
[8] C. Ohmann et al., Diagnostic scores for acute appendicitis, *Eur. J. Surg.* **161** (1995) 273-281.

Medical Informatics Europe '97
C. Pappas et al. (Eds.)
IOS Press, 1997

A second generation of terminological systems is coming

Angelo Rossi Mori, Fabrizio Consorti, Elena Galeazzi, Paolo Merialdo

Reparto Informatica Medica, ITBM-CNR, Roma
IV Clinica Chirurgica, Università La Sapienza, Roma
Dottorato in Informatica Medica, Università La Sapienza, Roma

Diverse achievements by recent computer-based terminological systems are outlining a new generation of systems (ie. a "second generation"). We collected the relevant features of various advanced terminological systems and we systematized these features into four components of a unique framework. We review a set of systems according to our framework, and we discuss how standardization activities can support the evolution of computer-based terminological systems towards a complete set of new performances.

1. Introduction

Advanced terminological systems — adapted or conceived for computer use — are coming. Designers of coding systems are independently enhancing their tools by a mix of new features that introduce computer-based processing of semantics; healthcare professionals will benefit of powerful interfaces to represent details on patients by flexible nomenclatures and to browse one or more nomenclatures according to multiple viewpoints.

For example, the module on surgical procedures of the Read Thesaurus (version 3 of Read Codes) adopted a compositional approach, based on a "formal frame of semantically defined attributes" [9], ie. a refinement of a standard structure [5]. All 16800 surgical procedures are systematically mapped to 1250 anatomical concepts; other "atomic" hierarchies are being developed and mapped; all the hierarchies are explicit and mutually aligned. Analogously, for laboratory results in LOINC [18], the terminological phrases are presented in a database, structured in "segments" and "subsegments" [19] that may correspond to a refinement of a standard structure [6]. An enhanced database was further produced according to a well-defined "template structure" [8] to allow direct processing of "atomic" concepts.

In a recent paper [12] we claimed that achievements by recent computer-based terminological systems are outlining a new generation of systems (ie. a **second generation**). We developed a comprehensive framework to describe terminological systems; in this paper we apply our framework to a set of systems, we show which advanced features they present, and we discuss how standards could assist their evolution.

2. Second generation: computer-based compositional systems

A set of computer-based terminological systems already in use or in a final development phase shows particular features that distinguish them from conventional paper-based systems. These systems were developed independently each other, and they have all a compositional approach and various other features, that envisage the establishment of a new generation of terminological systems; in order to describe them (see § 3), we first have to establish criteria and a vocabulary for that description.

2.1. The four components of a second-generation system

In our view, a second-generation system is made of four interdependent components [12]:

1. a *categorial structure* describes semantic categories, semantic links and most relevant structural patterns [2]; an interim release can be produced by a modest amount of resources in a short time; it can be the topic for a standard;

2. a *cross-thesaurus* organises a set of descriptors according to categories in 1.; it requires initially a modest amount of resources to work out most descriptors (for an example, see

[7]); complete development is complex as a standardization initiative, but results produced elsewhere may be included in a standard;

3. a family of structured *sub-systems of phrases* (various lists of classes, of real terminological phrases, ...); it requires continuous maintenance and local adaptations; it is not suitable for standardization bodies (except for ancillary sub-systems, as a "reference taxonomy", a "reference classification" and a "reference nomenclature");

4. a *knowledge base of "dissections"* (ie. where each phrase of 3. is represented by descriptors from the cross-thesaurus 2., according to a structural pattern from 1.). The production of the knowledge base has to rely on independent initiatives [eg. 3, 25], from sponsors external to the standardization environment.

Cross-thesaurus and knowledge base should not be intended as a new coding system or terminology, but as tools to produce, validate and exploit the family of sub-system in 3. .

The components of a second-generation system are developed by an iterative process of refinement, up to an adequate level of complexity and robustness.

2.2. Presentation and use of the second-generation systems

New terminological systems, conceived for computer use, process explicit details and are mappable one to the other by comparing dissections (if based on the same cross-thesaurus).

By appropriate design, diverse functionalities (previously typical of isolated classifications or nomenclatures) can thrive on the same background, ie. various lists of different granularity and flexibility can originate from a given categorial structure and cross-thesaurus.

Typically complexity and evolution rate preclude presentation on paper.

- *presentation:* categorial structure + cross-thesaurus + lists + knowledge base of dissections
- *organisation:* dynamic (multiple, hierarchical)
- *purposes:* multiple
- *flexibility and extension:* new atoms can be added by users, new combinations can be made by users
- *processing on semantics, using categorial structure and dissections:* cluster phrases according to criteria; extend a list in structured way; extract and arrange details; suggest details in structured input interfaces,...

---

3. Analysis of some existing systems

In table 1 we analyse a set of terminological systems according to the above framework; note that they are not academic experiments, but systems intended for practical use in real world.

The table and the following comments should not be intended as a *criticism* on the adequacy of individual systems for their tasks: we want to *demonstrate* that advanced features are present in a relevant number of actual systems; our intent is also to show that enhancements are within reach, by adding functionalities to existing systems at a relatively low cost.

Table 1. Presence of components of second-generation systems in some existing terminological systems

system	subject field	component			
		categorial structure	cross-thesaurus	family of lists	KB of dissections
LOINC-LAB [18]	laboratory properties	XXX	XX	XX	XXX
IUPAC-NPU [20]	laboratory properties	XX	XX	XX	XXX
DICOM-SDM [21]	structured reports on imaging	XX	XXX	-	-
MCTGE [22]	observations in digestive endoscopy	XX	XXX	XX	XX
SNOMED Int'l [1]	disease module	X	XX	XX	XX
RCC [13, 9]	module on surgical procedures	XXX	XX	XXX	XX
ICD-10-PCS [23]	surgical procedures	X	X	XX	XXX
ICNP [10]	nursing phenomena and interventions	XX	XX	XX	XX
CEN PT2-015 [7]	medical devices	XXX	XX	-	-
ECRI-UMDNS [11]	medical devices	X	X	XX	-

LOINC-LAB provides a clear categorial structure, but it does not distribute a cross-thesaurus, even if many collections of "answers" (valid concepts admitted for a field) are embedded in the database; only one list is provided (on lab results) even if the compositional approach allows to prepare and distribute a set of coherent lists (eg. on lab orders).

IUPAC-NPU provides extensive lists of descriptors (also according to external authoritative sources) and rules for systematic names according to a categorial structure, but does not provide an explicit list of allowed modifiers and the related structural patterns.

DICOM-SDM (SNOMED DICOM Microglossary) is a detailed cross-thesaurus built on SNOMED International and extending it with the necessary atomic descriptors, clustered by category. Categories are very detailed (eg. <radiographic contrast agent>, <body position with respect to gravity>) and correspond to the items of the DICOM messages. But a comprehensive model with the relations between categories is still implicit; the user has a complete freedom/responsibility of combining the atoms, because reference lists with most relevant (composite) terminological phrases for each major task is not provided.

The Minimum Common Terminology for Gastrointestinal Endoscopy (MCTGE) was developed by the European Society for Gastrointestinal Endoscopy (ESGE) and OMED from the extensive Maratka Terminology. It provides a simple mechanism for the controlled generation of detailed terminological phrases, ie. the list is presented as a set of structural patterns plus constraints on the allowed (pre-defined) values.

The disease module of SNOMED International provides for most entries a "references" field with a set of descriptors (as pointers to more atomic modules); unfortunately links among descriptors are not (yet) explicit and dissections are not systematized; categorial structure and structural patterns are implicit. SNOMED International (including the G-module of general modifiers) can be considered as a promising precursor for a universal cross-thesaurus, although atoms within each module are not yet separated from composite concepts.

The surgical procedure module of the Read Thesaurus is becoming perhaps the first example of a second-generation system; at the moment, only the anatomical hierarchy is completely mapped and synchronized with the surgical hierarchy, but work is in progress.

Surgical procedures in ICD-10-PCS have a fixed structural pattern, that creates a strong constraint on expressiveness; the related cross-thesaurus is limited, also in depth. It is a powerful structured *classification*, but intrinsic limitations decided in the design of the system (as it is now) cannot support a detailed *nomenclature* for routine use in the patient record.

The alpha version of ICNP is based on ontological work, but the categorial structure is not completely explicit. The cross-thesaurus was produced only for a part of the system. Together with existing systems on nursing, it is a concrete example of interlingua for the systematic mapping across systems. An initial knowledge base with dissections from existing systems (using ICNP as cross-thesaurus) is distributed.

The extensive experience of ECRI in developing their UMDNS on medical devices produced internal skills and guidelines on systematic construction of terminological phrases and selection of atomic terms. The list, robust and cross-referenced, is already used for multiple purposes. UMDNS could be enhanced using the CEN Prestandard to perform a systematic revision and producing the Knowledge Base of dissections. Repeating the analysis for other existing systems and refining the cross-thesaurus, this domain could be perhaps the first concrete application of the CEN approach to the integration of different systems.

4. Discussion

The "universal solution" (ie. a unique huge all-purpose nomenclature) seems impossible and inadequate. Expressive needs of healthcare professionals require the extreme flexibility of natural language, to represent unpredictable details; to achieve a well-accepted practical compromise, expressiveness of terminological systems has to be very high.

4.1. Coexistence of terminological systems and re-use of data

Management of semantics by second-generation systems allows mapping, conversion, rearrangement of details between first-generation coding systems.

It can accomodate for coexistence and integration of multiple coherent systems on the same subject field in the same information system (including local vocabularies, coherent lists of classes and terminological phrases for particular purposes).

Multiple uses of the same data are possible; in particular, appropriate recognition and conversion of relevant details — *scattered in various fields of a database or in segments of a message* — allow to construct ad hoc terminological phrases with appropriate details for any given task (eg. according to various reference classifications and nomenclatures).

These features will be amplified in formal systems (eg. GALEN [3]) that are able to exploit dynamically a concept model (by an appropriate formalism and a software engine).

4.2. Role of standards in the development process

Diffusion of computer applications and increase of electronic communication in healthcare is calling urgently for specific standards [14]. The process of standardization on terminology is far behind the needs. Many initiatives are comparing existing terminological systems and promoting their integration [15, 16, 17].

CEN/TC251/WG2[1] [26] anticipated the movement that is influencing the evolution of various terminological systems, with the production of a set of standards [2, 5, 6, 7] aiming at facilitating their gradual and *spontaneous* convergence. In the *medium term*, standard categorial structures and cross-thesauri on individual topics can be used in many ways:

1. to upgrade individual systems;
2. to support spontaneous convergence and systematic development of terminological systems about that topic;
3. to support convergence across subject fields;
4. more in general, to clarify expectations about the content of a coding system in the design of information systems. In fact, categorial structures allow the integration of concept systems within patient record and data interchange messages, by matching the items of terminological systems with the items in the information model.

In the *long term*, the categorial structures on the different (overlapping) topics should be harmonized on a deep ontological basis, and an integrated cross-thesaurus should be produced. Individual categorial structures will be made coherent by referring to a unique metastructure, facilitating also the development of "universal" formal models of third generation. The ultimate goal is the cooperative development of a standard on this *"shared ontology"* for healthcare [24], and thus of an integrated (universal) system of concepts.

5. Conclusions

Categorial structures are a powerful tool to synthetically describe the content of large concept systems, to allow their comparison and to facilitate future convergence by a more systematic design, even independently from computer-based applications.

Diversity of terminological systems is needed to satisfy a wide range of needs, but unnecessary diversity — ambiguities, inconsistencies, incompleteness — should be avoided.

Higher performances of terminological systems (eg. on expressiveness, granularity, flexibility, structure-driven processing) require more complexity and more resources during the utilization of the systems, but also in development of terminological systems and development of applications. Simpler and more economic solutions (ie. requiring more elementary software but providing limited functionalities) should co-exist with more complex and complete solutions; also during development, second- and third-generation systems could be used to prepare and distribute respectively first- and second-generation systems.

---

[1] ie. the Working Group 2 on "Terminology, semantics and knowledge bases" of the Technical Committee TC251 on "Medical Informatics" of CEN, the European Committee for Standardization

It is important to understand the potentialities and the limitations of each class of systems, in order to apply them in the most adequate contexts. Awareness of limitations and description of potentialities allows to adapt expectations and to evaluate adequacy to a particular task.

Acknowledgements. Work partially supported by contract HC1018 "GALEN-IN-USE" from European Union. The paper presents the view of the Authors, and should not be intended as official position of TC251/WG2.

6.   References

1   Rothwell DJ, Coté RA, Brochu L (eds), *SNOMED International*, Northfield, IL: College of American Pathologists, 1993, 3rd ed.; *see also* http://dumccss.mc.duke.edu/standards/termcode/snomed.htm

2   CEN ENV 12264:1995. Medical Informatics — Categorial structure of systems of concepts — Model for representation of semantics. Brussels: CEN, 1995

3   GALEN and GALEN-IN-USE documentation, available from the main contractor AL Rector, Medical Informatics Group, Dept. Computer Science, Univ. Manchester, Manchester M13 9 PL, UK (e-mail galen@cs.ac.man.uk; *see also home page at* http://www.cs.man.ac.uk/mig/galen)

4   Campbell K, Musen MA. Representation of clinical data using Snomed III and conceptual graphs. In: *Proceedings of the 16th Symposium Computer Applications in Medical Care.* November 1992 pp 354-8

5   CEN ENV 1828:1995. Health care informatics — Structure for classification and coding of surgical procedures. Brussels: CEN, 1995

6   CEN ENV 1614:1994. Health care informatics — System of concepts for systematic names, classification, and coding for properties, including quantities, in laboratory medicine. Brussels: CEN, 1994

7   CEN/TC251/PT2-015. Medical informatics — Categorial structure of systems of concepts — Medical devices (First Working Document). Brussels: CEN, 1995

8   Rocha RA, Stanley MH. Coupling Vocabularies and Data Structures: Lesson from LOINC. JAMIA 1996;symp. suppl.:90-94

9   Price C, et al. Anatomical Characterization of Surgical Procedures in the Read Thesaurus. JAMIA 1996;symp. suppl.:110-114; *see* http://dumccss.mc.duke.edu/standards/termcode/read.htm

10   Mortensen RA (ed). The International Classification for Nursing Practice ICNP with TELENURSE introduction. Copenhagen: The Danish Institute for Health and Nursing Research, 1996

11   ECRI, Universal medical device nomenclature system: product category thesaurus. Plymouth Meeting (PA): ECRI, 1996; *see* http://dumccss.mc.duke.edu/standards/termcode/ecri.htm

12   Rossi Mori A. Towards a new generation of terminologies and coding systems. In: Brender J et al, eds. *Medical Informatics Europe '96.* Amsterdam: IOS Press, 1996: 208-212

13   NHS Centre for Coding and Classification, The Read Codes Version 3. NHS-CCC-TP1200, July 1994

14   Board of Directors of the AMIA. Standards for medical identifiers, codes, and messages needed to create an efficient computer-stored medical record, JAMIA 1994;1,1-7

15   Chute CG, et al. The content coverage of clinical classifications. JAMIA 1996; 3:224-233

16   Shortliffe EH, et al. Collaborative Medical Informatics Research Using the Internet and the World Wide Web. JAMIA, 1996;symp. suppl.:125-129

17   UMLS: *see* http://dumccss.mc.duke.edu/standards/termcode/umls.htm

18   LOINC: *see* http://dumccss.mc.duke.edu/standards/termcode/loinc.htm

19   LOINC Manual, available at http://dumccss.mc.duke.edu/standards/termcode/loinclab/LOINMAN1.DOC

20   IUPAC: *see* http://dumccss.mc.duke.edu/standards/termcode/iupac.htm

21   DICOM: *for the standard in general see* http://www.xray.hmc.psu.edu/dicom/dicom_home.html or http://dumccss.mc.duke.edu/standards/HL7/sigs/image-management/HTML/dicom-home.html; *on SDM, see* http://dumccss.mc.duke.edu/standards/HL7/sigs/image-management/SNOMED/sdm101.html

22   ESGE/ASGE Minimum Common Terminology for Gastrointestinal Endoscopy (MCTGE): *see* http://www.hsc.missouri.edu/ASGE/docs/asge.html

23   Averill RA, Mullin RL, Steinbeck BA, Goldfield NI, Grant T (1995). *The development of the ICD-10 Procedure Coding System (ICD-10-PCS).* available from: 3M Health Information Systems, 100 Barnes Road, Wallingford CT 06492.

24   Steve G, Gangemi A. ONIONS Methodology and the Ontological Commitment of Medical Ontology ON8.5. Presented at KAW 96; *see* http://saussure.irmkant.rm.cnr.it/KAW/introduction.html

25   Galeazzi E, Rossi Mori A, Consorti F, Errera A. A cooperative methodology to build conceptual models in medicine (submitted to MIE 97)

26   CEN/TC251/WG2: *see* http://miginfo.rug.ac.be:8001/centc251/prestand/wg2/wg2.htm

Medical Informatics Europe '97
C. Pappas et al. (Eds.)
IOS Press, 1997

Using the GRAIL Language for Classification Management

P.E. Zanstra[1], E.J. van der Haring[1] , F. Flier[2], J.E. Rogers[3] , W.D. Solomon[3]

[1]*Dept. Medical Informatics, Epidemiology and Statistics, University of Nijmegen, NL*
[2]*WCC, National Centre for Medical Terminology, Zoetermeer, NL*
[3]*Medical Informatics Group; University of Manchester UK*
http://www.ehm.kun.nl/mi/galen or email:Galen@mie.kun.nl

Abstract. This paper describes a novel approach in classification management where a formal model of medical semantics is being used for manipulations on existing classification systems. The paper addresses the issue of semi-automatically making specialist classifications that are compatible with the source classification. The examples in this paper are from a limited domain. At the time of the presentation results will be shown of the present modelling work within the GALEN-In-Use project. The model will then contain several thousands of medical procedures from four different classification centres.

1. Introduction

In medicine, standard classifications, such as ICD and ICPM, are typically intended for a wide range of users and settings. Consequently they are not adapted to the needs of any particular user or the circumstances of any particular setting. To make standard classifications more attractive to users, they often have to be adapted in some way. Adaptation may involve selection of relevant classes, refinement of the classification by adding relevant subclasses, and rearrangement of classes in a more appealing order. Rearrangement, in particular, has to be done with care, to avoid breaching the compatibility with the standard classification. To date, production of compatible adaptations is mainly done manually, by means of a word processor, which can be a very time-consuming and thus costly task. The last version of ICD has taken 15 years to come to deployment. The translation and local adaptation takes an additional number of years, and a lot of effort. Consequently new ways are being sought to support this presently mainly manual craftsmanship.

Within the GALEN-In-Use-project a Classification Manager (ClaM) is being developed to assist Classification centres with their task of producing compatible adaptations and reliable conversions between different classifications. In addition the ClaM will support the translation of classifications.

In the third year of the GALEN-In-Use project a major validation of this approach will take place by nine Classification Centres in nine different countries

2. The Core Reference Model

GALEN aims to build a compositional generative model for medical terminology. This model comprises a well defined ontology of atomic medical entities with rules to combine these entities such that all and only sensible medical expressions can be generated. This means that with a relatively small model in principle billions of medically sensible expressions about patients can be made. Ultimately it is the intention that GALEN covers all of medicine. The language in which this knowledge is represented is called GRAIL, the GALEN Representation And Integration Language. The model of this knowledge is called the Common Reference Model, or CRM for short. The present version of the CRM comprises some 7000 elementary entities with about 15000 links. It is expected that to cover a general layer of medicine some 25000 elementary entities are required. [1,2,3]

3. Classification Schemes

The ClaM stores a classification scheme in a hierarchy consisting of *classes*. Each class consists of a *code* and one or more rubrics. A rubric can be further specified by its *kind* (e.g. *preferred, includes, excludes*) and a *language* (e.g. *Dutch, English*). For example the ICD-10 class A18.61 could have the rubrics:
Dutch preferred "Tuberculeuze otitis media"
Dutch synonym "Tuberculeuze middenoorontsteking"
Dutch note "Not sure whether the Dutch synonym is OK"
English preferred "Tuberculosis of ear"

A class in one classification scheme can reference a class in another classification scheme. This can, for example, be used to link a class in an existing classification scheme to a specialist classification scheme. Similarly, a class in a classification scheme can reference a concept in the CRM. The latter references are called *mappings* to differentiate them from references between classes in classification schemes. Both *references* and *mappings* are specified by their *kind*, e.g. *isEquivalentTo, isBroaderThen*, etcetera.

The ClaM supports the following functionality:
- *Activities involving a single classification scheme*
  - de novo creation
  - creating, modifying, moving and/or deleting classes
- *Activities involving multiple classification schemes*
  - creating and maintaining relationships between different classification schemes and/or different versions of one classification scheme
  - copying classes from one classification scheme to another
- *Activities involving a classification scheme and the GALEN CRM*
  - mapping classes of a classification scheme to concepts in the CRM
  - making selections of existing classification schemes knowledge in the CRM
  - extending existing classification schemes using knowledge in the CRM
  - rearranging existing classification schemes using knowledge in the CRM

4. Operations on a Classification Scheme

Medical specialists have specific requirements for the terminologies they use. They find the existing systems mostly not sufficiently detailed, or having a lack of precision. They also do not want to be bothered by terminology outside their own field of specialty, at least they do not want all the high detail outside their own domain. Making specialist classifications is tedious and therefor expensive, as it mostly can not be performed solely on the basis of the classifications own structure, nor by simple string matching procedures. Experience at WCC has shown that such approaches yield only 60% of the target specialist classification scheme (5). The remaining parts arc gathered by hard work.

Below we will outline a number of operations that are performed using the CRM as a backbone for manipulations. The examples here are meant to be illustrative for the kind of operations that are possible with this formalism. In the presentation we will show real examples of manipulations on the classifications of medical procedures. At the time of this writing four classification centres are working on the analysis of those classifications.

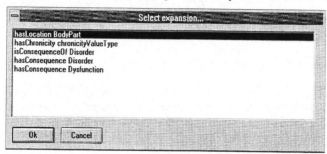

figure 1. The sensible statements for the refinement of the concept *Cellulitis of the external ear* (ICD-10) according to the GALEN CRM.

4.1 Refinement of a Classification Scheme

The ClaM can automatically create sub-classes for a class in a classification scheme based upon the concept in the CRM to which the class is mapped, and its sensible particularisation's in the CRM. For example suppose the class *H60.1 Cellulitis of the external ear* (ICD10) is mapped to the concept *(Cellulitis which < hasLocation ExternalEar >)* in the CRM. You can then select a statement from the list of sensible statements for the concept (figure 1) which will be used to create refined sub-classes for *H60.1*.

The entry *hasChronicity chronicityValueType* for example means that it is sensible for the concept *(Cellulitis which < hasLocation ExternalEar >)* to be refined using criteria of the form *hasChronicity chronicityValueType*. Upon selection of *hasChronicity chronicityValueType* the ClaM will generate the corresponding refinements e.g.,

- (Cellulitis which < hasLocation ExternalEar hasChronicity chronic >)
- (Cellulitis which < hasLocation ExternalEar hasChronicity acute >)
- (Cellulitis which < hasLocation ExternalEar hasChronicity subacute >)

In addition, the ClaM will generate subclasses below *H60.1 Cellulitis of the external ear* and map them to the new concepts. The rubrics of these new classes will be generated by the ClaM's natural language generator. This will result in these classes:

- H60.1.0 Chronic cellulitis of the external ear
- H60.1.1 Acute cellulitis of the external ear
- H60.1.2 Subacute cellulitis of the external ear

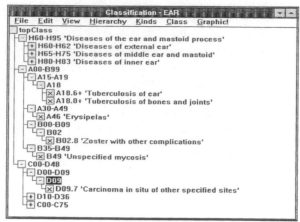

figure 2. En example of a selection from ICD10 based upon (Disorder which hasLocation ear). In the hierarchy an 'x' in the square box means this is a leaf node. Squares having a '+' mean that they have children underneath, which may be shown with a single click of the mouse on that box.

4.2 Selection from a Classification Scheme

The ClaM can select a number of classes from an existing classification scheme and copy them into a new classification scheme. An example of making a selection is to copy all the classes in the ICD10 that involve a disorder of the ear (figure 2) to a new classification. The ClaM collects all the descendants of e.g., *(Disorder which < hasLocation Ear >)* from the CRM, this will all be disorders that involve the ear or parts of the ear. Then the ClaM looks up all the classes in the source classification that map to any of these concepts. These classes and their ancestors will be copied to the target classification. The ClaM will also create the mappings between the classes in the new classification scheme and the CRM. You can modify the new classification as required, e.g., by adding or removing classes and rubrics.

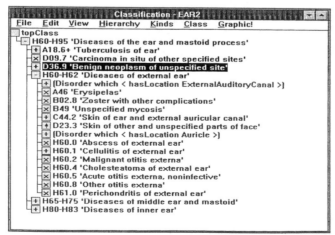

figure 3. An example of a re-arranged part of the ICD10 based upon the concept hierarchy below 'Disorder which hasLocation Ear'. Where there is no rubric in the original classification ClaM fills in the Grail concept (e.g.(Disorder which <hasLocation Auricle)). The next version will generate a natural language string for that GRAIL concept

4.3 ReArranging a Classification Scheme

This is similar to the previous operation, the main difference is that in *Selection from a classification scheme* the hierarchical structure of the original classification scheme is preserved in the new classification scheme. When the ClaM rearranges a classification scheme, the hierarchical structure of the new classification scheme reflects the structure in the CRM. For example, you could rearrange all the classes of the ICD10 that involve disorders of the ear. In ICD10 you will find such classes in several chapters. Again, the ClaM first collects all the descendants of *(Disorder which < hasLocation Ear >)*. The hierarchical structure of these concepts is copied to the new classification scheme. Then the ClaM looks up the classes in the source classification that map to these concepts, and copies their codes and rubrics to the new classification scheme.

In the example all the classes involving disorders of the ear from the ICD10 have been rearranged on the basis of the subsumption hierarchy in the CRM. Note that this is a multi-axial hierarchy. It contains a hierarchy by type of disorder (A18.6+; D09.7; D36.9) , and a hierarchy by topography (H60-H62; H65-H75; H80-H83).

5. Conclusions and Future Developments

The results given in this paper suggest that the GALEN CRM can be used for selection and refinement of specialist classification schemes. It must however be realised that the present CRM is only covering a small portion of medicine. Also there are only small sections of systems like ICD and SNOMED being mapped to the CRM. Therefor it is too early now to draw final conclusions. Present work on medical procedures in the GALEN-In-Use project should however give the answers of the usefulness of the GALEN approach for classification management purposes.

Future developments in the ClaM are that it will support the generation and analysis of natural language expressions. Natural language generation will take place in the present project period, analysis is pending on separate funding. Later this year the ClaM will be integrated with existing GRAIL based natural language generators. In the second quarter of 1997 we will assess the first results of language generation with the individual centres. By the end of 1997 natural language generation is planned for Dutch, English, Finnish, French, German, and Italian. This will allow the ClaM to automatically translate a classification scheme from one language into another.

6. References

1. Rector, A. (1994). Compositional models of medical concepts: towards re-usable application-independent medical terminologies. in Knowledge and Decisions in Health Telematics P. Barahona and J. Christensen (ed.). IOS Press. 133-142.

2. Rector, A., W. Solomon, W. Nowlan; T. Rush; W. Claassen; and P.E. Zanstra (1995). A Terminology Server for Medical Language and Medical Information Systems. Methods of Information in Medicine, Vol. 34, 147-157

3. Rector, A. and W.A. Nowlan (1993). The GALEN Representation and Integration Language (GRAIL) Kernel, Version 1. The GALEN Consortium for the EC AIM Programme. (Available from Medical Informatics Group, University of Manchester).

4. Anonymous (1995) Draft WCC Methodology for the development of specialist classifications.(in Dutch)

5. Anonymous(1993) Draft WCC standard classification on behalf of Ear, Nose and Throat Medicine, adaptation of the ICD-10 (in Dutch)

Medical Informatics Europe '97
C. Pappas et al. (Eds.)
IOS Press, 1997

Numerical Proposal for a Semiological Classification of Clinical Findings

Ramón BOOM-ANGLADA, Cesar COLINA, Antonio CERRITOS,
Cesar MONTEVERDE and Guzman TOLEDANO
School of Medicine, UNAM

Margaritas 312-25, 01030 México, D.F.

Abstract. The principal goal of this paper is to present a numerical classification of the characteristics of symptoms and signs. This classification begins with the ICD9 code and takes into account the semiological aspects of the already mentioned symptoms an signs, in such a way, that a digit represents, in cases of abdominal pain, site, another: radiating to, and the followings: aggravating, relieving factors, progresss, duration and type.
This way of representing data, with only a digit for each characteristic facilitates registration and elaboration of data bases, as well as, electronic data interchange.

Introduction

It has been a very difficult task to decide which clinical data will be classified and stored for future analysis in a patient record.

In spite of important progress made lately in hospital information systems, a universal agreement for this important point has not been reached.

Some authors prefer to mantain the traditional natural language in the medical record. When this occur, physicians use free-text to make their medical notes, and it is extremely difficult and cumbersome to extract useful clinical information from this material.

Others, use long and tedious questionaires. Aspects particularly important to make a differential diagnosis in a patient are completely irrelevant in another.

The process of selection of the relevant symptoms and signs, an their characteristics a particular patient, for decison making, is unconciously made by the medical expert.

Now, it is necessary to study this process and look for methods which will facilitate selection of the clinical material that will be saved.

Zvarova[1] proposed an intelligent approach with her "stochastic dependence for the constitution and reduction of data".

Besides, the material published by experts, about signs and symptoms, in different medical fields, using Bayes' theorem, discriminant and multivariate analysis, logical regression and fuzzy Sets to obtain a differential diagnosis must considerably help as an starting point.

The purpose of this paper is to facilitate the storage and transmission of medical data through a numerical designation and classification of clinical findings.

This numerical code classifies only relevant aspects of signs and symptoms and contributes to the necessary standarization, whenever two or more systems need to interchange data[2]

Material and Methods

As an starting point, we use the International Classification of Diseases (ICD 9) and will be using, in the near future the ICD 10.

The best way to explain the code system is through an example:

(ICD 9) for abdominal pain is 789.0 and we add another 0 to specify that we are dealing with and acute abdominal pain (less than one week duration).

789.00
Acute Abdominal Pain

1	2	3	4	5	6	7	8	9	0

1 SITE AT ONSET
  2 SITE AT PRESENT
    3 SITE AT PHYSICAL EXAMINATION
      4 RADIATING TO
        5 SEVERITY
          6 AGGRAVATING FACTORS
            7 RELIEVING FACTORS
              8 PROGRESS
                9 DURATION
                  0 TYPE

V.g. Patient with 36 hs of severe upper half pain at onset, actual pain in the right lower quadrant, radiating to the loin, aggravated by movement, colcky and getting worse would be.

789.00
5301210331

5	3	0	1	2	1	0	3	3	1
1	2	3	4	5	6	7	8	9	0
1 RUQ	1 RUQ	1 RUQ	1 *LOIN*	1 MOD	1 *MOV*	1 LYI	1 EQU	1 <12 h	1 *COL*
2 LUQ	2 LUQ	2 LUQ	2 GROI	2 *SEV*	2 COU	2 VOM	2 BET	2 12-24	2 HOU
3 RLQ	3 *RLQ*	3 RLQ	3 BUTT		3 BRE	3 ANT	3 *WOR*	3 *24-48*	3 DAY
4 LLQ	4 LLQ	4 LLQ	4 SHOU		4 GRE	4 FOO		4 >48 h	4 MON
5 *UPH*	5 UPH	5 UPH	5 ISCA		5 MIL	5 MIL		5 >1 W	5 CON
6 INH	6 INH	6 INH			6 ALC	6 ALC			
7 RH	7 RH	7 RH			7 BOW	7 BOW			
8 LH	8 LH	8 LH			8 SUP	8 THF			
9 CTR/G	9 CTR/G	9 CTR/G			9 STR	9 GAS			
0	0	0	0	0	0	0	0	0	0

RUQ=RIGHT UPPER QUADRANT; LUQ=LEFT UPPER QUADRANT; RLQ=RIGHT LOWER QUADRANT; LLQ=LEFT LOWER QUADRANT; UPH=UPPER HALF; INH=INFERIOR HALF; RH=RIGHT HALF; LH=LEFT HALF; CTR/G=CENTRAL OR GENERALIZED; LOIN=LOIN; GROI=GROIN; BUT=BUTTOCKS; SHO=SHOULDER; ISCA=INTERSCAPULOVERTEBRAL; MOD=MODERATE; SEV=SEVERE; MOV=MOVEMENT, COU=COUGHING; BRE=BREATHING; GRE=GREASY FOODS, MIL=MILK; ALC=ALCOHOL; BOW=BOWEL MOVEMENTS; SUP=SUPINE; STR=STRESS, THF=THORAX FLEXION; GAS=GAS EXPULSION, OTH=OTHER, EQU=EQUAL; BET=BETTER; WOR=WORSE; > 1 W MORE THAN A WEEK, COL=COLICKY PAIN, HOUR=RECURRENT LASTING HOURS, DAY=RECURRING LASTING DAYS, MON=RECURRENT LASTING MONTHS, CON= CONSTANT OR CONTINUOUS.

Results

We will present several cases to exemplify how to use the coding system
In cases of jaundice, the ICD 9 would be 782.4

782.4 JAUNDICE

```
1      2      3      4      5      6      7      8      9      0
1 PAIN (ACCOMPANIED BY)
     2 BILIARY COLIC ANTEC OR PRESENT
          3 FEVER OR RIGOR (ACCOMPANIED BY)
               4 ANOREXIA OR FLU LIKE (PRECEDING)
                    5 DYSPEPSIA ANTEC OR PRESENT
                         6 JAUNDICE PROGRESS
                              7 DURATION
                                   8 PRURITUS
                                        9 DARK URINE
                                             0 PALE STOOLS
```

V.g. Young female with light jaundice, 3 days duration, preceded by flu-like symptoms, light pain in upper abdomen, pruritus, dark urine and pale stools.

782.4
1001011111

1	0	0	1	0	1	1	1	1	1
1	2	3	4	5	6	7	8	9	0
1 *MOD*	1 BIL	1 FEV	1 *ANO*	1 DYS	1 *LIG*	1 <*IW*	1 *PRU*	1 *DAR*	1 *PALE STOOLS*
2 SEV		2 RIG			2 AUG	2 <IM			
		3 FE/RI			3 FLU	3 <IY			
						4 >IY			

0	0	0	0	0	0	0	0	0	0

MOD=MODERATE, SEV=SEVERE, BIL=BILIARY COLIC, FEV=FEVER, RIG=RIGORS, FE/RI=FEV AND RIGORS, ANO=ANOREXIA OF FLU-LIKE SYMPTOMS, DYS=DYSPEPSIA, LIG=LIGHT, AUG=AUGMENTING, FLU=FLUCTUATING, > 1W=LESS THAN ONE WEEK DURATION, LESS THAN 1 MONTH, LESS THAN 1 YEAR, > 1Y=MORE THAN 1 YEAR, PRU=PRURITUS, DAR=DARK URINE, PAL=PALE STOOLS.

UPPER G-1 BLEEDING
772.4

```
1      2      3      4      5      6      7      8      9      0
1 PAIN (ACCOMPANIED BY)
     2 DRUGS (PRECEDING)
          3 SHOCK (ACCOMPANIED BY)
               4 COMORBID DISEASE (ACCOMPANIED BY)
                    5 VOMITING (PRECEDING)
                         6 PROCESS
                              7 DURATION
                                   8 HEMATEMESIS
                                        9 MELENA
                                             0 DEHYDR
```

V.g. Patient with upper g-i bleeding of 12 hs duration, hematemessis (coffee ground) and melena, getting worse, without pain. The last 48 hs ingested 4 tablets of aspirin. He is Known of having Diabetes Mellitus

772.4
0100031210

0	1	0	0	0	3	1	2	1	0
1	2	3	4	5	6	7	8	9	0
1 MOD	1 *DRU*	1 SHO	1 CIR	1 VOM	1 EQU	1 *<12 h*	1 FRE	1 *MEL*	1 DEH
2 SEV	2 ALC		2 DM		2 BET	2 12-24	2 *COF*		
			3 HYP		3 *WOR*	3 24-48			
			4 HF			4 >48 h			
			5 PU			5 >1 W			
			6 GAS						
			7 REN						
			8 RES						
			9 CVA						
0	0	0	0	0	0	0	0	0	0

MOD=MODERATE, SEV=SEVERE, DRU=DRUGS, ALC=ALCOHOL, SHO=SHOCK, CIR=CIRRHOSIS, DM=DIABETES MELLITUS, HYP=HYPERTENSION, HF=HEART FAILURE, PU=PEPTIC ULCER, GAS=GASTRITIS, REN=RENAL INSUFFICIENCY, RES=RESPIRATORY INSUFF, CVA=CEREBROVASCULAR ACCIDENT, VOM=VOMITING PRECEDING HEMATEMESIS, EQU=EQUAL, BET=BETTER WOR=WORSE, <12 HS=LESS THAN 12 HS,ETC. FRE=FRESH BLOOD, COF=COFFE GROUND, MEL=MELENA, DEH=DEHYDRATATION.

CHEST PAIN
786.51

1	2	3	4	5	6	7	8	9	0
1 ONSET									

2 SITE OF PAIN
      3 NUMBNESS
            4 RADIATING TO
                  5 SEVERITY
                        6 AGGRAVATING FACTORS
                              7 RELIEVING FACTORS
                                  8 PROGRESS
                                    9 DURATION
                                      0 TYPE

V.g Male with a sudden, severe epigastric pain, radiating to left arm, of more than 48 hs. duration, improved by nytroglicerine:
786.51
1501201340

1	5	0	1	2	0	1	3	4	0
1	2	3	4	5	6	7	8	9	0
1 *SUD*	1 CTR	1 NUM	1 *LAR*	1 MOD	1 MOV	1 *NIT*	1 EQU	1 <12 h	1 CON
2 GRA	2 ACR		2 RAR	2 *SEV*	2 COU	2 RES	2 BET	2 12-24	2 INT
	3 LS		3 BAR		3 BRE	3 WAL	3 *WOR*	3 24-48	
	4 RS		4 BAC		4 OTH	4 OTH		4 *>48 h*	
	5 *EPI*		5 SHO					5 > 1 W	
	6 OTH		6 NEC						
			7 JAW						
			8 OTH						
0	0	0	0	0	0	0	0	0	0

SUD=SUDDEN, GRA=GRADUAL, CTR=CENTRAL, ACR=ACROSS, LS=LEFT SIDE, RS=RIGHT SIDE, EPI=EPIGASTRIC, OTH=OTHER, NUM=NUMBNESS, LAR=LEFT ARM, RAR=RIGHT ARM, BAR=BOTH ARMS, BAC=BACK, SHO=SHOULDER, NEC=NECK, JAW=JAW, MOD=MODERATE, SEV=SEVERE, MOV=MOVEMENT, COU=COUG, BRE=BREATHIN, NIT=NITROCLYCERINE. RES=RESTING, WAL=WALKING, EQU=EQUAL, BET=BETTER, WOR=WORSE, CON=CONTINOUS,

Discussion

As consensus is absolutely necessary, in our semiological classification, we give particular importance to those aspects emphasized by authors which are involved in the area under analysis.[3]

For codification of acute abdominal pain, as well as, in chest pain, we follow de Dombal's questionnaires.[3,4] In cases of chest pain we also took into account material from Sox,[5] Goldman,[6] Decora and Fisherkeller.[7]

Extraordinary efforts have been made by several groups[1,8] trying to arrive to standard in different fields of medicine, but a semiological classification, as the one presente here, is lacking.

Bibliography

1.　Zvarova A, Studeny M. Preiss J. On extracting relevant information from medical d Brender J, Christensen JP, Scherer JP and McNair P. Ioss Press 1966:649-653

2.　Hammond WE. Medinfo 95 HL7 Workshop. Livingstone: 1995 July 27.

3.　de Dombal FT. Diagnosis of acute abdominal pain. 2nd. Ed. Edimburgh Churchill.

4.　de Dombal FT. Chest pain questionnaire. Personal communication.

5.　Sox HC, Margulies Y, Sox CH. Psichological mediated effect of diagnosis tests. Personal communication.

6.　Goldman L et al. A computed derived protocol to aid in the diagnosis of emergency room patients with acute chest pain. New England J Med 1982;307:588-596

7.　Decora M and Fisherkeller. Computed assited diagnosis of chest pain. Report 1019 Naval Submarine USA 1984.

8.　Cote RA, Protti DJ, Scherer JR (eds). Role of informatics in health data and classification systems. Proc of IFIP-IMIA WG6. Intl Conference. Ottawa: 1984:(se 26-28).

Medical Informatics Europe '97
C. Pappas et al. (Eds.)
IOS Press, 1997

Medico-economical use of the medical record or the bridge between minimal and detailed data

F. Borst, Ch. Lovis, G. Thurler, P. Maricot, J.-R. Scherrer
Division d'Informatique Médicale
Hôpital Cantonal Universitaire - 1211 Geneva 14 - Switzerland

Medico-economical use of the medical record: the title encloses two different notions which represent two different trends within medical informatics. The first trend is worried about weighting aspects of health resources consumption, mainly about hospital acute care; their key-words are "DRG (Diagnostic Related Groups), Case-Mix, reimbursement by pathology, measurement of indicators (severity or outcome), costs". The other trend is looking for deeper understanding of the medical process and for better diffusion of relevant information helping the day-to-day care process; they speak of "CPR (Computerized patient record), full text reports and corresponding retrieval, detailed data, medical records on Internet, large access to literature and databases". It is mandatory to realize a bridge between these two trends for facing the information technology revolution entering into a self-revolutioning medicine. The purpose of this paper is to begin this bridge by showing what the DRG people expect from the CPR people and what the latter should receive from the former.

The DRG people and the CPR people

These two trends correspond to two different approaches of the reality. The DRG people tend to simplify the reality by looking at it throughout a set of predefined variables. They miss some proper characteristics of the patient but they are able to build an operational system. They can perform a arithmetic about patients with some operations like : "Is this patient more expensive than another ?" or "Does this set of patients consume the same amount of resources ?".
One could raise other questions such like "Is the patient going better ?" or "What will be his health state within 10 years ?". Present systems of the DRG trend cannot answer to these questions because they lack precise and detailed information. The answer is most probably somewhere within a CPR database (which potentially contains all the figures, reports and images of the patient record), but is still hidden, diluted, not directly extractable. In other world, DRG trend provide a measurable approach, but have too few information. On the opposite, CPR systems contain a lot information, but with a lack of structure.
The following examples illustrate that the full text reports of the CPR contain information about quality of care (risk of readmission) and severity of cases.
A study has been recently performed in our hospital with the intent to classify **readmissioned** patients into a) planned readmissions (e.g. for elective surgery, for iterative treatment such like chemotherapy) and into b) those who could have been potentially avoided with a better initial management. Preliminary results show that such a classification process requires more data than the encoded summary alone (36% of unclassified cases). The analysis of the discharge letters, on the opposite, leaves only 3% of unclassified cases.
Sager was able to automatically classify patients into three level of **complexity** on the basis on the text analysis of the discharge letters. performed an automatic classification of surgical discharge letters into three categories of complexity [1].

The urgency of the bridge

The discrepancy between the importance of some healthcare policy decisions and the relative weakness of the information justifying these decisions is impressive. As it would be totally unacceptable to treat a patient on the only basis of its age, sex and diagnostic, without taking into account its severity stage, medico-surgical past history, it should be as well unacceptable to close a hospital or decrease its budget on the basis of the same few information.

It is even unacceptable to get the same amount of money for treating patients considered as similar on the unique basis of their diagnoses (as it is the case in the reimbursement by pathology); especially if these data are not exact, as shown by Steinum [2] "In Sweden several studies have pointed to this problem of database input error and in recent years three publications from the Swedish Institute for Health Services Development (Spri) have shown that diagnosis/procedure errors lead to errors in DRG allocation in 18% of cases at surgical clinics; 9% at gynaecological clinics and 15% at clinics for infectious diseases."

Important decisions have to be taken on faithful and detailed information. With the increasing economical restrictions on healthcare, the realization of this bridge has become an emergency.

New problems, new solutions

Beyond daily increasing economical restrictions, medicine is confronted to a deep intern revolution based on new problems :
- increasing number of chronic patients (due to both aging and transformation of "killing diseases" into chronic diseases),
- dispersion of the healthcare system (from remote access to specialists to regionalisation of hospital care),
- rapid development of ambulatory care, home care, without any acceptable definition of episode of care,
- opposition between global cost control and need to treat individuals as best as possible,
- opposition between needs of large communication and to respect individual privacy,
- relative immaturity of tools for measuring quality regarding tools for computing expenses,
- lack of definition of hospital product based on outcome measurement, including initial measure of severity (beyond hospital product still on groups of diagnoses-procedures),
- increasing control of economical arguments on daily practice (throughout e.g. expansion of guidelines).

At the end of this century, information technology brings tools that potentially provide solutions impossible to imagine even 10 years ago :
- cheap and powerful archival, allowing to definitely eliminate the too restrictive notion of means for keeping the detailed data of all original individuals. These detailed data build Case-Based Reasoning retrieval, as illustrated by Shortliffe : "Dukes University's Coronary Artery Disease Data Bank allows a physician to indicate certain parameters of a patient, to instruct the system to identify past patients that had the same characteristics, and to request a display of how those patients did under various therapeutic options. The practitioner can then evaluate what the benefits of medical management versus bypass surgery or angioplasty would be in this particular case" [3].
- retrieval of information in the full text reports, as illustrated by MEDLINE or DOMED (DOMED is a computerized patient record developed in our hospital, with a detailed access to the whole patient record including searching in free text within the reports),
- retrieval of specific medical concepts among several thousands, as shown by LUCID (LUCID is a semi automatic encoding tool based on natural language processing concepts, helping the physician to choose the right expression among thousands of an international classification [4]).
- communication network disseminating information between several healthcare providers, sharing multimedia data (codes, figures, texts, images, sounds, etc.) along time, up to the patient himself, as illustrated by Ferrara [5] : "By nature, healthcare organisational structure in European countries is distributed, being a geographical spread of centers at different levels of complexity: from the general hospitals down to individual GPs. Also the structure of the individual healthcare center, and particularly of the hospitals, is evolving from a vertical, aggregate organisation, towards the integration of a set of specialised departments, which are characterised by diverse logistic, organisational and clinical requirements and aspects."

The bridge as a solution

The bridge is needed in order to enrich the quality, precision, level of details of the routine coded summaries. Adequacy regarding the specific state of the patient has also to be increased, as well as information describing the quality of care. Routinely collected data have to be recorded in an readily queriable form for performing statistical analysis. Data have to be exhaustive, without missing information. New technologies of information, including natural language processing and artificial intelligence, have to be oriented for obtaining these goals,

Such an approach is shown by Adelhard in the field of a cancer registry [6]. "Cancer is a chronic disease, its care an interdisciplinary long-term process. In many respects patient oriented care and scientific analysis of the data share the same demands. Correctness and completeness of data is crucial for both areas. High quality data is essential for the survival of a registry. A combination of scientific and patient oriented usage of the data is an optimal prerequisite for the generation of high quality information."

The bridge may be built of several components where CPR technology and information content helps to enrich the coded summary of the DRG system .

The first component is the **definition of the relevant information** that should be recorded on a routine basis for enriching the coded summaries. A typical example is provided by Hannan, who has shown that the addition of three cardiac risk factors (ejection fraction, reoperation, narrowing of the left main trunk) into a summary administrative database significantly improves its predictive power of mortality for coronary artery bypass graft surgery [7].

The component **quality of care indicators** may be defined on an operational basis. Quality indicators become based on the evolution of the patient severity **stage** regarding performed **actions**, followed by the **outcome** measurement. Bandon has a similar approach [8]: "The first state is the [...] diagnosis aiming the therapy selection. The second one is the therapy itself while the third is the follow-up of this therapy.".

For **chronic diseases**, quality of care measurement is based more specifically on the **outcome** by the follow-up of specific parameters. For Boye [9], "To assure quality of the care provided in government hospitals out-patient clinics the Danish Endocrine Society intends to set up a central database (DADIVOX) for medical audit in Hillerrd, Denmark. The clinics, which participate, report 47 essential and 28 optional parameters on each diabetic patient to the register annually. [...] Quality of patient care is pursued through optimization of treatment, incentives to self-care and self-monitoring of blood-glucose, and monitoring of eye, kidney, blood-vessel and nerve-function by means of clinical and para-clinical tests."

Natural language techniques may dramatically **improve the user-acceptance** of the data recording tool, as shown by the use of LUCID ([4], cf supra). One step further is to use artificial intelligence techniques for asking to the user the very specific question at the very adequate moment (depending on very specific context of the patient).

A mechanism of **alerts** could be set up for controlling and enriching the content of the coded summary on the automatic analysis of the discharge letter, as proposed by Lyman [10], who automatically detect the presence or absence of specific items in the text, and may trigger the recording of supplementary data.

The state in Geneva

In Geneva, several pieces of both DRG system and CPR system have already been developed,

On the basis of the **distributed hospital information system Diogene2**, an integrated database system called Archimed has been set up. **Archimed** acts as the permanent memory of the patients information, by gathering and uniforming data from several remote applications (ADT, Financing, Laboratory and Radiology information systems, MODCOD-LUCID encoding system [11] and DRGs). Beyond this archiving aspect, Archimed furthermore contains decision support systems.

A model of **computing cost of hospitalization** has been developed on Archimed, based on the reattribution of the total expenses of the hospital to each patient, mainly according to the time spent in each type of care unit. Medico-technical resources are directly attributed to the individual patient. First tests are mostly satisfactory; the validation phase has been planed.

A **complete medical record** is under development, called DOMED (cf supra), based on full text search of reports, archival of coded summaries [11], reports within Unidoc [12] and other patients data. Unidoc gathers all the hospital patient reports, providing an structured access into the network to each patient in free text, as dictated by the physician and typed by a secretary.

Several projects have been set up around the "Medical direction " with the intent to measuring and maintaining the quality of care. Among these, detailed structured clinical databases (firstly in the field of obstetrics and neonatology) have been integrated, building the first steps on the bridge. For example, the obstetrics clinical database records for each delivery the quality of care indicators as defined by the American College of Obstetricians and Gynecologists.

Conclusion

The discrepancy between the importance of healthcare policy decisions and the relative weakness of the information justifying these decisions is impressive. This discrepancy explains the emergency to develop a bridge between the Computerized Patient Record technology and its information content and the "DRG recording system", in order to enrich the quality, precision, level of details of the routinely collected data.
Several steps have been demonstrated, particularly in the definition and integration of quality of care and outcome indicators.

References

[1]   Sager N. et al "Clinical knowledge bases from natural language patient documents", in MEDINFO'92, Proceedings of the Seventh World Congress on Medical Informatics, Geneva, K.C. Lun et al (eds). Elsevier Science Publisher B.V. (North-Holland), IMIA 1992, 1375-1381.

[2]   Steinum O. "A correct DRG allocation presupposes correct diagnoses", in Proceedings of the 11th Conference of PCS/E, Oslo, Norway, 1995, 43-49.

[3]   Shortliffe EH. The Networked Physician : practitioner of the Future. In : "Healthcare Information Management Systems", Ball Douglas, O'Destry, Albright (eds), Springer-Verlag, 1991, pp 3-18.

[4]   Ch. Lovis et al "Medico-Economic Patient Encoding in the University Hospital of Geneva" in Medical Informatics Europe '96, Brender, Christenson, Scherrer, McNair (eds), IOS Press Publ. Comp. 159-163 1996.

[5]   Ferrara F.F. "The middleware-based architectural approach for opening and evolving healthcare information systems." in Medical Informatics Europe '96, Brender, Christenson, Scherrer, McNair (eds), IOS Press Publ. Comp. 264-270, 1996.

[6]   Adelhard K. et al "Interactive Access to Clinical and Epidemiological Cancer Data" in Medical Informatics Europe '96, Brender, Christenson, Scherrer, McNair (eds), IOS Press Publ. Comp. 113-117 1996

[7]   Hannan E.L. et al "Clinical Versus Administrative Data Bases for CABG Surgery - Does it Matter ?" Medical Care, Oct. 1992, 30:10, 892-907.

[8]   Bandon D,, Kanz R., Wehenkel Cl. "Anticipation by Learning of Image Retrieval", in Medical Informatic Europe '96, Brender, Christenson, Scherrer, McNair (eds), IOS Press Publ. Comp. 639-643, 1996.

[9]   Boye N. "DADIVOX Integration of Medical Audit and an Electronic Patient Record for use in Diabete Mellitus Out-patient Clinics in Denmark", in Medical Informatics Europe '96, Brender, Christenson Scherrer, McNair (eds), IOS Press Publ. Comp. 369-373, 1996.

[10]   Lyman M.S. "Health Care Evaluation", and "Audit Criteria for Healthcare Evaluation" in Medical Language Processing, Sager, Friedman, Lyman (eds), Addison-Wesley Publ. Comp. Reading, 1987, 29-3 and 317-323.

[11]   Borst F. et al "Fifteen Years of Medical Encoding in the Diogene HIS", in MEDINFO'95, Proceedings c the Eighth World Congress on Medical Informatics, Vancouver, Greenes, Peterson, Protti (eds Healthcare Computing & Communications Canada (Publ Comp), Edmonton 1995, 43-46.

[12]   Scherrer J.-R. et al "Medical Office Automation Integrated into the Distributed Architecture of the HIS DIOGENE 2", Methods Inf Med 1994;33:174-9, Reprinted in IMIA Yearbook of Medical Informatics 9. Schattauer ed comp, Stuttgart, 1995, 283-8.

Medical Informatics Europe '97
C. Pappas et al. (Eds.)
IOS Press, 1997

Case mix of elderly in-patients in the 29 hospitals in Lorraine in 1994 and 1995

Pierre GILLOIS, Hervé GARIN, Olivier BODENREIDER, François KOHLER
GRAIH de Lorraine - SPI EAO Faculté de Médecine de Nancy B.P. 184 - 54505
Vandoeuvre les Nancy Cedex France

Abstract : The creation of regional standardized medical information databases in relation with the French anonymous discharge dataset allows the study of the geriatric case mix processed in the Lorraine region for patients over 69. The age histogram (69 to 107 years) presents a two mode distribution with an important dip centered on 79 years probably in connection with the demography of Lorraine and the consequences of the First World War. These geriatric patients represent 17% of hospitalisations in public and private hospitals participating in the public sector. The case mix is related to the size of the hospital and to its juridical status. The bigger the size of an hospital, the less its activity is concentrated on a small number of disorders. Lung and heart diseases represent the first cause of hospitalisation in all hospitals. It is necessary to underline the limitation of an approach which uses the patients' individual hospitalisations, and which does not allow different stays of a given patient in the same hospital or between different hospitals to be linked. This approach prevents from appreciating the care network for this elderly population suffering from chronic diseases.

1. Introduction

The generalisation of the French 'Programme de Médicalisation du Système d'Information' (PMSI) and the setting up of regional medical databases about an in-patient dataset in public and private hospitals participating in the public sector, allows the study of hospital case mix [1]. Since 1993, the Lorraine region, has been one of the first experimental regions to transmit the summary of anonymous discharge (RSA) and is the test region for the MAHOS software. The regional group of hospital information (GRAIH) has been allowed to consult this database in order to carry out the study on elderly people hospitalisation in 1994-1995 with a good exhaustiveness of the records. In this survey, the emphasis has been put on the link between the size of hospitals and the kind of diseases. This first study can be justified by the ageing of the population, the chronicity of many medical diseases and the economical burden resulting from this hospitalisation [2]. Solution acting as an alternative to hospitalisation can also justify it. Several points have been taken into account : specificities of the Lorraine region, strategic aspects, setting up of a specific data system, money allowances [3, 4]... but we are also aware of some limitations such as the impossibility of linking the different hospitalisations for the same patient, which would be useful to trace the patient through the medical network.

2. Material and method

2.1 Data used

The data used come from the French RSA regional database of Lorraine of 1994-1995. Among the given information we have selected the type of hospital (according to size, juridical entity), sex and age of patient, principal diagnosis, French major diagnosis category (CMD), French diagnosis related group version 3 (GHM) and the surgical or medical aspect of the GHM [5].

2.2 *Groups of hospitals*

According to the status of the GRAIH in Lorraine and in order to preserve the anonymity of the hospital, such a study cannot be carried out solely on hospital. Therefore our study takes into account the grouping of hospitals as the one used for cost scale by the French Ministry of Health [6]. The only cancer centre in the Lorraine region has been associated with the private hospitals participating in the public sector. The public hospitals have been divided into 4 groups according to their sizes and all the private hospitals participating to the public sector make up a fifth group. This last group has quite a mixed character due to the size of the different hospitals, their degree of specialisation and their way of working such as in the specific social insurance of the mining region. Group number 1 includes the public hospitals which are not CHR (regional hospital) CHU (university hospital) and with more than 14 000 in-patients a year. Group number 2 includes, the public hospitals which are not CHR or CHU and with 7 000 to 14 000 inpatients a year. Group number 3 consists of non CHR or CHU public hospitals with less than 7 000 inpatients a year. Group 4 consists of the private hospitals participating in the public sector as well as the cancer centre. Group 5 is made up of the CHR and the CHU of the region. Table 1 shows how the twenty five hospitals in Lorraine are split up into these 5 groups.

2.3 *Medical grouping of patient hospital stays*

Taking into account the given data, we have set up pathological groups by subdividing the main categories of diagnoses (CMD) into sub medical categories according to the surgical or medical characteristics of the GHM classified in each CMD. Thus we have obtained 44 groups called CMDms. The French category 24 is excluded from this study as well as CMD 14 and CMD 15 which are specific to pregnancy and perinatal pathology. CMD 20 is composed of only one sub medical group. Finally we have obtained 41 CMDms sub groups (Table 2)

2.4 *Data reliability*

The 29 hospitals have been subject to compulsory internal and external controls of quality consisting in re coding 200 in-patients chosen at random for each year.

2.5 *Statistical analysis*

Besides the traditional descriptive statistics, the statistical analysis includes a study of the groups of hospitals and the case mix. This study is completed with a study of the GHM and a study of the principal diagnoses encountered in each of the CMDms.

3. Results

The database includes 855 636 hospital admissions. By selecting the patients over 69, having been admitted for a traditional stay (classified in CMD 1 to 23) we obtained 147 227 geriatric stays that is to say 17.2% of the total data.

In 1994 the RSA represented 49.2% of the database. This rise is not the result of an increase of hospitalisations but comes from a better exhaustiveness of the records in 1995. Table 3 shows how geriatric stays are distributed among the hospital: 31% are taken in charge by CHU and CHR; 43.4% are equally divided among highly-busy and moderately-busy hospitals. Female geriatric cases are majority (56.8%). The number of imprecisely coded diagnoses (_.9) is not significantly different according to the size of hospitals. Patient ages

Table 1 : Hospitals in their group

Number of Hospitals	GROUPS
4 hospitals	Large sized > 14 000 in-patients / year
8 hospitals	Medium sized between 7 and 14 000 in-patients / year
4 hospitals	Small sized < 7 000 in-patients / year
11 hospitals	Private
2 hospitals	CHU-CHR

Table 2 : Major diagnosis categories (CMDms)

CMD		CMD	
1	Nervous system group M/S	12	Male reproduction system group M/S
2	Eye group M/S	13	Female reproduction system group M/S
3	ENT group M/S	16	Haemo system M/S
4	Resporatory system group M/S	17	Myeloprolif system group M/S
5	Circulatory system group M/S	18	Infection group M/S
6	GI system group M/S	19	Psych group M/S
7	Hepatic system group M/S	21	Injury/Poisonning group M/S
8	Muscular skeletal system group M/S	22	Burns group M/S
9	Skin and brest group M/S	23	Other factors group M/S
10	Endocrine system group M/S	20	Substance abuse group M
11	Renal system group M/S		

Table 3 : Distribution of the geriatric stays

Hospitals	Number of stays	Percentage
Large-size	33 802	22,96%
Medium-size	30 073	20,43%
Small-sized	8 998	6,11%
Private	28 142	19,13%
CHU-CHR	46 165	31,36%
	TOTAL	147 180

Table 5 : Comparison 2 by 2 of the hospital groups (Khi^2)

	Medium	Large	Private	CHU-CHR
Small	592,6***	798,8***	2375,3***	1629,6***
Medium		548,6***	3591,8***	2618,8***
Large			2540,2***	2100,6***
Private				5140,4***

*** $p<0,0001$ df = 43

Table 4 : Distribution of the CMDms

CMD		Small	Medium	Large	Private	CHU CHR	Total	CMD		Small	Medium	Large	Private	CHU CHR	Total
5	M	2032	6368	6729	3266	8421	26816	11	S	50	133	339	483	439	1444
4	M	1101	3897	4114	3408	4176	16696	12	M	54	218	245	211	586	1314
1	M	668	2423	2951	1425	4011	11478	7	S	49	212	275	301	316	1153
6	M	900	2654	2517	2383	2991	11445	18	M	91	272	244	147	320	1074
23	M	837	1669	1914	1356	2951	8727	13	S	66	290	249	282	123	1010
8	M	484	1686	1894	1851	2440	8355	2	M	15	165	148	51	335	714
8	S	317	1428	1676	2856	1554	7831	13	M	30	141	120	236	105	632
2	S	2	766	699	688	2812	4967	1	S	4	69	66	118	369	626
10	M	257	869	1107	721	1954	4908	4	S	2	33	49	91	209	384
19	M	281	1199	1062	554	1310	4406	3	S	37	41	43	50	140	311
11	M	285	829	1084	754	1288	4240	20	M	13	63	73	36	90	275
6	S	223	702	927	1116	985	3953	23	S	2	22	47	55	148	274
9	M	241	720	819	655	1238	3673	21	S	4	28	67	65	78	242
5	S	54	250	605	788	1837	3534	10	S	10	16	23	53	102	204
17	M	75	426	833	1216	841	3391	17	S	11	34	26	50	60	181
7	M	170	498	694	516	1058	2936	16	S	1	7	10	17	15	50
3	M	185	676	571	399	994	2825	18	S	1	17	10	11	11	50
16	M	168	396	495	420	531	2010	22	M	0	6	8	3	23	40
12	S	64	259	455	712	446	1936	19	S	1	3	5	3	10	22
21	M	128	329	319	288	506	1570	22	S	0	2	2	0	14	18
9	S	85	257	288	507	328	1465			8998	30073	33802	28142	46165	147180

range from 69 to 107; the histogram has a two-mode distribution with an important dip centered at 79. (Figure 1).

The geriatric case mix is mainly concentrated in five medical CMDms: cardiology, pneumology, neurology, gastrology and other factor groups . These five groups represent 51% of the stays (Table 4). 14 CMDms out of the 41 CMDms represent more than 82% of the hospital activity.

The GHM analysis shows that 31 GHM gather more than 50% of the geriatric stays and that 88 GHM gather 80% of the stays. The five most frequent GHM include 16% of the stays. GHM 184 (cardiac insufficiency and circulatory trouble shock) and GHM 256 (gastro-enteritis and various digestive track disorders, patients over 69 and/or major associated co-morbidity (CMA)), GHM 675 (other factors causing health troubles), GHM 195 (arrhythmia and cardiac conduction troubles patients over 69 and/or major associated co-morbidity (CMA)), GHM 018 (cerebral ischemic stroke). The study of the principal diagnoses allow us to find 3471 different diagnosis ICD codes. The most frequent code is senile cataract (366.1: 2.3% of the stays). 79 principal diagnoses represent 50% of the stays. Therefore in the geriatric case mix, 22% of the GHM concern 80% of the stays and 10.3% of the principal diagnosis concern 80% of the stays.

We found a close relation between the type of the hospital and its case mix. (Khi^2 = 10 309, df 172, p< 0.0001). The hospital do not deal with the same kind of pathologies in elderly people. By comparing two by two the different groups of hospitals and whatever the comparisons may be, all the relationships are significant (Table 5). Table 6 show the most frequent geriatric case mix in relation to the type of hospital. For every hospital the most frequent pathologies are cardiac and pneumological diseases. In small-sized hospitals, the activity is concentrated on a very small variety of pathologies whereas in large-sized hospitals a larger number of pathologies are taken into account.

Table 6 : Required CMDms to obtain 50% of the case mix

CMDms	Small	Medium	Large	Private	CHU-CHR
1st	5 M	5 M	5 M	4 M	5 M
2nd	4 M	4 M	4 M	5 M	4 M
3rd	6 M	6 M	1 M	8 C	1 M
4th	23 M	1 M	6 M	6 M	6 M
5th	-	-	23 M	8 M	23 M
6th	-	-	-	1 M	2 S

Figure 1

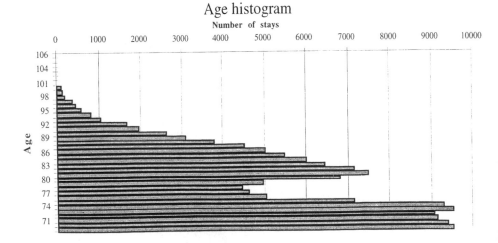

Age histogram

4. Discussion

The geriatric population represents more than 17% of the total hospitalisation with big variation from 3.8%(mental disorders and poisoning) to 45.9% (cardiological and vascular diseases) according to CMD. These results are similar to those observed in the rest of France. The two-mode age distribution can be superposed with the French age pyramid with a dip centered between 75 and 80 resulting from the First World War. We must stress the fact that in the coming years this dip will disappear. For the elderly population it is usual to observe an exponential increase in the rate of hospitalisation linked with the age from the 20s [7]. In our survey, comparing the number of hospitalisations with the Lorraine demography, we can observe the same facts. Moreover the medical consumption increases exponentially with ageing [9,10]. The French valorisation in economical points (ISA) for these elderly inpatients shows that they represent 31.7% of the total ISA in Lorraine. That is why the GHM housing inpatients are a burden for the economy. It would be interesting to study the medical procedures of these stays but the actual records do not allow us to do so [8]. In the private hospitals the rank of cardiology and pneumology diseases is inversed compared with the other groups. It can be explained by the specific social insurance of the mining region [11-12]. This survey confirms the importance of PMSI, to acquire a better knowledge of inpatients even though important limitations must be underlined. The lack of link between hospitalisation of specific patients in the same or in different hospitals prevent us from tracing them in the network, which is quite a trouble since these patients suffer from poly chronical diseases requiring the cares from different kinds of hospitals. The extension of the French PMSI will soon enable us to find a solution to this problem.

References

[1] HENNEN J., KRUMHOLZ H.M., RADFORD M.J., MEEHAN T.P., Readmission rates, 30 days and 365 days postdischarge, among the 20 most frequent DRG groups, Medicare inpatients age 65 or older in Connecticut hospitals, fiscal years 1991, 1992 and 1993. Conn. Med. 1995;59: 263-270

[2] BOCOGNANO A., GRANDFILS N., LE FUR PH., MIZRAHI AN., MIZRAHI AR. Santé, soins et protection sociale en 1993 - Enquête sur la santé et la protection sociale France 1993. CREDES, n° 1037, 1994

[3] PÉNIN F., MAYEUX D., JEANDEL C., SCHMAL-LAURAIN M.C., CUNY G. Réflexions à propos de quelques problèmes posés par l'hospitalisation des personnes âgées en « court séjour gériatrique ». Ann. Méd. de Nancy et de l'Est 1993; 32: 105-108

[4] VERGNENEGRE A;, CHALE J.J., GROUCHKA C.,SENE E., POUS J., BONNAUD F. Indicateurs explicatifs de la durée de séjour dans un service de Pneumologie. Rev. Mal. Respir. 1995;12:479-488

[5] Bulletin Officiel n° 94 - 2 bis. Manuel des groupes homogènes de malades version 2. Direction des Journaux Officiels

[6] Bulletin Officiel n° 95 - 5 bis. L'échelle nationale des coûts relatifs par groupes homogènes de malades Direction des Journaux Officiels

[7] FLAMER H.E., CHRISTOPHIDIS N., MARGETTS C., UGONI A., MCLEAN A.J. Extended hospital stays with incresing age : the impact of an acute geriatric unit

[8] SCHREIBER T.L., ELKHATIB A., GRINES C.L., O'NEILL W.W. Cardiologist versus internist management of patients with unstable angina : treatment patterns and outcomes. J. Am. Coll. Cardiol. 1995;26:577-582

[9] MEUNIER R. Vieillissement et consommation de santé. Le coût de la vieillesse, Société de Gérontologie de l'Est, 1995, pp 5-28

[10] PRICE M.A. Casemix classification and health care of the elderly. Med. J. Aust 1994;161:S23-26

[11] DIEZ A., TOMAS R., VARELA J., CASAS M., GONZALEZ-MACIAS J. Internal medicine in a group of 52 Spanish hospitals. Analysis of a case series and efficiency. Med. Clin. 1996;106:361-367

[12] HENNEN J., KRUMHOLZ H.M., RADFORD M.J. Twenty most frequent DRG groups among Medicare inpatients age 65 or older in Connecticut hospitals, fiscal years 1991, 1992 and 1993. Conn. Med. 1995;59:11-15

Medical Informatics Europe '97
C. Pappas et al. (Eds.)
IOS Press, 1997

A 3D ultrasound scanner : real time filtering and rendering algorithms

D. Cifarelli[1], C. Ruggiero[1], M. Brusacà[2], and M. Mazzarella[2]

1 - DIST Department of Information Systems and Telematic - University of Genova, Via All'opera Pia 13, 16145 Genova, Italy, Fax +39103532948
2 - ESAOTE BIOMEDICA Ultrasound Division, Via Siffredi 58, 16145 Genova, Italy, Fax +39106547275

Abstract
The work described here has been carried out within a collaborative project between DIST and ESAOTE BIOMEDICA aiming to set up a new ultrasonic scanner performing 3D reconstruction . A system is being set up to process and display 3D ultrasonic data in a fast , economical and user friendly way to help the physician during diagnosis. A comparison is presented among several algorithms for digital filtering , data segmentation and rendering for real time , PC based , three-dimensional reconstruction from B-mode ultrasonic biomedical images .Several algorithms for digital filtering have been compared as relates to processing time and to final image quality . Three-dimensional data segmentation techniques and rendering has been carried out with special reference to user friendly features for foreseeable applications and reconstruction speed .

1. Introduction

Nowadays there is a great interest toward ultrasonic imaging due to its versatility .
Ultrasonic scanners are very easy and fast to use and they are cheap compared to other tomographic devices . Moreover , ultrasounds is the only imaging technique available today which is non invasive without restrictions .Three dimensional ultrasonic imaging is at present one of the most interesting fields for industries . A collaborative project between DIST and ESAOTE BIOMEDICA is being carried out , aiming to realize a new high-performance 3D ultrasonic scanner . The present work focuses on the algorithmic aspect of the system . Whereas three-dimensional reconstruction from tomographic data is a very common and widely studied technique for several imaging methods like X-CT , MRI and PET , this is not the case for B-mode ultrasonic data which is regarded as a difficult and challenging field , due to strong limitations in the imaging system compared with other tomographic techniques. In ultrasonic imaging there are several noise sources and aberrations which cause great difficulties in the image processing and data segmentation steps , before rendering . Signal to noise ratio is very low compared to other imaging methods , ultrasonic biomedical images are corrupted by speckle and thermal noise , there is a general lack of contrast and several parts of the field of view are often out of focus .
In image processing of ultrasound data linear filters are generally useless , so we have considered different types of median filters such as 3D median and adaptive median filtering [1] which represent a good trade off between computational complexity , noise cleaning and edge preserving ability. Regarding data segmentation we have developed an almost totally automatic algorithm based on pseudo-3D *region growing* to simplify the reconstruction process for the physician and to maintain three-dimensional coherence between the different structures in the data set . For the last step in the reconstruction process we have used two different classes of rendering algorithms : solid voxel based photorealistic techniques like *Back to Front* [2] and *Front to Back* , together with *depth shading* and *gradient shading* [3,4] to enhance final image quality , and non photorealistic techniques based on direct features mapping [5] like *mean value projection* , *maximum value projection* and

transparent gradient shading .The reason why we have followed both approaches is that solid techniques are useful for morphology analysis on reconstructed structures , whereas direct feature mapping rendering gives a look-thru projection in some way similar to X-ray because all the information coming from the 3D data set is condensed using transparency on a two-dimensional view plane .

This semi-transparent representation is appreciated by physicians because it is closer to their cultural background than the photorealistc solid reconstruction .

2. Materials and methods

To acquire the data set in the beginning we used a conventional bidimensional ultrasonic probe operating in free hand mode . With this setup it was only possible to perform parallel acquisitions because there was no information about the spatial relationship between the different slices acquired. Later we have used a 6 degree of freedom position sensor , Polhemus Flock of Bird , directly attached on the ultrasonic probe .This makes it possible to acquire the sections of the data set with any position and orientation for the probe , then with a three-dimensional interpolation algorithm it is possible to give the data set homogeneous density filling the missing voxels .

For processing and rendering steps we have used a conventional , hi-end personal computer based either on a Pentium or on a Pentium Pro CPU with Windows 95 operating system .

3. Filtering

Working with ultrasonic images , linear filters are almost useless , the main result is a big information loss due to an excessive blurring which modifies the edge content of the processed image . A good filter for ultrasonic data must have a strong noise suppression ability without affecting edges , wich in ultrasound tomography are often not very visible . Therefore non linear filters have to be considered . We have examined several kinds of *median filters* and scale space filtering based on *anisotropic diffusion* [6] . The next step will be *wavelet* filtering , which will be compared with median filtering and anisotropic diffusion . Computational complexity for anisotropic diffusion is too heavy for a real time application based on commercial hardware , like in our case . Since this kind of filtering is an iterative process , the number of iterations required to get good results is too high for our case , although it's a powerful method well suited for ultrasonic data , and for applications without strong time constraints . We have focused on median filters , which represent a good trade off between CPU time , noise suppression and edge preserving ability. It's possible to obtain pretty good results even using the bidimensional median filter with a 5 by 5 or a 7 by 7 mask , but as we are working in a three-dimensional environment it is possible to get better results using a 3D median filter with a 3 by 3 by 3 or a 5 by 5 by 5 mask . The advantage in using the 3D median instead of the 2D one is due to the fact that spatial correlation for noise between different sections of the data set is much lower compared to real signal correlation , thus working with a 3D filter we gain noise suppression ability .

 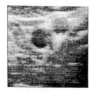

Figure 1 Left , original ultrasonic image of a carotid . Right , same image filtered with a 3 by 3 by 3 median.

Normal median filters are able to preserve ideal edges while modifying noise corrupted ones , so even with 3D median filter there is edge blurring , which can be a problem for the segmentation and rendering steps. There is a possible extension of the median filter [1] which is able to preserve image detail also increasing noise suppression .This filter is an adaptive median which can modify its mask size depending on the local statistical image content . In large and homogeneous areas the largest possible window is used , obtaining maximun noise suppression , in detail areas the window size is reduced so to retain important structures present in the image .The parameter used to fix the window size is $\dfrac{\sigma_x^2}{\bar{x}}$ where variance and mean are calculated on the maximum window , which is 2k+1 by 2k+1.

For each pixel the size of the window for the median used is given by $n = \left[k\left(1 - c\dfrac{\sigma_x^2}{\bar{x}}\right)\right]$,

where c is a scaling factor. The parameter c regulates the filter bandwidth , consequently noise suppression and edge preserving capability , and also processing time . For values of c close to 0 the filter behaviour is similar to the one of a pure median , so the maximum window size is always used , obtaining a high noise suppression but the processing time is long and the edges are not preserved to a good extent , for higher values of c noise suppression is lower , but edge preserving ability is higher . As a good compromise between speed and final image quality , we have used c=0.30 and maximum size 9 for the mask.

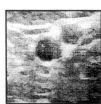

Figure 2 Same image filtered with adaptive median c=0.30 , mask size 9.

For a good 3D reconstruction the whole data set must have at least 64 sections .On a Pentium 120 PC with the 3D median filtering is performed in about 1 minute , with the variable window median it takes about three minutes , which are both reasonable times , since filtering is needed only once per acquisition , whereas segmentation and rendering can be repeated and modified without need of preprocessing . We will also consider the use of *wavelets* as low computational complexity non linear filtering , to gain speed in the noise cleaning step for 3D reconstruction .

4. Segmentation

Segmentation is important to choose the structure to be reconstructed from the whole data set . We have developed an almost totally automatic segmentation technique based on *region growing* , which is able to classify the 3D data set into regions assigning the same label to corresponding parts in different sections . The only parameter needed for segmentation is the number of regions that we want to use to segment the data set .

Region seeds are chosen in the same way for the whole data set , to give three-dimensional coherence to the segmented data . To increase noise immunity seeds are not chosen from real voxels in the data set , but the gray level range , 0 ... 255 , is partitioned depending on the number of regions chosen for segmentation . Regions are then created on the basis of minimum gray level distance from one of the available seeds . Practically using different data

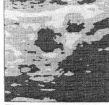

Figure 3 figure 1 image segmented with 4 regions

sets we have found that for ultrasonic images 4 or 6 regions are enough to obtain good reconstructions , anyway for a general data set the right number of regions for segmentation can be found with few trials . Regions found with this technique are generally not connected and often contain both interesting and unwanted structures ; great improvements can be obtained first using *spatial clipping* and then filtering among the remaining structures those whose area is below a threshold.

This algorithm is simple and requires low processing times , so it's well suited for a fast reconstruction application . The whole data set is processed in a few seconds and with very good results for the final rendering .

5. Rendering

Due to cheap commercial hardware and high speed constraints we have focused on voxel based rendering algorithms because their computational complexity is much lower than surface based or ray tracing algorithms . We have implemented both photorealistic solid methods and non photorealistic transparent algorithms . The first technique we have used is *Back to front* [2] . Voxels are projected on the screen and the data set is transversed with decreasing distance from the observer , so voxels far from the observer are covered by closer ones . The first depth cue used is depth shading : the intensity of each voxel projected on the screen is inversely proportional to view plane distance , voxels close to the observer are given a high intensity while a low intensity is chosen for far voxels . To gain more details depth shaded images have been processed with two different *gradient shading* algorithms based on the *Z-buffer* [3,4], using Phong illumination model [3] . The depth shaded image is completed in 2 seconds , the first gradient shading algorithm

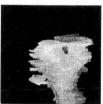
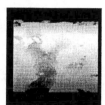

Figure 4 Left reconstruction of a carotid with gradient shading , right reconstruction of a carotid section with depth shading, both using back to front.

requires less than 1 second , while the second , which is more complex but gives better results , requires between 4 and 6 seconds depending on the parameters used .

The second method used is *Front to Back* , which gives the same kind of reconstruction of Back to front but it's faster is some cases . The data set is transversed with increasing distance from the observer using rays which are normal to the view plane , the data set is often not completely analyzed resulting in a faster processing time for reconstruction .In addition depth shading and gradient shading techniques are used to get more structural details . With front to back it's possible to save about 30 percent of processing time. Solid rendering algorithms are useful to analyze organ structure looking for deformations or to check organs for correct dimensions . Moreover , physicians are particularly interested in transparent methods which make look-thru projection possible .Using this kind of imaging technique , which is much more similar to X-ray , it's possible to compare data coming from different imaging methods . For instance , in digital mammography interesting results are sometimes obtained by comparison with ultrasounds .The first transparent rendering technique we have used is *mean value projection* [5] , in which the data set is transversed with rays which are normal to the view plane like in the front to back case and the mean value of all the voxels along each ray is calculated and then projected onto the screen .

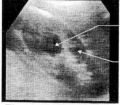

Cyst

Cyst

Figure 5 Mean value projection of a kidney with two Cysts .

This technique can also be modified to provide the user with a better depth feeling : the mean value is computed weighting each voxel on the basis of distance from the view plane , in this way the voxels nearer to the observer contribute more than the others to the final reconstructed image.Mean value projection images are generally not very detailed . Animation is a good technique to resolve visual ambiguities and to achieve a better trasparency feeling. From the computational point of view mean value projection is heavier than former methods requiring about 20 to 30 seconds for a reconstruction . *Maximum value projection* has the same structure of the previous algorithm but the maximum value along each ray is projected instead of the mean value . It's useful to underline strong acoustic impedance discontinuities in the ultrasonic data set , like bone structures , but it's a very noise sensitive method .

The last technique we have tried is *transparent gradient shading* in which there is a transparent projection of gradients magnitude along each ray rather than a projection of the data set voxels. The aim is to make a look-thru representation of the different surfaces between different tissues in the data set . Since when dealing with ultrasound to extract surfaces from the data set is very difficult , gradient calculation is used to enhance discontinuities due to surfaces .

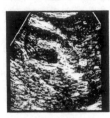

We have used a threshold to suppress small gradients along rays because these are often only noisy patterns which can cause great disturbance for final results after being integrated all along the ray. A better view of spatial relationship between tissues surfaces is achieved trough animation . Regarding processing time , this method is the heaviest among the algorithms we have tried , due to gradient calculation for each voxel , reconstruction time is about 30 to 40 seconds on a Pentium 120 .

Figure 6 Previous figure kidney rendered with transparent gradient shading .

6. Future work

For the future we will focus our attention first of all on the preprocessing step which is the main bottleneck of the system . We will work on fast and edge preserving filtering techniques based on wavelets . We are also planning to speed up all rendering algorithms . Moreover , we will focus on transparent rendering not only from the speed point of view , but also from the feature significance point of view . This will be performed in close connection with physicians , considering the high resemblance between transparent rendering and X-ray image representation .

7. References

[1] An Adaptive Weighted Median Filter for Speckle Suppression in Medical Ultrasonic Images
T.Loupas , W.N. MCDicken and P. Allan , IEEE Transaction on Circuits and Systems vol 36 , no 1 , January 1989
[2] Back to Front Display of Voxel Based Objects
Gideon Frieder , Dan Gordon and R. Anthony Reynolds , IEEE CG&A January 1985
[3] Investigation of Medical 3D-Rendering Algoritms
Ulf Tiede et alteri , IEEE CG&A March 1990
[4] Pseudo Shading Technique in the Two-Dimensional Domain : a post processing algorithm for enhancing the Z-buffer of a three-dimensional binary image .
A.C. Tan and Robin Richards , Medical Informatics vol 14 , no 2 , 1989
[5] Volume Rendering of 3D Medical Ultrasound Data Using Direct Feature Mapping
Erik Steen and Bjorn Olstad , IEEE Transaction on Medical Imaging vol 13 , no 3 , September 1994.
[6] Scale Space and Edge Detection Using Anisotropic Diffusion
Pietro Perona and Jitendra Malik IEEE trans. On Pattern Analysis and Machine Intelligence vol 12,no 7, July 1990
[7] Preprocessing and Volume Rendering of 3D Ultrasonic Data
Georgios Sakas et alteri , IEEE CG&A July 1995